NURSING
A GUIDE TO
DIAGNOSIS
PLANNING CARE
HANDBOOK

NURSING
A GUIDE TO
DIAGNOSIS
PLANNING CARE
HANDBOOK

SECOND EDITION

Betty J. Ackley MSN, EdS, RN

Gail B. Ladwig MSN, RN

and 38 Contributors

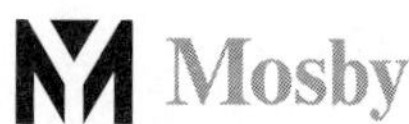

St. Louis Baltimore Boston Carlsbad Chicago Naples New York Philadelphia Portland
London Madrid Mexico City Singapore Sydney Tokyo Toronto Wiesbaden

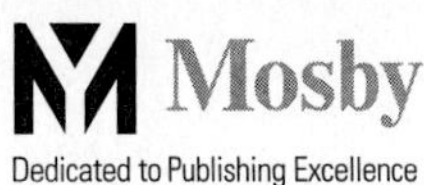

Dedicated to Publishing Excellence

A Times Mirror Company

Publisher: Nancy Coon
Editor: Loren Wilson
Associate Developmental Editor: Brian Dennison
Project Manager: Deborah Vogel
Production Editor: Jodi Willard
Manufacturing Supervisor: Theresa Fuchs
Designer: Susan Lane

A NOTE TO THE READER:
The author and publisher have made every attempt to check dosages and nursing content for accuracy. Because the science of pharmacology is continually advancing, our knowledge base continues to expand. Therefore we recommend that the reader always check product information for changes in dosage or administration before administering any medication. This is particularly important with new or rarely used drugs.

SECOND EDITION

Printed in the United States of America
Composition by Shepherd, Inc.
Printing/binding by R.R. Donnelley & Sons Company

Mosby-Year Book, Inc.
11830 Westline Industrial Drive
St. Louis, Missouri 63146

International Standard Book Number 0-8151-0342-5

95 96 97 98 99 / 9 8 7 6 5 4 3 2 1

Contributors

Betty J. Ackley MSN, EdS, RN
Professor of Nursing,
Jackson Community College,
Jackson, Michigan

Victoria L. Cole-Schonlau DNSc, MPA, RN
Director, Emergency Shelter and Assessment Center;
Director, Health Care Services,
Children's Institute International;
Assistant Professor, Nursing Care of Children,
California State University;
Nursing Supervisor,
Kenneth Norris, Jr. Cancer Hospital and Comprehensive Research Center,
University of Southern California,
Los Angeles, California

Sandra K. Cunningham MS, RN, CCRN, CS
Clinical Nurse Specialist,
St. Joseph Mercy Hospital,
Ann Arbor, Michigan

Jane Maria Curtis MSN, CNA, RN
Consultant,
Santa Fe, New Mexico

Gwethalyn B. Edwards MSN, RN
Director of Nursing Education,
W.A. Foote Memorial Hospital,
Jackson, Michigan

Pamela M. Emery BS, RNFA, CNOR, RN
Academic Clinical Coordinator of Education, Surgical Technology,
Baker College,
Flint, Michigan

Nancy English PhD, CS, RN
Consultant in Nursing Education;
Professor of Nursing,
Golden West College,
Huntington, California

Roslyn Fine MS, CCC, SLP
Speech Language Pathologist,
Nova Care Incorporated,
North East Division,
Grand Rapids, Michigan

Mary A. Fuerst-DeWys BS, RN
Infant Developmental Specialist,
Devos Children's Hospital at Butterworth,
Grand Rapids, Michigan

J. Keith Hampton MSN, RN, CS
Nurse Manager, Dialysis Services,
University of Minnesota Hospital and Clinic;
Adjunct Faculty, School of Nursing,
University of Minnesota,
Minneapolis, Minnesota

Mary Henrikson MN, RNC, ARNP
Director of Nursing, Maternal,
Salem Hospital,
Salem, Oregon

Kathie D. Hesnan BSN, RN, CETN
Continence Nursing, ET Nurse,
VNA of Greater Philadelphia,
Langhorne, Pennsylvania

Leslie Kalbach MN, RN, CNRN
Clinical Nurse Specialist,
Group Health Cooperative of Puget Sound,
Seattle, Washington

Helen Kelley MSN, RN
Psychiatric Nurse Consultant,
University of Michigan Medical Center,
Ann Arbor, Michigan

Diane Krasner MS, RN, CETN
ET Nurse Consultant;
Doctoral Student,
University of Maryland School of Nursing,
Baltimore, Maryland

Gail B. Ladwig MSN, RN
Professor of Nursing;
Department Chairperson,
Jackson Community College,
Jackson, Michigan

Marcia LaHaie BSN, RN, OCN
Oncology Education Coordinator,
St. Joseph Mercy Hospital,
Ann Arbor, Michigan

Margaret Lunney PhD, RN, CS
Associate Professor of Nursing,
Hunter-Bellevue School of Nursing,
New York, New York

Leslie Lysaght MS, RN, CCRN, CS
Clinical Nurse Specialist,
Medical Intensive Care Unit and Noninvasive Respiratory Care Unit,
St. Joseph Mercy Hospital,
Ann Arbor, Michigan

Marty J. Martin MSN, RN
Associate Professor of Nursing,
Jackson Community College;
Staff Nurse, Mental Health,
St. Lawrence Hospital,
Jackson, Michigan

Michelle Masta RN, BSN, CCRN
Agency Administrator,
ABC Home Health Services,
Coldwater, Michigan

Margo McCaffery MS, RN, FAAN
Consultant in the Nursing Care of Patients with Pain,
Los Angeles, California

Cathy McClean RN
Staff Nurse,
W.A. Foote Memorial Hospital,
Jackson, Michigan

Vicki E. McClurg MN, RN
Assistant Professor of Nursing,
Seattle Pacific University,
Seattle, Washington

Kathy A. Stimac O'Brien MSN, RN
Pediatric Home Health,
Kid's Club of Illinois,
Lombard, Illinois

Christine L. Pasero BSN, RN
Pain Management Consultant,
Rocklin, California

Beverly Pickett MA, BS, RN
Laboratory Assistant, Department of Nursing,
Jackson Community College,
Jackson, Michigan

Nancee Bender Radtke MSN, RN
Administrative Director,
Ambulatory Care Department,
W.A. Foote Hospital,
Jackson, Michigan

Judith S. Rizzo MS, RN, CS
Clinical Nurse Specialist,
Psychiatric Emergency Services,
University of Michigan Medical Center,
Ann Arbor, Michigan

Pam Bifano Schweitzer MS, RN, CS
Clinical Nurse Specialist,
Anxiety Disorders Program,
University of Michigan Psychiatric Hospitals,
Ann Arbor, Michigan

Suzanne Skowronski MSN, RN
Visiting Instructor in Nursing,
Oakland University,
Rochester, Michigan

Linda L. Straight MA, CES, RN
Manager Cardiac Rehabilitation,
W.A. Foote Memorial Hospital,
Jackson, Michigan

Terry VandenBosch MS, RN, CS
Research Specialist,
St. Joseph Mercy Hospital,
Ann Arbor, Michigan

Catherine Vincent MSN, RN
Assistant Professor, School of Nursing,
Oakland University,
Rochester, Michigan

Virginia R. Wall MN, RN, IBCLC
Lactation Specialist,
University of Washington Medical Center,
Seattle, Washington

Peggy A. Wetsch MSN, RN, CNA
Coordinator Computer and Learning Resources,
Los Angeles County Medical Center School of Nursing,
Los Angeles, California

Linda Williams MSN, RN, C, CS
Associate Professor of Nursing;
Gerontological Clinical Nurse Specialist,
Jackson Community College;
Staff Nurse, PACU,
W.A. Foote Hospital
Jackson, Michigan

Fran Wistom MSN, RN, CSW, CPN
Nurse Psychotherapist, Private Practice,
White Lake Counseling,
Whitehall, Michigan

Janet Woodruff BSN, RN
Charge Nurse, Neuro ICU,
University of Utah,
Salt Lake City, Utah

Kathy Wyngarden MSN, RN
Director of Clinical Practice Model,
Butterworth Hospital,
Grand Rapids, Michigan

Dedication

This book is dedicated to:

- Dale Ackley, the greatest guy in the world without whose support this book would have never happened; Dawn Ackley, who with Dale has been the joy of my life;
- Jerry Ladwig, my wonderful husband who after 28 years is still supportive and patient—I couldn't have done it without him; my children and their spouses, Jerry, Kathy, and Alexandra, Chrissy and John, Jenny and Jim and Amy—the greatest family anyone could ever hope for;
- and our nursing faculty colleagues; friends are one of life's most precious gifts.

Acknowledgments

We would like to thank the following people at Mosby: Loren Wilson, Nursing Editor, who supported us with this second edition of the text with intelligence and kindness; Brian Dennison, Associate Developmental Editor, who was a great resource in our endeavor; Terry Van Schaik, previous Nursing Editor, who championed the first edition; and all of the people in the production editing department who finalized the production of this edition, especially Jodi Willard.

We acknowledge with gratitude the nursing students and graduates of Jackson Community College, who made us think and shared a very special time with us; Linda Straight, Marcy Keefe Slager, and Joy Frizzel, who kindly reviewed care plans and made excellent suggestions; the nurses at W.A. Foote Memorial Hospital, Doctors Hospital in Jackson, Community Mental Health and the Community Nursing Agencies, who have helped us educate students and served as role models for excellence in nursing care; and, finally, each other, for perseverance, patience, and friendship.

Preface

Nursing Diagnosis Handbook: A Guide to Planning Care is a convenient reference to help the practicing nurse or nursing student make a nursing diagnosis and write a care plan with ease and confidence. This handbook helps the nurse correlate nursing diagnoses with what is known about the client on the basis of assessment findings, established medical or psychiatric diagnoses, and the current treatment plan.

Making a nursing diagnosis and planning care are complex processes that involve diagnostic reasoning and critical thinking skills. Nursing students and practicing nurses cannot possibly memorize over 1000 defining characteristics, related factors, and risk factors for the 128 diagnoses approved by the North American Nursing Diagnosis Association (NANDA). This book correlates suggested nursing diagnoses with what the nurse knows about the client and offers a care plan for each nursing diagnosis.

Section I, Nursing Diagnosis and the Nursing Process, explains how the nurse formulates a nursing diagnosis statement using assessment findings and other data. In Section II, Guide to Nursing Diagnoses, the nurse can look up symptoms and problems and their suggested nursing diagnoses for over 1000 client symptoms, medical and psychiatric diagnoses, diagnostic procedures, surgical interventions, and clinical states. In Section III, Guide to Planning Care, the nurse can find care plans for all nursing diagnoses suggested in Section II.

Nursing Diagnosis Handbook: A Guide to Planning Care includes medical diagnoses because nurses find them useful in suggesting appropriate nursing diagnoses. For example, under the medical diagnosis of AIDS, the user will find the nursing diagnosis **Body image disturbance** related to chronic contagious illness, cachexia. The nurse who is using this text needs to determine if this suggested nursing diagnosis is appropriate to the client.

Special features of the second edition of *Nursing Diagnosis Handbook: A Guide to Planning Care* include the following:

- Nineteen new nursing diagnoses recently adopted by NANDA
- Suggested nursing diagnoses for over 1000 clinical entities including 300 signs and symptoms, 300 medical diagnoses, 120 surgeries, 200 maternal-child disorders, 100 mental health disorders, and 50 geriatric disorders
- Rationales for nursing interventions that are based on nursing research and literature
- Nursing references identified for each care plan
- Major clinical practice guidelines of the Agency for Health Care Policy and Research (AHCPR) used in appropriate care plans
- Nursing care plans that contain many holistic interventions
- Care plans for **Pain** written by national experts on pain, Margo McCaffery and Christine Pasero, which includes Appendix D on pain rating scales and equianalgesic medication doses
- Care plans on **Skin integrity** written by national expert Diane Krasner, who has lectured and written extensively on the topic

The following features of *Nursing Diagnosis Handbook: A Guide to Planning Care* are included from the first edition:

- A format that facilitates a process nurses already use—analyzing signs and symptoms, which are defining characteristics of nursing diagnoses—to make a diagnosis

- Use of NANDA terminology and approved diagnoses, including revisions of existing nursing diagnoses as recommended at the Eleventh NANDA Conference in 1994
- Inclusion of two additional nursing diagnoses; **Grieving** and **Altered comfort**, because of their usefulness in caring for many clients
- An alphabetical format for Section II, Guide to Nursing Diagnoses and Section III, Guide to Planning Care, which allows rapid access to information in the text
- Nursing care plans for all nursing diagnoses listed in Section II
- Specific geriatric interventions in appropriate plans of care
- Specific client/family teaching interventions in each plan of care
- Inclusion of commonly used abbreviations (e.g., AIDS, MI, CHF) and cross-referencing to the complete term in Section II
- Contributions by 38 nurse experts from throughout the United States, who together represent all of the major nursing specialties and have extensive experience with nursing diagnosis and the nursing process

We acknowledge the work of NANDA, which is used extensively throughout this text. In some cases the authors and contributors have modified the NANDA work to increase ease of use. The original NANDA work can be found in *NANDA Nursing Diagnoses: Definitions and Classification 1995-1996.*

Several contributors are the original authors of the nursing diagnoses established by NANDA. These contributors include the following:

Mary Fuerst-DeWys

- **Disorganized infant behavior**
- **Potential for enhanced organized infant behavior**
- **Risk for disorganized behavior**

Nancy English

- **Impaired environmental interpretation syndrome**

Margaret Lunney

- **Effective management of therapeutic regimen**
- **Ineffective community coping**
- **Ineffective management of therapeutic regimen**
- **Ineffective management of therapeutic regimen: community**
- **Ineffective management of therapeutic regimen: families**
- **Potential for enhanced community coping**

Vicki McClurg, Mary Henrikson, and Virginia Wall

- **Effective breast-feeding**
- **Ineffective breast-feeding**
- **Interrupted breast-feeding**

Kathy Wyngarden

- **Risk for altered parent/infant/child attachment**

We and the contributors trust that the nurse finds the second edition of *Nursing Diagnosis Handbook: A Guide to Planning Care* to be a valuable tool that simplifies the process of diagnosing clients and planning for their care and thus allows the nurse more time to provide care that speeds the client's recovery.

Betty J. Ackley
Gail B. Ladwig

How to Use Nursing Diagnosis Handbook: A Guide to Planning Care

1. Assess the client, using the format provided by the clinical setting. Collect data, including client symptoms, clinical states, and known medical or psychiatric diagnoses.
2. Turn to Section II, Guide to Nursing Diagnoses, an alphabetical listing. Locate the client's symptoms, clinical state, medical or psychiatric diagnoses, anticipated or prescribed diagnostic studies, or surgical intervention. Note suggestions for appropriate nursing diagnoses.
3. Use Section III, Guide to Planning Care to evaluate each suggested nursing diagnosis and "related to" (etiology) statement. Section III is an alphabetical listing of care plans for each nursing diagnosis found in Section II. Determine the appropriateness of each nursing diagnosis by comparing the defining characteristics and risk factors to the data collected on the client.
4. Continue to use Section III to determine appropriate Client Outcomes/Goals and Nursing Interventions and Rationales.

Contents

NURSING
A GUIDE TO
DIAGNOSIS
PLANNING CARE
HANDBOOK

Section I

Nursing Diagnosis and the Nursing Process

The nursing process is an organizing framework for professional nursing practice. Components of the process include performing a nursing assessment, making nursing diagnoses, writing outcome/goal statements, determining appropriate nursing interventions, and evaluating the nursing care that has been given. An essential part of this process is the nursing diagnosis.

> A nursing diagnosis is a clinical judgment about individual, family, or community responses to actual or potential health problems or life processes. Nursing diagnoses provide the basis for selection of nursing interventions to achieve outcomes for which the nurse is accountable (NANDA, 1990).

ASSESSMENT

Before determining appropriate nursing diagnoses, the nurse must perform a thorough holistic nursing assessment of the client. The nurse may use the assessment format adopted by the facility in which he or she is practicing. Several organizational approaches to assessment are available, including Gordon's Functional Health Patterns and head-to-toe and body systems approaches. Regardless of the approach used, the nurse assesses for client symptoms to help formulate a nursing diagnosis.

To elicit as many symptoms as possible, the nurse uses open-ended, rather than yes/no, questions during the assessment. The nurse also obtains information via physical assessment and diagnostic test results. If the client is critically ill or unable to respond verbally, the nurse obtains most of the data from physical assessment and diagnostic test results and possibly from the client's significant others. The nurse can use data from each of these sources to formulate a nursing diagnosis.

NURSING DIAGNOSTIC STATEMENT

A working nursing diagnostic statement has three parts:

1. The nursing diagnosis
2. "Related to" phrase or Etiology
3. Defining characteristics phrase

Nursing Diagnosis

The nurse makes a nursing diagnosis by categorizing symptoms as common patterns of response to actual or potential health problems. After completing the assessment, the nurse lists all identified symptoms and clusters similar symptoms together. For example, the following symptoms may be identified in the assessment of a client with an admitting medical diagnosis of asthma: dyspnea, anxiety, hypertension, respiratory rate of 28, temperature of 99° F. Of these signs and symptoms, dyspnea and respiratory rate of 28 (tachypnea) would be clustered because they are related. Using Section II Guide to Nursing Diagnoses, the nurse can then look up dyspnea or tachypnea and find the nursing diagnosis **Ineffective breathing pattern** suggested for each symptom.

To validate that the diagnosis **Ineffective breathing pattern** is appropriate for the client, the nurse then turns to Section III Guide to Planning Care, and reads through its definition and its list of defining characteristics. The definition should describe the condition that the nurse is observing in the client. Many of the nursing diagnoses in Section III differentiate between major and minor defining characteristics or specify critical defining characteristics. For a diagnosis to be accurate, NANDA suggests that the client should have most of the major or critical defining characteristics.

To help verify the diagnoses made on the basis of client signs and symptoms, the nurse may look up the client's medical diagnoses in Section II Guide to Nursing Diagnoses. For example, one of the nursing diagnoses listed under the medical diagnosis asthma is **Ineffective breathing pattern.**

The process of identifying significant symptoms, clustering them into logical patterns, and then choosing an appropriate nursing diagnosis involves diagnostic reasoning skills (critical thinking) that must be learned in the process of becoming a nurse. Our text serves as a tool to help the nurse in this process.

"Related to" Phrase or Etiology

The second part of the nursing diagnosis statement is the "related to" (r/t) phrase. This phrase states what may be causing, or contributing to, the nursing diagnosis, or the etiology. Pathophysiological and psychosocial changes, such as developmental age and cultural and environmental situations, may be causative factors.

Ideally, the etiology, or cause, of the nursing diagnosis is something the nurse can treat. A carefully written, individualized r/t statement enables the nurse to plan nursing interventions that will assist the client in accomplishing goals and returning to optimum health.

For each suggested nursing diagnosis, the nurse should refer to the statements listed under the heading "Related Factors (r/t)" in Section III. These r/t factors may or may not be appropriate for the individual client. If they are not appropriate, the nurse should write an appropriate r/t statement.

Defining Characteristics Phrase

The third part of the nursing diagnostic statement consists of defining characteristics (signs and symptoms) that the nurse has gathered during the assessment phase. The phrase as evidenced by (aeb) may be used to connect the etiology (r/t) and defining characteristics. The use of defining characteristics is similar to the process the physician uses when making a medical diagnosis. For example, for the medical diagnosis of asthma, the physician may observe the following signs and symptoms: wheezing, chest retractions, and abnormalities with pulmonary function testing. The nurse uses the same process.

Examples of Writing a Nursing Diagnostic Statement

To write a nursing diagnostic statement for a client with the symptom of alopecia, the nurse should use Section II. Listed under the heading *alopecia* is the following information:

> **Alopecia**
> **Body image disturbance** (nursing diagnosis) r/t loss of hair, change in appearance (etiology).

To the information found in Section II, the "defining characteristics" phrase is added: aeb verbalization of fear of rejection by others because of hair loss.

With the above information, the nurse is able to make the following nursing diagnosis statement:

> **Body image disturbance** r/t loss of hair, change in appearance aeb verbalization of fear of rejection by others because of hair loss.

To use Section II to write a nursing diagnostic statement for a client who has peritonitis, the nurse should look up the diagnosis *peritonitis.* Listed under this medical diagnosis is the following information:

Peritonitis
Fluid volume deficit (nursing diagnosis) r/t retention of fluid in the bowel with loss of circulating blood volume (etiology).

To the information in Section II, the "defining characteristics" phrase is added: aeb dry mucous membranes, poor skin turgor.

With the above information, the nurse is able to make the following nursing diagnostic statement:

Fluid volume deficit r/t retention of fluid in the bowel with loss of circulating blood volume aeb dry mucous membranes, poor skin turgor.

PLANNING

For most clients the nurse will make more than one nursing diagnosis. Therefore the next step in the nursing process is to determine the priority for care from the list of nursing diagnoses. The nurse can determine the highest priority nursing diagnoses by using Maslow's Hierarchy of Needs. In this Hierarchy, highest priority is generally given to immediate problems that may be life threatening. For example, **Ineffective airway clearance** would have a higher priority than **Ineffective individual coping.** Refer to Appendix A, "Nursing Diagnoses Arranged by Maslow's Hierarchy of Needs" for assistance in prioritizing nursing diagnoses.

Outcomes/Goals

After determining the appropriate priority of the nursing diagnoses, the nurse writes client outcome/goal statements. Section III lists suggested choices of outcomes/goals for each nursing diagnosis. If at all possible, the nurse involves the client in determining appropriate outcomes/goals. Following discussion with the client, the nurse plans nursing care that will assist the client to accomplish the outcome/goal.

After the client's outcomes/goals are selected, the nurse establishes a means to accomplish the outcomes/goals. The usual means are by nursing interventions.

INTERVENTIONS

Interventions are like a road map directing nursing care and the best ways to provide it. The more clearly a nurse writes the intervention, the easier it will be to complete the journey and arrive at the destination of successful client outcomes/goals.

Section III supplies choices of interventions for each nursing diagnosis. The nurse may choose the ones appropriate for the client and individualize them accordingly or determine additional interventions.

Putting It All Together—Writing the Care Plan

The final planning phase is writing the actual care plan, including prioritized nursing diagnostic statements, outcomes/goals, and interventions. The care plan must be written and shared with all health care personnel caring for the client to ensure continuity of care.

IMPLEMENTATION

The implementation phase of the nursing process is the actual initiation of the nursing care plan. Client outcomes/goals are achieved by the performance of the nursing interventions. During this phase the nurse continues to assess the client to determine if the interventions are effective. An important part of this phase is documentation. The nurse should use his or her facility's tool for documentation and record the results of implementing nursing interventions. Documentation is also necessary for legal reasons because in a legal dispute, "If it wasn't charted, it wasn't done."

EVALUATION

Although evaluation is listed as the last phase of the nursing process, it is actually an integral part of each phase that the nurse does continuously. When evaluation is performed as the last phase, the nurse refers to the client's outcomes/goals and determines if they were met. If the outcomes/goals were not met, the nurse begins again with assessment and determines why they were not met. Were the goals attainable? Was the wrong nursing diagnosis made? Should the interventions be changed? At this point, the nurse can look up any new symptoms or conditions that have been identified in the client and then adjust the care plan as needed.

Many health care providers are using critical pathways to plan nursing care. The use of nursing diagnoses should be an integral part of any critical pathway to ensure that nursing care needs are being assessed and appropriate nursing interventions are planned and implemented.

The use of nursing diagnoses ensures that nurses are speaking a common language when taking care of client problems. This system is also easily computerized for easier documentation and analysis of patterns of care. Nursing diagnosis is the essence of nursing to ensure that clients receive excellent, holistic nursing care.

Section II

Guide to Nursing Diagnoses

A

Abdominal Distention

Altered nutrition: less than body requirements r/t nausea, vomiting
Constipation r/t decreased activity, decreased fluid intake, pathological process
Pain r/t retention of air and gastrointestinal secretions

Abdominal Hysterectomy

Refer to Hysterectomy

Abdominal Pain

Altered nutrition: less than body requirements r/t unresolved pain
Pain r/t injury, pathological process
Refer to cause of Abdominal Pain

Abdominal Perineal Resection

Risk for perioperative positioning injury r/t prolonged surgery and lithotomy position
Refer to Abdominal Surgery; Colostomy

Abdominal Surgery

Altered health maintenance r/t knowledge deficit regarding self-care following surgery
Altered nutrition: less than body requirements r/t high metabolic needs, decreased ability to digest food
Constipation r/t decreased activity, decreased fluid intake, anesthesia, narcotics
Pain r/t surgical procedure
Risk for altered tissue perfusion: peripheral r/t immobility and abdominal surgery resulting in stasis of blood flow
Risk for infection r/t invasive procedure
Refer to Surgery

Abortion—Induced

Altered health maintenance r/t knowledge deficit regarding self-care following abortion
Health-seeking behaviors r/t desire to control fertility
Ineffective family coping: compromised r/t unresolved feelings about decision
Risk for infection r/t open uterine blood vessels, dilated cervix
Self-esteem disturbance r/t feelings of guilt
Spiritual distress r/t perceived moral implications of decision

Abortion—Spontaneous

Altered family processes r/t unmet expectations for pregnancy and childbirth
Altered health maintenance r/t knowledge deficit regarding self-care following abortion
Body image disturbance r/t perceived inability to carry pregnancy, produce child
Fear r/t implications for future pregnancies
Ineffective family coping: disabling r/t unresolved feelings about loss
Ineffective individual coping r/t personal vulnerability
Pain r/t uterine contractions, surgical intervention
Risk for dysfunctional grieving r/t loss of fetus
Risk for fluid volume deficit r/t hemorrhage
Risk for infection r/t septic or incomplete abortion of products of conception, open uterine blood vessels, dilated cervix
Self-esteem disturbance r/t feelings of failure, guilt

Abruptio Placenta (>36 weeks)

Altered family processes r/t unmet expectations for pregnancy/childbirth
Altered health maintenance r/t knowledge deficit regarding self-care with disorder
Anxiety r/t unknown outcome, change in birth plans
Fear r/t threat to well-being of self and fetus
Pain r/t irritable uterus, hypertonic uterus
Risk for altered tissue perfusion (fetal) r/t uteroplacental insufficiency
Risk for fluid volume deficit r/t hemorrhage
Risk for infection r/t partial separation of the placenta
Risk for injury (fetal) r/t hypoxia
Risk for injury (maternal) r/t uterine rupture

Abscess Formation

Altered health maintenance r/t knowledge deficit regarding self-care with an abscess
Altered protection r/t inadequate nutrition, abnormal blood profile, drug therapy or treatment
Impaired tissue integrity r/t altered circulation, nutritional deficit/excess

Abuse, Child

Refer to Child Abuse

Abuse, Spouse, Parent, or Significant Other

Altered family process: alcoholism r/t inadequate coping skills
Anxiety r/t to threat to self-concept, situational crisis of abuse
Caregiver role strain r/t chronic illness, self-care

deficits, lack of respite care, extent of caregiving required

Defensive coping r/t low self-esteem

Impaired verbal communication r/t psychological barriers of fear

Ineffective family coping: compromised r/t abusive patterns

Post-trauma response r/t history of abuse

Powerlessness r/t life-style of helplessness

Risk for self-directed violence r/t history of abuse

Self-esteem disturbance r/t negative family interactions

Sleep pattern disturbance r/t psychological stress

Accessory Muscle Use (to breathe)

Ineffective breathing pattern r/t neuromuscular impairment, pain, musculoskeletal impairment, perception/cognitive impairment, anxiety, decreased energy, fatigue

Refer to COPD; Asthma; Bronchitis; Respiratory Infections, Acute Childhood

Accident Prone

Acute confusion r/t altered level of consciousness

Ineffective individual coping r/t personal vulnerability, situational crises

Risk for injury r/t history of accidents

Achalasia

Impaired swallowing r/t neuromuscular impairment

Ineffective individual coping r/t chronic disease

Pain r/t stasis of food in the esophagus

Risk for aspiration r/t nocturnal regurgitation

Acidosis, Metabolic

Altered nutrition: less than body requirements r/t inability to ingest, absorb nutrients

Altered thought processes r/t central nervous system depression

Decreased cardiac output r/t dysrhythmias from hyperkalemia

Impaired memory r/t electrolyte imbalance

Pain: headache r/t neuromuscular irritability

Risk for injury r/t disorientation, weakness, stupor

Acidosis, Respiratory

Activity intolerance r/t imbalance between oxygen supply and demand

Altered thought processes r/t central nervous system depression

Impaired gas exchange r/t ventilation perfusion imbalance

Impaired memory r/t hypoxia

Risk for decreased cardiac output r/t arrhythmias associated with respiratory acidosis

Acquired Immune Deficiency Disorder

Refer to AIDS

Activity Intolerance

Activity intolerance r/t bedrest/immobility, generalized weakness, sedentary life-style, imbalance between oxygen supply/demand, pain

Activity Intolerance, Potential to Develop

Risk for activity intolerance r/t deconditioned status, presence of circulatory/respiratory problems, inexperience with the activity

Acute Abdomen

Fluid volume deficit r/t fluids trapped in bowel, inability to drink

Pain r/t pathological process

Refer to cause of Acute Abdomen

Acute Back

Altered health maintenance r/t knowledge deficit regarding self-care with painful back

Anxiety r/t situational crisis, back injury

Colonic constipation r/t decreased activity

Impaired physical mobility r/t pain

Ineffective individual coping r/t situational crisis, back injury

Pain r/t back injury

Acute Confusion

Acute confusion r/t being over 60 years of age, dementia, alcohol abuse, drug abuse, delirium

Adams-Stokes Syndrome

Refer to Dysrhythmias

Addiction

Refer to Alcoholism; Drug Abuse

Addison's Disease

Activity intolerance r/t weakness, fatigue

Altered health maintenance r/t knowledge deficit

Altered nutrition: less than body requirements r/t chronic illness

Fluid volume deficit r/t failure of regulatory mechanisms

Risk for injury r/t weakness

Adenoidectomy

Altered comfort r/t effects of anesthesia, nausea and vomiting
Altered health maintenance r/t knowledge deficit of postoperative care
Ineffective airway clearance r/t hesitation/reluctance to cough secondary to pain
Pain r/t surgical incision
Risk for altered nutrition: less than body requirements r/t hesitation/reluctance to swallow
Risk for aspiration/suffocation r/t postoperative drainage and impaired swallowing
Risk for fluid volume deficit r/t decreased intake secondary to painful swallowing, effects of anesthesia

Adhesions, Lysis of

Refer to Abdominal Surgery

Adjustment Disorder

Anxiety r/t inability to cope with psychosocial stressor
Impaired adjustment r/t assault to self-esteem
Personal identity disturbance r/t psychosocial stressor (specific to individual)
Situational low self-esteem r/t change in role function

Adjustment Impairment

Impaired adjustment r/t disability requiring change in life-style, inadequate support systems, impaired cognition, sensory overload, assault to self-esteem, altered locus of control, incomplete grieving

Adolescent, Pregnant

Altered family processes r/t unmet expectations for adolescent, situational crisis
Altered growth and development r/t pregnancy
Altered health maintenance r/t knowledge deficit with denial of pregnancy, desire to keep pregnancy secret, fear
Altered nutrition: less than body requirements r/t lack of knowledge of nutritional needs during pregnancy and as a growing adolescent
Altered role performance r/t pregnancy
Anxiety r/t situational and maturational crisis, pregnancy
Body image disturbance r/t pregnancy superimposed on developing body
Decisional conflict: keeping child vs giving up child vs abortion r/t lack of experience with decision making, interference with decision making, multiple or divergent sources of information, lack of support system
Family coping: disabling r/t highly ambivalent family relationships, chronically unresolved feelings of guilt, anger, or despair
Fear r/t labor and delivery
Health-seeking behaviors r/t desire for optimal maternal and fetal outcome
Impaired social interaction r/t self-concept disturbance
Ineffective denial r/t fear of consequences of pregnancy becoming known
Ineffective individual coping r/t situational and maturational crisis, personal vulnerability
Noncompliance r/t denial of pregnancy
Risk for injury (fetal and maternal) r/t limitations of maturational age
Situational low self-esteem r/t feelings of shame and guilt over becoming and being pregnant

Adoption, Giving Child Up for

Decisional conflict r/t unclear personal values or beliefs, perceived threat to value system, support system deficit
Grieving r/t loss of child, loss of role of parent
Potential for enhanced spiritual well-being r/t harmony with self regarding final decision

Adrenal Crisis

Altered protection r/t inability to tolerate stress
Refer to Addison's Disease; Shock

Adult Respiratory Distress Syndrome

Refer to ARDS

Advance Directives

Anticipatory grieving r/t possible loss of self, significant other
Decisional conflict r/t unclear personal values or beliefs, perceived threat to value system, support system deficit
Potential for enhanced spiritual well-being r/t harmonious interconnectedness with self, others, and higher power/God

Affective Disorders

Altered health maintenance r/t lack of ability to make good judgments regarding ways to obtain help
Chronic low self-esteem r/t repeated unmet expectations
Colonic constipation r/t inactivity, decreased fluid intake
Dysfunctional grieving r/t lack of previous

resolution of former grieving response
Fatigue r/t psychological demands
Hopelessness r/t feeling of abandonment, long-term stress
Ineffective individual coping r/t dysfunctional grieving
Risk for loneliness r/t pattern of social isolation and feelings of low self-esteem
Risk for violence: self-directed r/t panic state
Self-care deficit: specify r/t depression, cognitive impairment
Sexual dysfunction r/t loss of sexual desire
Sleep pattern disturbance r/t inactivity
Social isolation r/t ineffective coping
Refer to specific disorder: Depression/Major; Dysthymic Disorder; Manic Disorder

Aggressive Behavior

Risk for violence: self-directed or directed at others r/t antisocial character, battered woman, catatonic excitement, child abuse, manic excitement, organic brain syndrome, panic states, rage reactions, suicidal behavior, temporal lobe epilepsy, toxic reactions to medication

Agitation

Acute confusion r/t side effect of medication, alcohol abuse or withdrawal, substance abuse or withdrawal, sensory deprivation, sensory overload

Agoraphobia

Anxiety r/t real or perceived threat to physical integrity
Fear r/t leaving home and going out in public places
Ineffective individual coping r/t inadequate support systems
Impaired social interaction r/t disturbance in self-concept
Social isolation r/t altered thought process

Agranulocytosis

Altered health maintenance r/t knowledge deficit of protective measures to prevent infection
Altered protection r/t abnormal blood profile

AIDS (Acquired Immune Deficiency Syndrome)

Altered family processes r/t distress over diagnosis of human immunodeficiency virus (HIV) infection
Altered health maintenance r/t knowledge deficit regarding transmission of infection, lack of exposure to information, misinterpretation of information
Altered nutrition: less than body requirements r/t decreased ability to eat and absorb nutrients secondary to anorexia, nausea, or diarrhea
Altered protection r/t risk for infection secondary to inadequate immune system
Anticipatory grieving: family/parental r/t potential/impending death of loved one
Anticipatory grieving: individual r/t loss of physio-psychosocial well-being
Body image disturbance r/t chronic contagious illness, cachexia
Caregiver role strain r/t unpredictable illness course, presence of situation stressors
Chronic pain r/t tissue inflammation and destruction
Diarrhea r/t inflammatory changes in bowel
Energy field disturbance r/t chronic illness
Fatigue r/t disease process, stress, poor nutritional intake
Fear r/t powerlessness, threat to well-being
Hopelessness r/t deteriorating physical condition
Risk for altered oral mucous membranes r/t immunological deficit
Risk for altered thought processes r/t infection in brain
Risk for fluid volume deficit r/t diarrhea, vomiting, fever, bleeding
Risk for infection r/t inadequate immune system
Risk for impaired skin integrity r/t immunological deficit or diarrhea
Risk for loneliness r/t social isolation
Situational low self-esteem r/t crisis of chronic contagious illness
Social isolation r/t self-concept disturbance, therapeutic isolation
Spiritual distress r/t challenged beliefs or moral system
Refer to Cancer; Pneumonia; AIDS in Child

AIDS Dementia

Impaired environmental interpretation syndrome r/t viral invasion of nervous system

AIDS in Child

Altered parenting r/t congenital acquisition of infection secondary to IV drug use, multiple sexual partners, history of contaminated blood transfusion
Refer to AIDS; Hospitalized Child; Child with Chronic Condition; Terminally Ill Child/Death of Child

Airway Obstruction/Secretions

Ineffective airway clearance r/t decreased energy; fatigue; tracheobronchial infection, obstruction, or secretions; perceptual/cognitive impairment;

trauma; decreased force of cough because of aging

Alcohol Withdrawal

Acute confusion r/t effects of alcohol withdrawal
Altered health maintenance r/t knowledge deficit regarding chronic illness or effects of alcohol consumption
Altered nutrition: less than body requirements r/t poor dietary habits
Altered thought processes r/t potential delirium tremors
Anxiety r/t situational crisis, withdrawal
Chronic low self-esteem r/t repeated unmet expectations
Ineffective individual coping r/t personal vulnerability
Risk for fluid volume deficit r/t excessive diaphoresis, agitation, decreased fluid intake
Risk for violence r/t substance withdrawal
Sensory/perceptual alterations: visual, auditory, kinesthetic, tactile, olfactory r/t neurochemical imbalance in brain
Sleep pattern disturbance r/t effect of depressants, alcohol withdrawal, anxiety

Alcoholism

Acute confusion r/t alcohol abuse
Altered family process: alcoholism r/t alcohol abuse
Altered nutrition: less than body requirements r/t anorexia
Altered protection r/t malnutrition, sleep deprivation
Anxiety r/t loss of control
Compromised/dysfunctional family coping r/t co-dependency issues
Impaired Environmental Interpretation Syndrome r/t neurological effects of chronic alcohol intake
Impaired home maintenance management r/t memory deficits, fatigue
Impaired memory r/t alcohol abuse
Ineffective individual coping r/t use of alcohol to cope with life events
Powerlessness r/t alcohol addiction
Risk for injury r/t alteration in sensory perceptual function
Risk for loneliness r/t unacceptable social behavior
Risk for violence r/t reactions to substances used, impulsive behavior, disorientation, impaired judgment
Self-esteem disturbance r/t failure at life events
Sleep pattern disturbance r/t irritability, nightmares, tremors
Social isolation r/t unacceptable social behavior, values

Alkalosis

Refer to Metabolic Alkalosis

Alopecia

Body image disturbance r/t loss of hair, change in appearance

Alzheimer Type Dementia

Altered health maintenance r/t knowledge deficit of caregiver regarding appropriate care
Altered thought processes r/t chronic organic disorder
Caregiver role strain r/t duration and extent of caregiving required
Chronic confusion r/t Alzheimer's disease
Fear r/t loss of self
Hopelessness r/t deteriorating condition
Impaired home maintenance management r/t impaired cognitive function, inadequate support systems
Impaired memory r/t neurological disturbance
Impaired physical mobility r/t severe neurological dysfunction
Ineffective family coping: compromised r/t altered family processes
Powerlessness r/t deteriorating condition
Risk for injury r/t confusion
Risk for loneliness r/t potential social isolation
Risk for violence: directed at others r/t frustration, fear, anger
Self-care deficit: specify r/t psychological-physiological impairment
Sleep pattern disturbance r/t neurological impairment and daytime naps
Social isolation r/t fear of disclosure of memory loss

Refer to Dementia

Amenorrhea

Risk for sexual dysfunction r/t altered body function

Refer to Sexuality, Adolescent

Amnesia

Impaired memory r/t excessive environmental disturbance, neurological disturbance
Post-trauma response r/t history of abuse, catastrophic illness, disaster, or accident

Amniocentesis

Decisional conflict r/t choice of treatment pending results of test

Amnionitis

Refer to Chorioamnionitis

Amniotic Membrane Rupture

Refer to Premature Rupture of Membranes

Amputation

Altered health maintenance r/t knowledge deficit of care of stump, rehabilitation
Altered tissue perfusion: peripheral r/t impaired arterial circulation
Body image disturbance r/t negative effects of amputation, response from others
Grieving r/t loss of body part and future life-style changes
Impaired physical mobility r/t musculoskeletal impairment and limited movement
Impaired skin integrity r/t poor healing, prosthesis rubbing
Pain r/t surgery, phantom limb sensation
Risk for fluid volume deficit: hemorrhage r/t vulnerable surgical site

Amyotrophic Lateral Sclerosis

Decisional conflict: ventilator therapy r/t unclear personal values or beliefs, lack of relevant information
Impaired swallowing r/t weakness of muscles involved in swallowing
Impaired verbal communication r/t weakness of muscles of speech, knowledge deficit of ways to compensate and alternative communication devices
Inability to sustain spontaneous ventilation r/t weakness of muscles of respiration
Risk for aspiration r/t impaired swallowing
Refer to Neurological Disorder

Anal Fistula

Refer to Fistulectomy

Anaphylactic Shock

Inability to maintain spontaneous ventilation r/t acute airway obstruction
Refer to Shock

Anasarca

Fluid volume excess r/t excessive fluid intake, cardiac/renal dysfunction, loss of plasma proteins
Risk for impaired skin integrity r/t impaired circulation to skin
Refer to cause of Anasarca

Anemia

Altered health maintenance r/t knowledge deficit of nutritional and medical treatment of anemia
Anxiety r/t cause of disease
Fatigue r/t decreased oxygen supply to the body
Impaired memory r/t anemia
Risk for injury r/t alteration in peripheral sensory perception

Anemia in Pregnancy

Altered health maintenance r/t knowledge deficit regarding nutrition in pregnancy
Anxiety r/t concerns about health of self and fetus
Fatigue r/t decreased oxygen supply to the body and increased cardiac workload
Risk for infection r/t reduction in the oxygen-carrying capacity of the blood

Anemia, Sickle Cell

Refer to Sickle Cell Anemia/Crisis; Anemia

Anencephaly

Refer to Neurotube Defects

Aneurysm, Abdominal Surgery

Risk for altered tissue perfusion: peripheral r/t impaired arterial circulation
Risk for fluid volume deficit: hemorrhage r/t potential abnormal blood loss
Risk for infection r/t invasive procedure
Refer to Abdominal Surgery

Aneurysm, Cerebral

Refer to Craniectomy/Craniotomy or Subarachnoid Hemorrhage if aneurysm has ruptured

Anger

Anxiety r/t situational crisis
Fear r/t environmental stressor, hospitalization
Grieving r/t significant loss
Impaired adjustment r/t assault to self-esteem, disability requiring change in life-style, inadequate support system
Powerlessness r/t health care environment
Risk for violence r/t history of violence, rage reaction

Angina Pectoris

Activity intolerance r/t acute pain, arrhythmias
Altered health maintenance r/t knowledge deficit of care of angina condition
Altered sexuality pattern r/t disease process, medications, loss of libido

Anxiety r/t situational crisis
Decreased cardiac output r/t myocardial ischemia, medication effect, arrhythmias
Grieving r/t pain and life-style changes
Ineffective individual coping r/t personal vulnerability to situational crisis of new diagnosis, deteriorating health
Pain r/t myocardial ischemia

Angiocardiography (Cardiac Cath)

Refer to Cardiac Catheterization

Angioplasty, Coronary Balloon

Altered health maintenance r/t knowledge deficit regarding care following procedures, measures to limit coronary artery disease
Fear r/t possible outcome of interventional procedure
Risk for altered tissue perfusion: peripheral/ cardiopulmonary r/t vasospasm, hematoma formation
Risk for decreased cardiac output r/t ventricular ischemia, dysrhythmias
Risk for fluid volume deficit r/t possible damage to coronary artery, hematoma formation, hemorrhage

Anomaly, Fetal/Newborn (Parent Dealing With)

Altered family processes r/t unmet expectations for perfect baby, lack of adequate support systems
Altered parenting r/t interruption of bonding process
Anxiety r/t threat to role functioning, situational crisis
Decisional conflict: interventions for fetus/newborn r/t lack of relevant information, spiritual distress, threat to value system
Fear r/t real or imagined threat to baby, implications for future pregnancies, powerlessness
Hopelessness r/t long-term stress, deteriorating physical condition of child, lost spiritual belief
Knowledge deficit r/t limited exposure to situation
Ineffective family coping: disabling r/t chronically unresolved feelings of loss of perfect baby
Ineffective individual coping r/t personal vulnerability in situational crisis
Parental role conflict r/t separation from newborn, intimidation with invasive or restrictive modalities, specialized care center policies
Powerlessness r/t complication threatening fetus/newborn
Risk for altered parent/infant/child attachment r/t ill infant who is unable to effectively initiate parental contact as a result of altered behavioral organization
Risk for altered parenting r/t interruption of bonding process; unrealistic expectations for self, infant, or partner; perceived threat to own emotional survival; severe stress; lack of knowledge
Risk for dysfunctional grieving r/t loss of perfect child
Self-esteem disturbance r/t perceived inability to produce a perfect child
Spiritual distress r/t test of spiritual beliefs

Anorexia

Altered nutrition: less than body requirements r/t loss of appetite, nausea, and vomiting
Fluid volume deficit r/t inability to drink

Anorexia Nervosa

Activity intolerance r/t fatigue, weakness
Altered nutrition: less than body requirements r/t inadequate food intake
Altered patterns of sexuality r/t loss of libido from malnutrition
Altered thought processes r/t anorexia
Body image disturbance r/t misconception of actual body appearance
Chronic low self-esteem r/t repeated unmet expectations
Constipation r/t lack of adequate food, fluid intake
Defensive coping r/t psychological impairment, eating disorder
Diarrhea r/t laxative abuse
Ineffective denial r/t fear of consequences of therapy and possible weight gain
Ineffective family coping: disabling r/t highly ambivalent family relationships
Ineffective management of therapeutic regimen: families r/t family conflict, excessive demands on family r/t complexity of condition and treatment
Risk for infection r/t malnutrition resulting in depressed immune system
Refer to Maturational Issues, Adolescent

Anosmia—Loss of Smell

Sensory/perceptual alteration: olfactory r/t altered sensory reception, transmission, and/or integration

Antepartum Period

Refer to Prenatal Care/Normal; Pregnancy

Anterior Repair—Anterior Colporrhaphy

Risk for perioperative positioning injury
Refer to Vaginal Hysterectomy

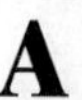

Anticoagulant Therapy

Altered health maintenance r/t knowledge deficit regarding precautions to take with anticoagulant therapy
Altered protection r/t altered clotting function from anticoagulant
Anxiety r/t situational crisis
Risk for fluid volume deficit: hemorrhage r/t altered clotting mechanism

Antisocial Personality Disorder

Impaired social interaction r/t sociocultural conflict, chemical dependence, inability to form relationships
Ineffective individual coping r/t frequently violating the norms and rules of society
Ineffective management of therapeutic regimen: families r/t excessive demands on family
Risk for altered parenting r/t inability to function as a parent or guardian, emotional instability
Risk for loneliness r/t inability to interact appropriately with others
Risk for violence directed at others r/t history of violence

Anuria

Refer to Renal Failure

Anxiety

Anxiety r/t unconscious conflict about essential values or goals of life, threat to self-concept, threat of death, threat to or change in health status, threat to or change in role functioning, threat to or change in environment, threat to or change in interaction patterns, situational or maturational crises, interpersonal transmission/contagion, unmet needs

Anxiety Disorder

Altered thought processes r/t anxiety
Anxiety r/t unmet security and safety needs
Decisional conflict r/t low self-esteem, fear of making a mistake
Energy field disturbance r/t hopelessness, helplessness, fear
Ineffective family coping: disabling r/t ritualistic behavior, actions
Ineffective individual coping r/t inability to express feelings appropriately
Powerlessness r/t life-style of helplessness
Self-care deficit r/t ritualistic behavior, activities
Sleep pattern disturbance r/t psychological impairment, emotional instability

Aortic Aneurysm Repair (Abdominal Surgery)

Refer to Aneurysm; Abdominal Surgery

Aortic Valvular Stenosis

Refer to Congenital Heart Disease/Cardiac Anomalies

Aphasia

Altered health maintenance r/t knowledge deficit regarding information on aphasia and alternative communication techniques
Anxiety r/t situational crisis of aphasia
Impaired verbal communication r/t decrease in circulation to brain
Ineffective individual coping r/t loss of speech

Apnea in Infancy

Refer to SIDS, Near Miss; Premature Infant

Apneustic Respirations

Impaired breathing pattern r/t perception/cognitive impairment, neurological impairment
Refer to cause of Apneustic Respirations

Appendectomy

Altered health maintenance r/t knowledge deficit regarding self-care following appendectomy
Fluid volume deficit r/t fluid restriction, hypermetabolic state, and nausea and vomiting
Pain r/t surgical incision
Risk for infection r/t perforation/rupture of appendix, surgical incision, peritonitis
Refer to Surgery; Hospitalized Child

Appendicitis

Fluid volume deficit r/t anorexia, nausea, and vomiting
Pain r/t inflammation
Risk for infection r/t possible perforation of appendix

Apprehension

Anxiety r/t threat to self concept, threat to health status, situational crisis

ARDS (Adult Respiratory Distress Syndrome)

Impaired gas exchange r/t damage to alveolar-capillary membrane, change in lung compliance
Inability to sustain spontaneous ventilation r/t damage to the alveolar capillary membrane

Ineffective airway clearance r/t excessive tracheobronchial secretions
Refer to Ventilator Client; Child with Chronic Condition

Arrhythmias

Refer to Dysrhythmias

Arterial Insufficiency

Altered tissue perfusion: peripheral r/t interruption of arterial flow

Arthritis

Activity intolerance r/t chronic pain, fatigue, weakness
Altered health maintenance r/t knowledge deficit regarding care of arthritis
Body image disturbance r/t ineffective coping with joint abnormalities
Chronic pain r/t progression of joint deterioration
Impaired physical mobility r/t musculoskeletal impairment
Self-care deficit: specify r/t pain, musculoskeletal impairment
Refer to Rheumatoid Arthritis, Juvenile

Arthrocentesis

Pain r/t invasive procedure

Arthroplasty—Total Hip Replacement

Activity intolerance r/t limitations from surgery
Constipation r/t immobility
Pain r/t tissue trauma associated with surgery
Risk for infection r/t invasive surgery, foreign object in body, anesthesia, immobility with stasis of respiratory secretions
Risk for injury r/t interruption of arterial blood flow, dislocation of prosthesis
Risk for perioperative positioning injury r/t immobilization, muscle weakness
Risk for peripheral neurovascular dysfunction r/t orthopedic surgery
Refer to Surgery

Arthroscopy

Altered health maintenance r/t knowledge deficit regarding procedure, postoperative restrictions

Ascites

Altered health maintenance r/t knowledge deficit of care with condition of ascites
Altered nutrition: less than body requirements r/t loss of appetite
Chronic pain r/t altered body function
Ineffective breathing pattern r/t increased abdominal girth
Refer to cause of Ascites; Cirrhosis; Cancer

Asphyxia, Birth

Altered tissue perfusion r/t poor placental perfusion or cord compression
Fear (parental) r/t concern over safety of infant
Impaired gas exchange r/t poor placental perfusion or lack of initiation of breathing by newborn
Inability to sustain spontaneous ventilation r/t brain injury
Ineffective breathing pattern r/t depression of breathing reflex secondary to anoxia
Risk for injury r/t lack of oxygen to brain

Aspiration, Danger of

Risk for aspiration r/t reduced level of consciousness; depressed cough or gag reflexes; presence of tracheostomy or endotracheal tube; incomplete lower esophageal sphincter; presence of gastrointestinal tubes or tube feedings; medication administration; situations hindering elevation of upper body; increased intragastric pressure; increased gastric residual; decreased gastrointestinal motility; delayed gastric emptying; impaired swallowing; facial, oral, or neck surgery or trauma; wired jaws

Assault Victim

Post-trauma response r/t assault
Rape-trauma syndrome r/t rape

Assaultive Client

Altered thought process r/t use of hallucinogenic substance, psychological disorder
Ineffective individual coping r/t lack of control of impulsive actions
Risk for violence r/t paranoid ideation
Risk for injury r/t confused thought process and impaired judgment

Asthma

Activity intolerance r/t fatigue, energy shift to meet muscle needs for breathing to overcome airway obstruction
Altered health maintenance r/t knowledge deficit regarding physical triggers, medications, treatment of early warning signs
Anxiety r/t inability to breathe effectively, fear of suffocation
Body image disturbance r/t decreased participation in physical activities

Impaired home maintenance management r/t knowledge deficit regarding control of environmental triggers
Ineffective airway clearance r/t tracheobronchial narrowing, excessive secretions
Ineffective breathing pattern r/t anxiety
Ineffective individual coping r/t personal vulnerability to a situational crisis
Refer to Child with Chronic Condition; Hospitalized Child

Ataxia

Anxiety r/t change in health status
Body image disturbance r/t staggering gait
Impaired physical mobility r/t neuromuscular impairment
Risk for injury r/t gait alteration

Atelectasis

Impaired gas exchange r/t decreased alveolar-capillary surface
Ineffective breathing pattern r/t loss of functional lung tissue, depression of respiratory function or hypoventilation because of pain

Athlete's Foot

Altered health maintenance r/t knowledge deficit regarding treatment and prevention of athlete's foot
Impaired skin integrity r/t effects of fungal agent

Atrial Septal Defect

Refer to Congenital Heart Disease/Cardiac Anomalies

Attention Deficit Disorder

Risk for altered parenting r/t lack of knowledge of factors contributing to child's behavior
Risk for loneliness r/t social isolation
Self-esteem disturbance r/t difficulty in participating in expected activities
Social isolation r/t unacceptable social behavior

Autism

Altered growth and development r/t inability to develop relations with other human beings, inability to identify own body as separate from those of other people, inability to integrate concept of self
Altered thought processes r/t inability to perceive self or others, cognitive dissonance, perceptual dysfunction
Identity disturbance r/t inability to distinguish between self and environment, inability to identify own body as separate from those of other people, inability to integrate concept of self
Impaired social interaction r/t communication barriers, inability to relate interpersonally to others
Impaired verbal communication r/t speech and language delays
Ineffective family coping: compromised/disabling r/t parental guilt over etiology of disease, inability to accept or adapt to child's condition, inability to help child and other family members seek treatment
Personal identity disturbance r/t inability to distinguish between self and environment, inability to identify own body as separate from those of other people, inability to integrate concept of self
Risk for self-mutilation r/t autistic state
Risk for violence: self- and other-directed r/t frequent destructive rages toward self or others secondary to extreme response to changes in routine, fear of harmless things
Refer to Mental Retardation; Child with Chronic Condition

Autonomic Hyperreflexia

Dysreflexia r/t bladder distention, bowel distention, or other noxious stimuli

B

Back Pain

Altered health maintenance r/t knowledge deficit regarding prevention of further injury, proper body mechanics
Anxiety r/t situational crisis, back injury
Impaired physical mobility r/t pain
Ineffective individual coping r/t situational crisis, back injury
Pain r/t back injury
Risk for colonic constipation r/t decreased activity
Risk for disuse syndrome r/t severe pain

Barrel Chest

Can also be associated with aging
Refer to COPD

Bathing/Hygiene Problems

Bathing/hygiene self-care deficit r/t intolerance to activity, decreased strength and endurance, pain, discomfort, perceptual or cognitive impairment, neuromuscular impairment, musculoskeletal impairment, depression, severe anxiety

B

Battered Child Syndrome

Altered family process: alcoholism r/t inadequate coping skills
Altered growth and development: regression vs delayed r/t diminished/absent environmental stimuli, inadequate caretaking, inconsistent responsiveness by caretaker
Altered nutrition: less than body requirements r/t inadequate caretaking
Anxiety/fear r/t (child) r/t threat of punishment for perceived wrongdoing
Chronic low self-esteem r/t lack of positive feedback or excessive negative feedback
Diversional activity deficit r/t diminished/absent environmental or personal stimuli
Impaired skin integrity r/t altered nutritional state, physical abuse
Pain r/t physical injuries
Post-trauma response r/t physical abuse, incest/rape/molestation
Risk for poisoning r/t inadequate safeguards, lack of proper safety precautions, accessibility of illicit substances secondary to impaired home maintenance management
Risk for self-mutilation r/t feelings of rejection, dysfunctional family
Risk for suffocation/aspiration r/t propped bottle, unattended child
Risk for trauma r/t inadequate precautions, cognitive or emotional difficulties
Sleep pattern disturbance r/t hypervigilance, anxiety
Social isolation: family imposed r/t fear of disclosure of family dysfunction and abuse

Battered Person

Refer to Abuse, Spouse, Parent, or Significant Other

Bedbugs, Infestation

Impaired home maintenance management r/t knowledge deficit regarding prevention of bedbug infestation
Impaired skin integrity r/t bites of bedbugs

Bedrest, Prolonged

Disuse syndrome r/t prolonged immobility

Bedsores

Refer to Pressure Ulcers

Bedwetting

Refer to Enuresis

Benign Prostatic Hypertrophy

Refer to BPH; Prostatic Hypertrophy

Bereavement

Grieving r/t loss of significant person

Biliary Atresia

Altered comfort r/t pruritis, nausea
Altered nutrition: less than body requirements r/t decreased absorption of fat and fat-soluble vitamins, poor feeding
Anxiety/fear r/t surgical intervention (Kasai procedure), possible liver transplantation
Risk for ineffective breathing patterns r/t enlarged liver, development of ascites
Risk for injury: bleeding r/t vitamin K deficiency, altered clotting mechanisms
Risk for impaired skin integrity r/t to pruritis
Refer to Hospitalized Child; Child with Chronic Condition; Terminally Ill Child/Death of Child; Cirrhosis as complication

Biliary Calculus

Refer to Cholelithiasis

Biliary Obstruction

Refer to Jaundice

Biopsy

Altered health maintenance r/t knowledge deficit regarding biopsy site, further needed health care
Fear r/t outcome of biopsy

Bipolar Disorder I (Most Recent Episode, Depressed or Manic)

Altered health maintenance r/t lack of ability to make good judgments regarding ways to obtain help
Chronic low self-esteem r/t repeated unmet expectations
Dysfunctional grieving r/t lack of previous resolution of former grieving response
Fatigue r/t psychological demands
Ineffective individual coping r/t dysfunctional grieving
Self-care deficit: specify r/t depression, cognitive impairment
Social isolation r/t ineffective coping
Refer to Depression; Manic Disorder

Birth Asphyxia

Refer to Asphyxia, Birth

Bladder Cancer

Urinary retention r/t clots obstructing urethra
Refer to TURP; Cancer

Bladder Distention

Urinary retention r/t high urethral pressure caused by weak detrusor, inhibition of reflex arc, blockage, strong sphincter

Bladder Training

Altered health maintenance r/t knowledge deficit on dealing with incontinence
Functional incontinence r/t altered environment; sensory, cognitive, or mobility deficit
Stress incontinence r/t degenerative change in pelvic muscles and structural supports
Urge incontinence r/t decreased bladder capacity, increased urine concentration, overdistention of bladder

Blepharoplasty

Altered health maintenance r/t knowledge deficit regarding postoperative care of surgical area
Body image disturbance r/t effects of surgery

Blindness

Sensory perceptual alteration: visual r/t altered sensory reception, transmission, and/or integration

Blood Disorders

Altered protection r/t abnormal blood profile
Refer to cause of Blood Disorder

Blood Pressure Alteration

Refer to Hypertension; Hypotension

Blood Transfusion

Anxiety r/t possibility of harm from transfusion
Refer to Anemia

Body Image Change

Body image disturbance r/t chronic illness, loss of body part, change in body appearance

Body Temperature, Altered

Risk for altered body temperature r/t extremes of age or weight, exposure to cold or hot environment, dehydration, change in activity, medication effect, dysfunction of body temperature regulation center

Bone Marrow Biopsy

Altered health maintenance r/t knowledge deficit of expectations following procedure, disease treatment following biopsy
Fear r/t unknown outcome of results of biopsy
Pain r/t bone marrow aspiration
Refer to disease necessitating Bone Marrow Biopsy such as Leukemia

Borderline Personality Disorder

Altered thought process r/t poor reality testing
Anxiety r/t perceived threat to self-concept
Defensive coping r/t difficulty with relationships, inability to accept blame for own behavior
Disturbance in self-concept r/t unmet dependency needs
Ineffective individual coping r/t use of maladjusted defense mechanisms (e.g., projection, denial)
Ineffective management of therapeutic regimen: families r/t manipulative behavior of client
Powerlessness r/t life-style of helplessness
Risk for caregiver role strain r/t inability of care receiver to accept criticism, care receiver takes advantage of others to meet own needs or has unreasonable expectations
Risk for self-mutilation r/t ineffective coping, feelings of self-hatred
Risk for violence: self-directed r/t feelings of need to punish self/manipulative behavior
Social isolation r/t immature interests

Boredom

Diversional activity deficit r/t environmental lack of diversional activity

Botulism

Altered health maintenance r/t knowledge deficit regarding prevention of botulism, care following episode
Fluid volume deficit r/t profuse diarrhea

Bowel Incontinence

Bowel incontinence r/t decreased awareness of need to defecate, loss of sphincter control, fecal impaction

Bowel Obstruction

Altered nutrition: less than body requirements r/t nausea, vomiting
Constipation r/t decreased motility, intestinal obstruction

Fluid volume deficit r/t inadequate fluid volume intake, fluid loss in bowel
Pain r/t pressure from distended abdomen

Bowel Resection

Refer to Abdominal Surgery

Bowel Sounds, Absent or Diminished

Constipation r/t decreased or absent peristalsis
Fluid volume deficit r/t inability to ingest fluids, loss of fluids in bowel

Bowel Sounds, Hyperactive

Diarrhea r/t increased gastrointestinal motility

Bowel Training

Altered health maintenance r/t knowledge deficit regarding treatment of bowel incontinence
Bowel incontinence r/t loss of control of rectal sphincter

BPH (Benign Prostatic Hypertrophy)

Altered health maintenance r/t knowledge deficit regarding self-care with prostatic hypertrophy
Risk for infection r/t urinary residual postvoiding, bacterial invasion of bladder
Sleep pattern disturbance r/t nocturia
Urinary retention r/t obstruction

Bradycardia

Altered health maintenance r/t knowledge deficit of condition, effects of cardiac medications
Altered tissue perfusion: cerebral r/t decreased cardiac output secondary to bradycardia
Decreased cardiac output r/t slow heart rate supplying inadequate amount of blood for body function
Risk for injury r/t decreased cerebral tissue perfusion

Bradypnea

Ineffective breathing pattern r/t neuromuscular impairment, pain, musculoskeletal impairment, perception/cognitive impairment, anxiety, decreased energy/fatigue, drug effect
Refer to cause of Bradypnea

Brain Injury

Refer to Intracranial Pressure, Increased

Brain Surgery

Refer to Craniectomy/Craniotomy

Brain Tumor

Altered thought processes r/t altered circulation or destruction of brain tissue
Anticipatory grieving r/t potential loss of physiosocial-psychosocial well-being
Decreased adaptive capacity: intracranial r/t presence of brain tumor
Fear r/t threat to well-being
Pain r/t neurological injury
Risk for injury r/t sensory-perceptual alterations, weakness
Sensory/perceptual alteration: specify r/t tumor growth compressing brain tissue
Refer to Craniectomy/Craniotomy; Cancer; Chemotherapy; Radiation Therapy; Hospitalized Child; Child with Chronic Condition; Terminally Ill Child

Braxton Hicks Contractions

Activity intolerance r/t increased perception of contractions with increased gestation
Altered sexuality patterns r/t fear of contractions
Anxiety r/t uncertainty about beginning labor
Fatigue r/t lack of sleep
Sleep pattern disturbance r/t contractions when lying down
Stress incontinence r/t increased pressure on bladder with contractions

Breast Biopsy

Altered health maintenance r/t knowledge deficit regarding appropriate postoperative care of breasts
Fear r/t potential for diagnosis of cancer

Breast Cancer

Disturbance in self-concept r/t surgery, possible side effects of chemotherapy and/or radiation
Fear r/t diagnosis of cancer
Ineffective coping r/t treatment and prognosis
Sexual dysfunction r/t loss of body part, partner's reaction to loss
Refer to Mastectomy

Breast-feeding, Effective

Effective breast-feeding r/t basic breast-feeding knowledge, normal breast structure, normal infant oral structure, infant gestational age greater than 34 weeks, support sources or maternal confidence

Breast-feeding, Ineffective

Ineffective breast-feeding r/t prematurity, infant anomaly, maternal breast anomaly, previous breast surgery, previous history of breast-feeding failure, infant receiving supplemental feedings with artificial nipple, poor infant sucking reflex, nonsupportive partner/family, knowledge deficit, interruption in breast-feeding, maternal anxiety or ambivalence

Refer to Painful Breasts—Engorgement; Painful Breasts—Cracked Nipples

Breast-feeding, Interrupted

Interrupted breast-feeding r/t maternal or infant illness, prematurity, maternal employment, contraindications to breast-feeding (e.g., drugs, true breastmilk jaundice), need to abruptly wean infant

Breast Lumps

Altered health maintenance r/t knowledge deficit regarding appropriate care of breasts

Fear r/t potential for diagnosis of cancer

Breast Pumping

Altered health maintenance r/t knowledge deficit regarding breast milk expression and storage

Anxiety r/t interrupted breast-feeding

Body image disturbance r/t individual response to breast-feeding process

Decisional conflict r/t infant feeding method

Risk for impaired skin integrity r/t high suction

Risk for infection r/t contaminated breast pump parts, incomplete emptying of breast

Breath Sounds, Decreased or Absent

Refer to Atelectasis; Pneumothorax

Breathing Pattern Alteration

Ineffective breathing pattern r/t neuromuscular impairment, pain, musculoskeletal impairment, perception/cognitive impairment, anxiety, decreased energy/fatigue

Breech Birth

Anxiety (maternal) r/t threat to self and infant

Impaired gas exchange (fetal) r/t compressed umbilical cord

Risk for aspiration (fetal) r/t birth of body before head

Risk for injury (fetal) r/t birth trauma

Risk for injury (maternal) r/t difficult birth

Bronchitis

Altered health maintenance r/t knowledge deficit regarding care of condition

Anxiety r/t potential chronic condition

Health-seeking behavior r/t wish to stop smoking

Ineffective airway clearance r/t excessive thickened mucus secretion

Bronchopulmonary Dysplasia

Activity intolerance r/t imbalance between oxygen supply and demand

Altered nutrition: less than body requirements r/t poor feeding, increased caloric needs secondary to increased work of breathing

Fluid volume excess r/t sodium and water retention

Refer to Respiratory Conditions of the Neonate; Child with Chronic Condition; Hospitalized Child

Bronchoscopy

Risk for aspiration r/t temporary loss of gag reflex

Risk for injury r/t complication of pneumothorax, laryngeal edema, hemorrhage if biopsy done

Bruits, Carotid

Altered tissue perfusion: cerebral r/t interruption of carotid blood flow

Risk for injury r/t loss of motor, sensory, or visual function

Bryant's Traction

Refer to Traction

Buck's Traction

Refer to Traction

Buerger's Disease

Refer to Peripheral Vascular Disease

Bulimia

Altered nutrition: less than body requirements r/t induced vomiting

Chronic low self-esteem r/t lack of positive feedback

Defensive coping r/t eating disorder

Disturbance in body image r/t misperception about actual appearance and body weight

Fear r/t food ingestion and weight gain

Ineffective family coping r/t chronically unresolved feelings of guilt, anger, and hostility

Noncompliance r/t negative feelings toward treatment regimen

Powerlessness r/t urge to purge self after eating

Refer to Maturational Issues, Adolescent

Bunion

Altered health maintenance r/t knowledge deficit regarding appropriate care of feet

Bunionectomy

Altered health maintenance r/t knowledge deficit regarding postoperative care of foot
Impaired physical mobility r/t sore foot
Risk for infection r/t surgical incision, advanced age

Burns

Altered nutrition: less than body requirements r/t increased metabolic needs, anorexia, protein and fluid loss
Altered tissue perfusion: peripheral r/t circumferential burns, impaired arterial/venous circulation
Anticipatory grieving r/t loss of bodily function, loss of future hopes and plans
Anxiety/fear r/t pain from treatments, possible permanent disfigurement
Body image disturbance r/t altered physical appearance
Diversional activity deficit r/t long-term hospitalization
Hypothermia r/t impaired skin integrity
Impaired physical mobility r/t pain, musculoskeletal impairment, contracture formation
Impaired skin integrity r/t injury of skin
Pain r/t injury and treatments
Post-trauma response r/t life-threatening event
Risk for fluid volume deficit r/t loss from skin surface, fluid shift
Risk for infection r/t loss of intact skin, trauma, invasive sites
Risk for ineffective airway clearance r/t potential tracheobronchial obstruction, edema
Risk for peripheral neurovascular dysfunction r/t eschar formation with circumferential burn
Refer to Safety, Childhood; Hospitalized Child

Bursitis

Impaired physical mobility r/t inflammation in joint
Pain r/t inflammation in joint

Bypass Graft

Refer to Coronary Artery Bypass Grafting

C

Cachexia

Altered nutrition: less than body requirements r/t inability to ingest food due to biological factors
Altered protection r/t inadequate nutrition

Calcium Alteration

Refer to Hypercalcemia; Hypocalcemia

Cancer

Activity intolerance r/t side effects of treatment, weakness from cancer
Altered health maintenance r/t knowledge deficit regarding prescribed treatment
Altered nutrition: less than body requirements r/t loss of appetite, difficulty swallowing, side effects of chemotherapy, obstruction by tumor
Altered oral mucous membranes r/t chemotherapy, oral pH changes, decreased/altered oral flora
Altered protection r/t cancer suppressing immune system
Altered role performance r/t change in physical capacity, inability to resume prior role
Anticipatory grieving r/t potential loss of significant others, high risk for infertility
Body image disturbance r/t side effects of treatment, cachexia
Chronic pain r/t metastatic cancer
Colonic constipation r/t side effects of medication, altered nutrition, decreased activity
Decisional conflict r/t selection of treatment choices, continuation/discontinuation of treatment, Do Not Resuscitate decision
Fear r/t serious threat to well-being
Hopelessness r/t loss of control, terminal illness
Impaired physical mobility r/t weakness, neuromusculoskeletal impairment, pain
Impaired skin integrity r/t immunological deficit, immobility
Ineffective denial r/t dysfunctional grieving process
Ineffective family coping: compromised r/t prolonged disease or disability progression that exhausts the supportive ability of significant others
Ineffective individual coping r/t personal vulnerability in situational crisis, terminal illness
Potential for enhanced spiritual well-being r/t desire for harmony with self, others, and higher power/God when faced with serious illness
Powerlessness r/t treatment, progression of disease
Risk for disuse syndrome r/t severe pain, change in level of consciousness
Risk for impaired home maintenance management r/t lack of familiarity with community resources
Risk for infection r/t inadequate immune system
Risk for injury r/t bleeding secondary to bone marrow depression
Self-care deficit: specify r/t pain, intolerance to activity, decreased strength

Sleep pattern disturbance r/t anxiety, pain
Social isolation r/t hospitalization, life-style changes
Spiritual distress r/t test of spiritual beliefs
Refer to Chemotherapy; Child with Chronic Condition; Hospitalized Child; Terminally Ill Child/Death of Child

Candidiasis, Oral

Altered health maintenance r/t knowledge deficit regarding care of infected mouth
Altered oral mucous membranes r/t overgrowth of infectious agent, depressed immune function

Capillary Refill Time, Prolonged

Altered tissue perfusion: peripheral r/t interruption of arterial or venous flow
Impaired gas exchange r/t ventilation perfusion imbalance
Risk for peripheral neurovascular dysfunction r/t vascular obstruction
Refer to Shock

Cardiac Catheterization

Altered comfort r/t postprocedure restrictions, invasive procedure
Altered health maintenance r/t knowledge deficit regarding procedure, postprocedure care, and treatment and prevention of coronary artery disease
Anxiety/fear r/t invasive procedure, uncertainty of outcome of procedure
Risk for altered tissue perfusion r/t impaired arterial or venous circulation
Risk for decreased cardiac output r/t ventricular ischemia, dysrhythmias
Risk for injury: hematoma r/t invasive procedure
Risk for peripheral neurovascular dysfunction r/t vascular obstruction

Cardiac Disorders

Decreased cardiac output r/t cardiac disorder
Refer to specific disorder

Cardiac Disorders in Pregnancy

Activity intolerance r/t cardiac pathophysiology, increased demand secondary to pregnancy, weakness, fatigue
Altered family processes r/t changes in role, hospitalization, maternal incapacitation
Altered health maintenance r/t knowledge deficit regarding treatment, restrictions with cardiac disorder
Altered role performance r/t changes in life-style, expectations secondary to disease process with superimposed pregnancy
Anxiety r/t unknown outcomes of pregnancy, family well-being
Fatigue r/t metabolic demands, psychological-emotional demands
Fear r/t potential maternal effects, potential poor fetal/maternal outcome
Ineffective family coping: compromised r/t prolonged hospitalization/maternal incapacitation that exhausts supportive capacity of significant others
Ineffective individual coping r/t personal vulnerability
Powerlessness r/t illness-related regimen
Risk for altered fetal tissue perfusion r/t poor maternal oxygenation
Risk for fetal injury r/t hypoxia
Risk for fluid volume excess r/t compromised regulatory mechanism with increased afterload, increased preload, and/or increased circulating blood volume
Risk for impaired gas exchange r/t pulmonary edema
Risk for maternal injury r/t thrombembolic episode secondary to valvular defect
Situational low self-esteem r/t situational crisis, pregnancy
Social isolation r/t limitations of activity, bedrest/hospitalization, separation from family and friends

Cardiac Dysrhythmias

Refer to Dysrhythmias

Cardiac Output Decrease

Decreased cardiac output r/t cardiac dysfunction

Cardiac Tamponade

Decreased cardiac output r/t fluid in pericardial sac
Refer to Pericarditis

Cardiogenic Shock

Decreased cardiac output r/t decreased myocardial contractility, dysrhythmias
Refer to Shock

Caregiver Role Strain

Caregiver role strain r/t pathophysiological factors; developmental factors; psychosocial factors; situational factors
Risk for caregiver role strain r/t pathophysiological factors; developmental factors; psychosocial factors; situational factors

Carious Teeth

Refer to Cavities in Teeth

Carotid Endarterectomy

Altered health maintenance r/t knowledge deficit regarding postoperative care
Fear r/t surgery in vital area
Risk for altered tissue perfusion: cerebral r/t hemorrhage, clot formation
Risk for ineffective breathing pattern r/t hematoma compressing trachea
Risk for injury r/t possible hematoma formation

Carpal Tunnel Syndrome

Impaired physical mobility r/t neuromuscular impairment
Pain r/t unrelieved pressure on median nerve

Carpopedal Spasm

Refer to Hypocalcemia

Casts

Altered health maintenance r/t knowledge deficit regarding cast care, personal care with cast
Diversional activity deficit r/t physical limitations from the cast
Impaired physical mobility r/t limb immobilization
Risk for peripheral neurovascular dysfunction r/t mechanical compression from cast
Risk for impaired skin integrity r/t unrelieved pressure on skin

Cataract Extraction

Altered health maintenance r/t knowledge deficit regarding postoperative restrictions
Anxiety r/t threat of permanent vision loss, surgical procedure
Risk for injury r/t increased intraocular pressure, accommodation to new visual field
Sensory/perceptual alteration: vision r/t edema from surgery

Cataracts

Sensory/perceptual alteration: vision r/t altered sensory input

Catatonic Schizophrenia

Altered nutrition: less than body requirements r/t decrease in outside stimulation, no perception of hunger, resistance to instructions to eat
Impaired memory r/t cognitive impairment
Impaired physical mobility r/t cognitive impairment, maintenance of rigid posture, inappropriate/bizarre postures
Impaired verbal communication r/t mutism
Social isolation r/t inability to communicate, immobility
Refer to Schizophrenia

Catheterization, Urinary

Altered health maintenance r/t knowledge deficit of normal sensation of catheter in place, care of catheter
Risk for infection r/t invasive procedure

Cavities in Teeth

Altered health maintenance r/t lack of knowledge regarding prevention of dental disease secondary to high sugar diet, giving infants/toddlers with erupted teeth bottles of milk at bedtime, lack of fluoride treatments, inadequate or improper brushing of teeth

Cellulitis

Altered tissue perfusion: peripheral r/t edema
Impaired skin integrity r/t inflammatory process damaging skin
Pain r/t inflammatory changes in tissues from infection

Cellulitis, Periorbital

Hyperthermia r/t infectious process
Impaired skin integrity r/t inflammation/infection of skin/tissues
Pain r/t edema and inflammation of skin/tissues
Sensory/perceptual alterations: visual r/t decreased visual fields secondary to edema of eyelids
Refer to Hospitalized Child

Central Line Insertion

Altered health maintenance r/t knowledge deficit regarding precautions to take when central line in place
Risk for infection r/t invasive procedure

Cerebral Aneurysm

Refer to Craniectomy/Craniotomy; Intracranial Pressure—Increased; Subarachnoid Hemorrhage

Cerebral Palsy

Altered nutrition: less than body requirements r/t spasticity, feeding or swallowing difficulties
Diversional activity deficit r/t physical impairments, limitations on ability to participate in recreational activities
Impaired physical mobility r/t spasticity, neuromuscular impairment/weakness

Impaired social interaction r/t impaired communication skills, limited physical activity, perceived differences from peers
Impaired verbal communication r/t impaired ability to articulate/speak words secondary to facial muscle involvement
Risk for injury/trauma r/t muscle weakness, inability to control spasticity
Self-care deficit: specify r/t neuromuscular impairments, sensory deficits
Refer to Child with Chronic Condition

Cerebrovascular Accident

Refer to CVA

Cervixitis

Altered health maintenance r/t knowledge deficit regarding care and prevention of condition
Altered pattern of sexuality r/t abstinence during acute stage
Risk for infection r/t spread of infection, recurrence of infection

Cesarean Delivery

Alteration in comfort: nausea, vomiting, pruritis r/t side effects of systemic or epidural narcotics
Altered family processes r/t unmet expectations for childbirth
Altered health maintenance r/t knowledge deficit regarding postoperative care
Altered role performance r/t unmet expectations for childbirth
Anxiety r/t unmet expectations for childbirth, unknown outcome of surgery
Body image disturbance r/t surgery, unmet expectations for childbirth
Fear r/t perceived threat to own well-being
Impaired physical mobility r/t pain
Pain r/t surgical incision, decreased or absent peristalsis secondary to anesthesia, manipulation of abdominal organs during surgery, immobilization, restricted diet
Risk for aspiration r/t positioning for general anesthesia
Risk for fluid volume deficit r/t increased blood loss secondary to surgery
Risk for infection r/t surgical incision, stasis of respiratory secretions secondary to general anesthesia
Risk for urinary retention r/t regional anesthesia
Situational low self-esteem r/t inability to birth child vaginally

Chemical Dependence

Refer to Alcoholism; Drug Abuse

Chemotherapy

Altered comfort: nausea and vomiting r/t effects of chemotherapy
Altered health maintenance r/t knowledge deficit regarding action, side effects, and how to integrate chemotherapy into life-style
Altered nutrition: less than body requirements r/t side effects of chemotherapy
Altered oral mucous membranes r/t effects of chemotherapy
Altered protection r/t suppressed immune system, decreased platelets
Body image disturbance r/t loss of weight, loss of hair
Fatigue r/t disease process, anemia, drug effects
Risk for altered tissue perfusion r/t anemia
Risk for fluid volume deficit r/t vomiting, diarrhea
Risk for infection r/t immunosuppression
Refer to Cancer

Chest Pain

Fear r/t potential threat of death
Pain r/t myocardial injury, ischemia
Risk for decreased cardiac output r/t ventricular ischemia
Refer to Angina; MI

Chest Tubes

Impaired gas exchange r/t decreased functional lung tissue
Ineffective breathing pattern r/t asymmetrical lung expansion secondary to pain
Pain r/t presence of chest tubes, injury
Risk for injury r/t presence of invasive chest tube

Cheyne-Stokes Respiration

Ineffective breathing pattern r/t critical illness
Refer to cause of Cheyne-Stokes Respiration

CHF (Congestive Heart Failure)

Activity intolerance r/t weakness, fatigue
Altered health maintenance r/t knowledge deficit regarding care of disease
Constipation r/t activity intolerance
Decreased cardiac output r/t impaired cardiac function
Fatigue r/t disease process
Fear r/t threat to one's own well-being
Fluid volume excess r/t impaired excretion of sodium and water

Impaired gas exchange r/t excessive fluid in interstitial space of lungs, alveoli

Refer to Congenital Heart Disease/Cardiac Anomalies; Hospitalized Child; Child with Chronic Condition

Chickenpox

Refer to Communicable Diseases, Childhood

Child Abuse

Altered family process: alcoholism r/t inadequate coping skills

Altered growth and development: regression vs delayed r/t diminished/absent environmental stimuli, inadequate caretaking, inconsistent responsiveness by caretaker

Altered nutrition: less than body requirements r/t inadequate caretaking

Altered parenting r/t psychological impairment, physical or emotional abuse of parent, substance abuse, unrealistic expectations of child

Anxiety/fear r/t (child) r/t threat of punishment for perceived wrongdoing

Chronic low self-esteem r/t lack of positive feedback or excessive negative feedback

Diversional activity deficit r/t diminished or absent environmental/personal stimuli

Impaired skin integrity r/t altered nutritional state, physical abuse

Ineffective management of therapeutic regimen: community r/t deficits in community regarding prevention of child abuse

Pain r/t physical injuries

Post-trauma response r/t physical abuse, incest, rape, molestation

Risk for poisoning r/t inadequate safeguards, lack of proper safety precautions, accessibility of illicit substances secondary to impaired home maintenance management

Risk for suffocation/aspiration r/t propped bottle, unattended child

Risk for trauma r/t inadequate precautions, cognitive or emotional difficulties

Sleep pattern disturbance r/t hypervigilance, anxiety

Social isolation: family imposed r/t fear of disclosure of family dysfunction and abuse

Childbirth

Refer to Labor—Normal; Postpartum—Normal

Child Neglect

Refer to Child Abuse; Failure to Thrive

Child with Chronic Condition

Activity intolerance r/t fatigue associated with chronic illness

Altered family processes r/t intermittent situational crisis of illness, disease, and hospitalization

Altered growth and development r/t regression or lack of progression toward developmental milestones secondary to frequent or prolonged hospitalization, inadequate or inappropriate stimulation, cerebral insult, chronic illness, effects of physical disability, prescribed dependence

Altered health maintenance r/t exhausting family resources (finances, physical energy, support systems)

Altered nutrition: less than body requirements r/t anorexia, fatigue secondary to physical exertion

Altered nutrition: more than body requirements r/t effects of steroid medications on appetite

Altered sexuality patterns (parental) r/t disrupted relationship with sexual partner

Chronic low self-esteem r/t actual or perceived differences, peer acceptance, decreased ability to participate in physical/school/social activities

Chronic pain r/t physical, biological, chemical, or psychological factors

Decisional conflict r/t treatment options, conflicting values

Diversional activity deficit r/t immobility, monotonous environment, frequent/lengthy treatments, reluctance to participate, self-imposed social isolation

Family coping: potential for growth r/t impact of crisis on family values, priorities, goals, or relationships; changes in family choices to optimize wellness

Hopelessness (child) r/t prolonged activity restriction, long-term stress, lack of involvement in or passively allowing care secondary to parental overprotection

Impaired home maintenance management r/t overtaxed family members (e.g., exhausted, anxious)

Impaired social interaction r/t developmental lag/delay, perceived differences

Ineffective family coping: compromised r/t prolonged disease or disability progression that exhausts supportive capacity of significant people

Ineffective family coping: disabling r/t prolonged overconcern for child; distortion of reality regarding child's health problem, including extreme denial about its existence or severity

Ineffective individual coping (child) r/t situational or maturational crises

Knowledge deficit: potential for enhanced health maintenance r/t knowledge/skill acquisition regarding health practices, acceptance of limitations, promotion of maximum potential of child and self-actualization of rest of family
Parental role conflict r/t separation from child due to chronic illness; home care of child with special needs; interruptions of family life due to home care regimen
Powerlessness (child) r/t health care environment; illness-related regimen; life-style of learned helplessness
Risk for altered parenting r/t impaired/disrupted bonding, child with perceived overwhelming care needs
Risk for infection r/t debilitating physical condition
Risk for noncompliance r/t complex or prolonged home care regimens; expressed intent to not comply secondary to value systems, health beliefs, and cultural/religious practices
Sleep pattern disturbance (child or parent) r/t time-intensive treatments, exacerbation of condition, 24-hour care needs
Social isolation: family r/t actual or perceived social stigmatization, complex care requirements

Chills

Hyperthermia r/t infectious process

Chlamydia Infection

Refer to Sexually Transmitted Disease

Choking/Coughing with Feeding

Impaired swallowing r/t neuromuscular impairment
Risk for aspiration r/t depressed cough and gag reflexes

Cholasma

Body image disturbance r/t change in skin color

Cholecystectomy

Altered health maintenance r/t knowledge deficit regarding postoperative care
Altered nutrition: less than body requirements r/t high metabolic needs, decreased ability to digest fatty foods
Pain r/t recent surgery
Risk for fluid volume deficit r/t restricted intake, nausea, vomiting
Risk for ineffective breathing pattern r/t proximity of incision to lungs resulting in pain with deep breathing
Refer to Abdominal Surgery

Cholelithiasis

Altered health maintenance r/t knowledge deficit regarding care of disease
Altered nutrition: less than body requirements r/t anorexia, nausea, vomiting
Pain r/t obstruction of bile flow, inflammation in gallbladder

Chorioamnionitis

Anticipatory grieving r/t guilt over potential loss of ideal pregnancy and birth
Anxiety r/t threat to self and infant
Hyperthermia r/t infectious process
Risk for injury (fetal) r/t infectious process, threat of preterm birth
Risk for injury (fetal) r/t transmission of infection from mother
Situational low self-esteem r/t guilt over threat to infant's health

Chovstek's Sign

Refer to Hypocalcemia

Chronic Lymphocytic Leukemia

Refer to Leukemia

Chronic Obstructive Pulmonary Disease

Refer to COPD

Chronic Pain

Refer to Pain, Chronic

Chronic Renal Failure

Refer to Renal Failure

Circumcision

Altered health maintenance r/t knowledge deficit (parental) regarding care of surgical area
Pain r/t surgical intervention
Risk for fluid volume deficit r/t hemorrhage
Risk for infection r/t surgical wound

Cirrhosis

Altered health maintenance r/t knowledge deficit regarding correlation between life-style habits and disease process
Altered nutrition: less than body requirements r/t loss of appetite, nausea, vomiting
Altered thought processes r/t chronic organic disorder with increased ammonia levels or substance abuse
Chronic low self-esteem r/t chronic illness
Chronic pain r/t liver enlargement
Diarrhea r/t dietary changes, medications

Fatigue r/t malnutrition
Ineffective management of therapeutic regimen r/t denial of severity of illness
Risk for altered oral mucous membranes r/t altered nutrition
Risk for fluid volume deficit: hemorrhage r/t abnormal bleeding from esophagus
Risk for injury r/t substance intoxication, potential delirium tremors

Cleft Lip/Cleft Palate

Altered health maintenance r/t lack of parental knowledge regarding feeding techniques, wound care, use of elbow restraints
Altered nutrition: less than body requirements r/t inability to feed with normal techniques
Altered oral mucous membranes r/t surgical correction
Fear (parental) r/t special care needs, surgery
Grieving r/t loss of perfect child, birth of child with congenital defect
Impaired physical mobility r/t imposed restricted activity, use of elbow restraints
Impaired skin integrity r/t incomplete joining of lip, palate ridges
Impaired verbal communication r/t inadequate palate function and possible hearing loss from infected eustachian tubes
Ineffective airway clearance r/t common feeding and breathing passage; postoperative laryngeal and/or incisional edema
Ineffective breast-feeding r/t infant anomaly
Ineffective infant feeding pattern r/t cleft lip, cleft palate
Pain r/t surgical correction, elbow restraints
Risk for aspiration r/t common feeding and breathing passage
Risk for body image disturbance r/t disfigurement, speech impediment
Risk for infection r/t invasive procedure, disruption of eustachian tube development, aspiration

Clotting Disorder

Altered health maintenance r/t knowledge deficit regarding treatment of disorder
Altered protection r/t clotting disorder
Anxiety/fear r/t threat to well-being
Risk for fluid volume deficit r/t uncontrolled bleeding
Refer to Hemophilia; Anticoagulant Therapy; DIC

Coarctation of the Aorta

Refer to Congenital Heart Disease/Cardiac Anomalies

Cocaine Abuse

Altered thought processes r/t excessive stimulation of nervous system by cocaine
Ineffective breathing pattern r/t drug effect on respiratory center
Ineffective individual coping r/t inability to deal with life stresses
Refer to Substance Abuse

Cocaine Babies

Refer to Crack Babies

Codependency

Caregiver role strain r/t codependency
Decisional conflict r/t support system deficit
Denial r/t unmet self-needs
Impaired verbal communication r/t psychological barriers
Ineffective individual coping r/t inadequate support systems
Powerlessness r/t life-style of helplessness

Cognitive Deficit

Altered thought processes r/t neurological impairment

Cold, Viral

Altered comfort: sore throat, aching, nasal discomfort r/t viral infection
Altered health maintenance r/t knowledge deficit regarding care of viral condition, prevention of further infections

Colectomy

Altered health maintenance r/t knowledge deficit regarding procedure, postoperative care
Altered nutrition: less than body requirements r/t high metabolic needs, decreased ability to ingest/digest food
Constipation r/t decreased activity, decreased fluid intake
Pain r/t recent surgery
Risk for infection r/t invasive procedure
Refer to Abdominal Surgery

Colitis

Diarrhea r/t inflammation in colon
Fluid volume deficit r/t frequent stools
Pain r/t inflammation in colon
Refer to Ulcerative Colitis; Crohn's Disease; Inflammatory Bowel Syndrome

Collagen Disease

Refer to specific disease: Lupus Erythematosus; Rheumatoid Arthritis

Colostomy

Altered health maintenance r/t knowledge deficit regarding care of stoma, integrating colostomy care into life-style
Body image disturbance r/t presence of stoma, daily care of fecal material
Risk for altered sexuality pattern r/t altered body image, self-concept
Risk for constipation/diarrhea r/t inappropriate diet
Risk for impaired skin integrity r/t irritation from bowel contents
Risk for social isolation r/t anxiety over appearance of stoma and possible leakage

Colporrhaphy, Anterior

Refer to Vaginal Hysterectomy

Coma

Altered family processes r/t illness/disability of family member
Altered thought processes r/t neurological changes
Ineffective management of therapeutic regimen: families r/t complexity of therapeutic regimen
Risk for altered oral mucous membranes r/t dry mouth
Risk for aspiration r/t impaired swallowing, loss of cough/gag reflex
Risk for disuse syndrome r/t altered level of consciousness impairing mobility
Risk for impaired skin integrity r/t immobility
Risk for injury r/t potential seizure activity
Self-care deficit: specify r/t neuromuscular impairment
Total incontinence r/t neurological dysfunction
Refer to the cause of client's comatose state

Comfort, Loss of

Altered comfort r/t injury agent

Communicable Diseases, Childhood (Measles, Mumps, Rubella, Chickenpox, Scabies, Lice, Impetigo)

Altered comfort r/t hyperthermia secondary to infectious disease process, pruritis secondary to skin rash or subdermal organisms
Altered health maintenance r/t nonadherence to appropriate immunization schedules, lack of prevention of transmission of infection
Diversional activity deficit r/t imposed isolation from peers, disruption in usual play activities, fatigue, activity intolerance
Pain r/t impaired skin integrity, edema
Risk for infection: transmission to others r/t contagious organisms
Refer to Meningitis/Encephalitis; Respiratory Infections, Acute Childhood; Reye's Syndrome

Communication Problems

Impaired verbal communication r/t decrease in circulation to brain, brain tumor, physical barrier (tracheostomy, intubation), anatomical defect, cleft palate, psychological barriers, cultural difference, developmental lag

Community Coping

Ineffective community coping r/t deficits in social support, inadequate resources for problem solving, powerlessness
Potential for enhanced community coping r/t available social supports, available resources for problem solving, community's sense of power to manage stressors

Community Management of Therapeutic Regimen

Ineffective management of therapeutic regimen: community r/t inadequate community resources

Compartment Syndrome

Altered tissue perfusion: peripheral r/t increased pressure within compartment
Fear r/t possible loss of limb, damage to limb

Compulsion

Refer to Obsessive Compulsive Personality Disorder

Conduction Disorders (Cardiac)

Refer to Dysrhythmias

Confusion, Acute

Acute confusion r/t process causing delirium

Confusion, Chronic

Altered thought processes r/t organic mental disorder, disruption of cerebral arterial blood flow, chemical imbalance, intoxication
Chronic confusion r/t Alzheimer's disease, Korsakoff's psychosis, multi-infarct dementia, cerebral vascular accident, head injury

Congenital Heart Disease/Cardiac Anomalies

Acyanotic: patent ductus arteriosus; atrial/ventricular septal defect; pulmonary stenosis; endocardial cushion defect; aortic valvular stenosis; coarctation of the aorta

Cyanotic: tetralogy of Fallot; tricuspid atresia; transposition of the great vessels; truncus arteriosus; total anomalous pulmonary venous return; hypoplastic left lung

Activity intolerance r/t fatigue, generalized weakness, lack of adequate oxygenation
Altered family processes r/t to ill child
Altered growth and development r/t inadequate oxygen and nutrients to tissues
Altered nutrition: less than body requirements r/t fatigue, generalized weakness, inability of infant to suck and feed, increased caloric requirements
Decreased cardiac output r/t cardiac dysfunction
Fluid volume excess r/t cardiac defect, side effects of medication
Impaired gas exchange r/t cardiac defect, pulmonary congestion
Ineffective breathing patterns r/t pulmonary vascular disease
Risk for disorganized infant behavior r/t invasive procedures
Risk for fluid volume deficit r/t side effects of diuretics
Risk for ineffective thermoregulation r/t neonatal age
Risk for poisoning r/t potential toxicity of cardiac medications
Refer to Hospitalized Child; Child with Chronic Illness

Congestive Heart Failure

Refer to CHF

Conjunctivitis

Pain r/t inflammatory process
Risk for injury r/t change in visual acuity
Sensory/perceptual alteration r/t change in visual acuity resulting from inflammation

Consciousness, Altered Level of

Altered thought processes r/t neurological changes
Altered tissue perfusion: cerebral r/t increased intracranial pressure, decreased cerebral perfusion
Decreased adaptive capacity: intracranial r/t brain injury
Disuse syndrome r/t impaired mobility resulting from altered level of consciousness
Impaired memory r/t neurological disturbances
Risk for altered oral mucous membranes r/t dry mouth
Risk for aspiration r/t impaired swallowing, loss of cough/gag reflex
Risk for impaired skin integrity r/t immobility
Self-care deficit: specify r/t neuromuscular impairment
Total incontinence r/t neurological dysfunction
Refer to the cause of client's change in level of consciousness

Constipation

Constipation r/t decreased fluid intake, decreased intake of foods containing bulk, inactivity, immobility, knowledge deficit of appropriate bowel routine, lack of privacy for defecation

Constipation, Colonic with Hard, Dry Stool

Colonic constipation r/t less than adequate fluid and/or dietary intake

Constipation, Perceived

Perceived constipation r/t cultural or family health beliefs, faulty appraisal, impaired thought processes

Continent Ileostomy (Kock Pouch)

Altered health maintenance r/t knowledge deficit regarding postoperative care
Altered nutrition: less than body requirements r/t malabsorption
Ineffective individual coping r/t stress of disease and exacerbations related to stress
Risk for injury r/t failure of valve, stomal cyanosis, intestinal obstruction
Refer to Abdominal Surgery

Contraceptive Method

Decisional conflict (method of contraception) r/t unclear personal values or beliefs, lack of experience or interference with decision making, lack of relevant information, support system deficit

Conversion Disorder

Altered role performance r/t physical conversion system
Anxiety r/t unresolved conflict
Hopelessness r/t long-term stress
Impaired physical mobility r/t physical conversion symptom
Impaired social interaction r/t altered thought process

Ineffective individual coping r/t personal vulnerability
Powerlessness r/t life-style of helplessness
Risk for injury r/t physical conversion symptom
Self-esteem disturbance r/t unsatisfactory or inadequate interpersonal relationships

Convulsions

Altered health maintenance r/t knowledge deficit regarding need for medication and care during seizure activity
Anxiety r/t concern over controling convulsions
Impaired memory r/t neurological disturbance
Risk for altered thought processes r/t seizure activity
Risk for aspiration r/t impaired swallowing
Risk for injury r/t seizure activity
Refer to Seizure Disorders, Childhood

COPD (Chronic Obstructive Pulmonary Disease)

Activity intolerance r/t imbalance between oxygen supply and demand
Altered family process r/t role changes
Altered health maintenance r/t knowledge deficit regarding care of disease
Altered nutrition: less than body requirements r/t decreased intake because of dyspnea, unpleasant taste in mouth left by medications
Anxiety r/t breathlessness, change in health status
Chronic low self-esteem r/t chronic illness
Health-seeking behavior r/t wish to stop smoking
Impaired gas exchange r/t ventilation-perfusion inequality
Impaired social interaction r/t social isolation secondary to oxygen use, activity intolerance
Ineffective airway clearance r/t bronchoconstriction, increased mucus, ineffective cough, and infection
Noncompliance r/t reluctance to accept responsibility for changing detrimental health practices
Powerlessness r/t progressive nature of the disease
Risk for infection r/t stasis of respiratory secretions
Self-care deficit: specify r/t fatigue secondary to increased work of breathing
Sleep pattern disturbance r/t dyspnea, side effect of medications

Coping Problems

Defensive coping r/t superior attitude toward others, difficulty establishing or maintaining relationships, hostile laughter or ridicule of others, difficulty in reality-testing perceptions, lack of follow-through or participation in treatment or therapy
Ineffective individual coping r/t situational crises, maturational crises, personal vulnerability
Refer to Family Problems; Community Coping

Corneal Reflex, Absent

Risk for injury r/t accidental corneal abrasion, drying of cornea

Coronary Artery Bypass Grafting

Altered health maintenance r/t knowledge deficit regarding postprocedure care, life-style adjustment after surgery
Decreased cardiac output r/t dysrhythmias, depressed cardiac function, increased systemic vascular resistance
Fear r/t outcome of surgical procedure
Fluid volume deficit r/t intraoperative fluid loss, use of diuretics in surgery
Pain r/t traumatic surgery
Risk for perioperative positioning injury r/t hypothermia, extended supine position

Costovertebral Angle Tenderness

Refer to Kidney Stones; Pyelonephritis

Cough, Effective/Ineffective

Ineffective airway clearance r/t decreased energy, fatigue, normal aging changes
Refer to Bronchitis; COPD; Pulmonary Edema

Crack Abuse

Refer to Cocaine Abuse

Crack Baby

Altered growth and development r/t effects of maternal use of drugs, neurological impairment, decreased attentiveness to environmental stimuli
Altered nutrition: less than body requirements r/t feeding problems; uncoordinated or ineffective suck and swallow; effects of diarrhea, vomiting, or colic
Altered parenting r/t impaired or lack of attachment behaviors, inadequate support systems
Altered protection r/t effects of maternal substance abuse
Diarrhea r/t effects of withdrawal, increased peristalsis secondary to hyperirritability
Disorganized infant behavior r/t lack of attachment, prematurity, pain
Ineffective airway clearance r/t pooling of secretions secondary to lack of adequate cough reflex

Ineffective infant feeding r/t prematurity, neurological impairment
Risk for infection (skin, meningeal, respiratory) r/t effects of withdrawal
Sensory-perceptual alteration r/t hypersensitivity to environmental stimuli
Sleep pattern disturbance r/t hyperirritability, hypersensitivity to environmental stimuli

Crackles in Lungs, Coarse

Ineffective airway clearance r/t excessive secretions in airways, ineffective cough
Refer to cause of Coarse Crackles

Crackles in Lungs, Fine

Ineffective breathing pattern r/t decreased energy, fatigue, surgery
If crackles cardiac in origin, refer to CHF; if from pulmonary infection, refer to Bronchitis or Pneumonia

Craniectomy/Craniotomy

Altered tissue perfusion: cerebral r/t cerebral edema, decreased cerebral perfusion, increased intracranial pressure
Decreased adaptive capacity: intracranial r/t brain injury, intracranial hypertension
Fear r/t threat to well-being
Impaired memory r/t neurological surgery
Pain r/t recent surgery, headache
Risk for altered thought processes r/t neurophysiological changes
Risk for injury r/t potential confusion
Refer to Coma if relevant

Crepitation, Subcutaneous

Refer to Pneumothorax

Crisis

Anticipatory grieving r/t potential significant loss
Anxiety r/t threat to or change in environment, health status, interaction patterns, situation, self-concept, or role-functioning; threat of death of self or significant other
Energy field disturbance r/t disharmony caused by crisis
Fear r/t crisis situation
Ineffective family coping: compromised r/t situational or developmental crisis
Ineffective individual coping r/t situational or maturational crisis
Situational low self-esteem r/t perception of inability to handle crisis
Spiritual distress r/t intense suffering

Crohn's Disease

Altered health maintenance r/t knowledge deficit regarding management of the disease
Altered nutrition: less than body requirements r/t diarrhea, altered ability to digest and absorb food
Anxiety r/t change in health status
Diarrhea r/t inflammatory process
Ineffective individual coping r/t repeated episodes of diarrhea
Pain r/t increased peristalsis
Powerlessness r/t chronic disease
Risk for fluid volume deficit r/t abnormal fluid loss with diarrhea

Croup

Refer to Respiratory Infections, Acute Childhood

Cryosurgery for Retinal Detachment

Refer to Retinal Detachment

Cushing's Syndrome

Activity intolerance r/t fatigue, weakness
Altered health maintenance r/t knowledge deficit regarding need care with disease
Body image disturbance r/t change in appearance from disease process
Fluid volume excess r/t failure of regulatory mechanisms
Risk for infection r/t suppression of the immune system secondary to increased cortisol
Risk for injury r/t decreased muscle strength, osteoporosis
Sexual dysfunction r/t loss of libido

CVA (Cerebrovascular Accident)

Altered family process r/t illness, disability of family member
Altered health maintenance r/t knowledge deficit regarding self-care following CVA
Altered thought processes r/t neurophysiological changes
Anxiety r/t situational crisis, change in physical or emotional condition
Body image disturbance r/t chronic illness, paralysis
Caregiver role strain r/t cognitive problems of care receiver, need for significant home care
Chronic confusion r/t neurological changes
Constipation r/t decreased activity
Grieving r/t loss of health
Impaired memory r/t neurological disturbances
Impaired physical mobility r/t loss of balance and coordination
Impaired social interaction r/t limited physical mobility, limited ability to communicate

Impaired swallowing r/t neuromuscular dysfunction
Impaired verbal communication r/t pressure damage, decreased circulation to the brain of the speech center informational sources
Ineffective individual coping r/t disability
Reflex incontinence r/t loss of feeling to void
Risk for aspiration r/t impaired swallowing, loss of gag reflex
Risk for disuse syndrome r/t paralysis
Risk for impaired skin integrity r/t immobility
Risk for injury r/t sensory-perceptual alteration
Self-care deficit: specify r/t decreased strength and endurance, paralysis
Sensory/perceptual alteration: visual, tactile, kinesthetic r/t neurological deficit
Total incontinence r/t neurological dysfunction
Unilateral neglect r/t disturbed perception from neurological damage

Cyanosis, Central with Cyanosis of Oral Mucous Membranes

Impaired gas exchange r/t alveolar-capillary membrane changes

Cyanosis, Peripheral with Cyanosis of Nailbeds

Altered tissue perfusion r/t interruption of arterial flow, severe vasoconstriction, or cold
Risk for peripheral neurovascular dysfunction r/t condition causing a disruption in circulation

Cystic Fibrosis

Activity intolerance r/t imbalance between oxygen supply and demand
Altered nutrition: less than body requirements r/t anorexia, decreased absorption of nutrients or fat, increased work of breathing
Anxiety r/t dyspnea and oxygen deprivation
Body image disturbance r/t changes in physical appearance and treatment of chronic lung disease (clubbing, barrel chest, home oxygen therapy)
Impaired gas exchange r/t ventilation perfusion imbalance
Impaired home maintenance management r/t extensive daily treatment, medications necessary for health, mist or oxygen tents
Ineffective airway clearance r/t increased production of thick mucus
Risk for caregiver role strain r/t illness severity of the care receiver, unpredictable course of illness
Risk for fluid volume deficit r/t decreased fluid intake and increased work of breathing
Risk for infection r/t thick, tenacious mucus; harboring bacterial organisms; debilitated state
Refer to Child with Chronic Condition; Hospitalized Child; Terminally Ill Child/Death of Child

Cystitis

Altered health maintenance r/t knowledge deficit regarding methods to treat and prevent urinary tract infections
Altered urinary elimination: frequency r/t urinary tract infection
Pain: dysuria r/t inflammatory process in bladder

Cystocele

Altered health maintenance r/t knowledge deficit regarding personal care, Kegel's exercises to strengthen perineal muscles
Stress incontinence r/t prolapsed bladder
Urge incontinence r/t prolapsed bladder

Cystoscopy

Altered health maintenance r/t knowledge deficit regarding postoperative care
Risk for infection r/t invasive procedure
Urinary retention r/t edema in urethra obstructing flow of urine

D

Deafness

Impaired verbal communication r/t impaired hearing
Sensory perceptual alteration: olfactory r/t alteration in sensory reception, transmission, and/or integration

Death, Oncoming

Anticipatory grieving r/t loss of significant other
Fear r/t threat of death
Ineffective family coping: compromised r/t client's inability to provide support to the family
Ineffective individual coping r/t personal vulnerability
Potential for enhanced spiritual well-being r/t desire of client and family to be in harmony with each other and higher power/God
Powerlessness r/t effects of illness, oncoming death
Social isolation r/t altered state of wellness
Spiritual distress r/t intense suffering
Refer to Terminally Ill Child/Death of Child

Decisions, Difficulty Making

Decisional conflict r/t unclear personal values or beliefs, perceived threat to value system, lack of experience or interference with decision making, lack of relevant information, support system deficit, multiple or divergent sources of information

Decubitus Ulcer

Refer to Pressure Ulcer

Deep Vein Thrombosis

Refer to DVT

Defensive Behavior

Defensive coping r/t nonacceptance of blame, denial of problems or weaknesses

Dehiscence, Abdominal

Fear r/t threat of death, severe dysfunction
Impaired skin integrity r/t altered circulation, malnutrition, opening in incision
Impaired tissue integrity r/t exposure of abdominal contents to external environment
Pain r/t stretching of abdominal wall
Risk for infection r/t loss of skin integrity

Dehydration

Altered health maintenance r/t knowledge deficit regarding treatment and prevention of dehydration
Altered oral mucous membranes r/t decreased salivation and fluid deficit
Fluid volume deficit r/t active fluid volume loss
Refer to cause of Dehydration

Delirium

Acute confusion r/t side effect of medication, response to hospitalization, alcohol abuse, substance abuse, sensory deprivation, or overload
Altered thought processes r/t head trauma, altered metabolic state, substance abuse, sleep deprivation, sensory deprivation or overload

Delirium Tremens (DTs)

Refer to Alcohol Withdrawal

Delivery

Refer to Labor—Normal

Delusions

Altered thought processes r/t mental disorder
Anxiety r/t content of intrusive thoughts
Impaired verbal communication r/t psychological impairment, delusional thinking
Ineffective individual coping r/t distortion and insecurity of life events
Risk for violence: self-directed or directed at others r/t delusional thinking

Dementia

Altered family process r/t disability of family member
Altered nutrition: less than body requirements r/t psychological impairment
Chronic confusion r/t neurological dysfunction
Impaired environmental interpretation syndrome r/t dementia
Impaired home maintenance management r/t inadequate support system
Impaired physical mobility r/t neuromuscular impairment
Risk for caregiver role strain r/t amount of caregiving tasks, duration of caregiving required
Risk for impaired skin integrity r/t altered nutritional status, immobility
Risk for injury r/t confusion, decreased muscle coordination
Self-care deficit: specify r/t psychological or neuromuscular impairment
Sleep pattern disturbance r/t neurological impairment, naps during the day
Total incontinence r/t neuromuscular impairment

Denial of Health Status

Ineffective denial r/t lack of perception about health status effects of illness
Ineffective management of therapeutic regimen r/t denial of seriousness of health situation

Dental Caries

Altered health maintenance r/t lack of knowledge regarding prevention of dental disease secondary to high sugar diet, giving infants or toddlers with erupted teeth bottles of milk at bedtime, lack of fluoride treatments, inadequate or improper brushing of teeth

Depression (Major Depressive Disorder)

Altered health maintenance r/t lack of ability to make good judgments regarding ways to obtain help
Chronic low self-esteem r/t repeated unmet expectations
Colonic constipation r/t inactivity, decreased fluid intake
Dysfunctional grieving r/t lack of previous resolution of former grieving response

Fatigue r/t psychological demands
Hopelessness r/t feeling of abandonment, long-term stress
Impaired environmental interpretation syndrome r/t severe mental functional impairment
Ineffective individual coping r/t dysfunctional grieving
Powerlessness r/t pattern of helplessness
Risk for violence: self-directed r/t panic state
Self-care deficit: specify r/t depression, cognitive impairment
Sexual dysfunction r/t loss of sexual desire
Sleep pattern disturbance r/t inactivity
Social isolation r/t ineffective coping

Dermatitis

Altered comfort: pruritis r/t inflammation of skin
Altered health maintenance r/t knowledge deficit methods to decrease inflammation
Anxiety r/t situational crisis imposed by illness
Impaired skin integrity r/t side effect of medication, allergic reaction

Despondency

Hopelessness r/t long-term stress
Refer to Depression

Destructive Behavior Toward Others

Ineffective individual coping r/t situational crises, maturational crises, personal vulnerability

Diabetes in Pregnancy

Refer to Gestational Diabetes

Diabetes Insipidus

Altered health maintenance r/t knowledge deficit regarding care of disease, importance of medications
Fluid volume deficit r/t inability to conserve fluid

Diabetes Mellitus

Altered health maintenance r/t knowledge deficit regarding care of diabetic condition
Altered nutrition: less than body requirements r/t inability to use glucose (Type I Diabetes)
Altered nutrition: more than body requirements r/t excessive intake of nutrients (Type II Diabetes)
Altered tissue perfusion: peripheral r/t impaired arterial circulation
Ineffective management of therapeutic regimen r/t complexity of therapeutic regimen
Noncompliance r/t restrictive life-style; changes in diet, medication, and exercise
Powerlessness r/t perceived lack of personal control
Risk for altered thought processes r/t hypoglycemia, hyperglycemia
Risk for impaired skin integrity r/t loss of pain perception in extremities
Risk for infection r/t hyperglycemia, impaired healing, circulatory changes
Risk for injury: hypoglycemia or hyperglycemia r/t failure to consume adequate calories, failure to take insulin
Sensory/perceptual alteration r/t altered tissue perfusion
Sexual dysfunction r/t neuropathy associated with disease

Diabetes Mellitus, Juvenile (IDDM Type I)

Altered health maintenance r/t parental/child knowledge deficit regarding dietary management, medication administration, physical activity, and interaction between the three; daily changes in diet, medications, and activity related to child's growth spurts and needs; need to instruct other caregivers and teachers regarding signs and symptoms of hypoglycemia or hyperglycemia and treatment
Altered nutrition: less than body requirements r/t inability of body to adequately metabolize and use glucose and nutrients, increased caloric needs of child to promote growth and physical activity participation with peers
Body image disturbance r/t to imposed deviations from biophysical and psychosocial norm, perceived differences from peers
Impaired adjustment r/t inability to participate in normal childhood activities
Pain r/t insulin injections, peripheral blood glucose testing
Risk for noncompliance r/t body image disturbance and impaired adjustment secondary to adolescent maturational crises
Refer to Diabetes Mellitus; Child with Chronic Illness; Hospitalized Child

Diabetic Coma

Altered thought processes r/t hyperglycemia, presence of excessive metabolic acids
Fluid volume deficit r/t hyperglycemia resulting in polyuria
Ineffective management of therapeutic regimen r/t lack of understanding of preventive measures and adequate blood sugar control

Risk for infection r/t hyperglycemia, changes in vascular system
Refer to Diabetes Mellitus

Diabetic Ketoacidosis

Refer to Ketoacidosis

Diabetic Retinopathy

Altered health maintenance r/t knowledge deficit regarding preserving vision with treatment if possible, use of low vision aids
Grieving r/t loss of vision
Sensory-perceptual alteration: visual r/t change in sensory reception

Dialysis

Refer to Hemodialysis; Peritoneal Dialysis

Diaphoresis

Altered comfort r/t excessive sweating

Diaphragmatic Hernia

Refer to Hiatus Hernia

Diarrhea

Diarrhea r/t infection, change in diet, gastrointestinal disorders, stress, medication effect, impaction

DIC (Disseminated Intravascular Coagulation)

Altered protection r/t abnormal clotting mechanism
Fear r/t threat to well-being
Fluid volume deficit: hemorrhage r/t depletion of clotting factors
Risk for altered tissue perfusion: peripheral r/t hypovolemia from profuse bleeding, formation of microemboli in vascular system

Digitalis Toxicity

Decreased cardiac output r/t drug toxicity affecting cardiac rhythm, rate
Ineffective management of therapeutic regimen r/t knowledge deficit regarding action, appropriate method of administration of digitalis

Dilation and Curretage (D & C)

Altered health maintenance r/t knowledge deficit regarding postoperative self-care
Pain r/t uterine contractions
Risk for altered sexuality patterns r/t painful coitus, fear associated with surgery on genital area
Risk for fluid volume deficit: hemorrhage r/t excessive blood loss during or after the procedure
Risk for infection r/t surgical procedure

Discharge Planning

Altered health maintenance r/t lack of material sources
Knowledge deficit r/t lack of exposure to information for home care
Impaired home maintenance management r/t family member's disease or injury interfering with home maintenance
Potential for enhanced community coping r/t support available in community for follow-up care and services

Discomforts of Pregnancy

Alteration in comfort r/t hormonal changes (nausea, ptyalism, leukorrhea, urinary frequency), enlarged uterus (shortness of breath, abdominal distention, pruritus, reduced bladder capacity), and increased vascularization (nasal stuffiness, varicosities)
Body image disturbance r/t pregnancy-induced body changes
Constipation r/t decreased gastrointestinal tract motility, pressure from enlarged uterus, supplementary iron
Fatigue r/t hormonal, metabolic, and body changes
Pain: indigestion and heartburn r/t decreased gastrointestinal tract motility, relaxed cardiac sphincter, enlarged uterus; hemorrhoids r/t enlarged uterus, constipation, pelvic venous stasis, decreased gastrointestinal tract motility; joint and backache r/t enlarged uterus, relaxation of joints; leg cramps r/t nerve compression and calcium/phosphorus/potassium imbalance; headache r/t vascular and hormonal changes
Risk for injury r/t faintness and/or syncope secondary to vasomotor lability or postural hypotension, venous stasis in lower extremities
Sleep pattern disturbance r/t psychological stress, fetal movement, muscular cramping, urinary frequency, shortness of breath
Stress incontinence r/t enlarged uterus and fetal movement

Dissecting Aneurysm

Fear r/t threat to own well-being
Refer to Aneurysm; Abdominal Surgery

Disseminated Intravascular Coagulation

Refer to DIC

Dissociative Disorder (Not Otherwise Specified)

Alteration in thought processes r/t repressed anxiety
Anxiety r/t psychosocial stress
Disturbance in self-concept r/t childhood trauma, childhood abuse
Impaired memory r/t altered state of consciousness
Ineffective individual coping r/t personal vulnerability in crisis of accurate self-perception
Personal identity disturbance r/t inability to distinguish self caused by multiple personality disorder, depersonalization, or disturbance in memory
Sensory/perceptual alteration: kinesthetic r/t underdeveloped ego

Distress

Anxiety r/t situational crises, maturational crises

Disuse Syndrome, Potential to Develop

Risk for disuse syndrome r/t paralysis, mechanical immobilization, prescribed immobilization, severe pain, altered level of consciousness

Diversional Activity, Lack of

Diversional activity deficit r/t environmental lack of diversional activity

Diverticulitis

Altered nutrition: less than body requirements r/t loss of appetite
Constipation r/t dietary deficiency of fiber and roughage
Diarrhea r/t increased intestinal motility secondary to inflammation
Knowledge deficit r/t diet needed to control disease, medication regimen
Pain r/t inflammation of bowel
Risk for fluid volume deficit r/t diarrhea

Dizziness

Altered tissue perfusion: cerebral r/t interruption of cerebral arterial blood flow
Decreased cardiac output r/t dysfunctional electrical conduction
Impaired physical mobility r/t dizziness
Risk for injury r/t difficulty maintaining balance

Down's Syndrome

Refer to Mental Retardation; Child with Chronic Illness

Dressing Self, Inability to Dress

Dressing/grooming self-care deficit r/t intolerance to activity, decreased strength and endurance, pain, discomfort, perceptual or cognitive impairment, neuromuscular impairment, musculoskeletal impairment, depression, severe anxiety

Dribbling of Urine

Stress incontinence r/t degenerative changes in pelvic muscles and structural supports

Drooling

Impaired swallowing r/t neuromuscular impairment, mechanical obstruction

Drug Abuse

Altered nutrition: less than body requirements r/t poor eating habits
Anxiety r/t threat to self-concept, lack of control of drug use
Ineffective individual coping r/t situational crisis
Noncompliance r/t denial of illness
Risk for injury r/t hallucinations, drug effects
Risk for violence r/t poor impulse control
Sensory/perceptual alterations: specify r/t substance intoxication
Sleep pattern disturbance r/t effects of drugs and/or medications

Drug Withdrawal

Acute confusion r/t effects of substance withdrawal
Altered nutrition: less than body requirements r/t poor eating habits
Anxiety r/t physiological withdrawal
Ineffective individual coping r/t situational crisis, withdrawal
Noncompliance r/t denial of illness
Risk for injury r/t hallucinations
Risk for violence r/t poor impulse control
Sensory/perceptual alterations: specify r/t substance intoxication
Sleep pattern disturbance r/t effects of drugs and/or medications

DTs (Delirium Tremens)

Refer to Alcohol Withdrawal

DVT—Deep Vein Thrombosis

Altered health maintenance r/t knowledge deficit regarding self-care needs, treatment regimen, outcome

Altered tissue perfusion: peripheral r/t interruption of venous blood flow
Colonic constipation r/t inactivity, bedrest
Impaired physical mobility r/t pain in extremity, forced bedrest
Pain r/t vascular inflammation, edema
Refer to Anticoagulant Therapy

Dying Client

Refer to Terminally Ill Adult

Dysfunctional Eating Pattern

Risk for altered nutrition: more than body requirements r/t observed use of food as a reward or comfort measure
Refer to Anorexia Nervosa; Bulimia

Dysfunctional Family Unit

Refer to Family Problems

Dysfunctional Grieving

Dysfunctional grieving r/t actual or perceived loss

Dysfunctional Ventilatory Weaning

Dysfunctional ventilatory weaning response r/t physical, psychological, or situational factors

Dysmenorrhea

Altered health maintenance r/t knowledge deficit regarding prevention and treatment of painful menstruation
Pain r/t cramping from hormonal effects

Dyspareunia

Sexual dysfunction r/t lack of lubrication during intercourse, alteration in reproductive organ function

Dyspepsia

Altered health maintenance r/t knowledge deficit regarding treatment of disease
Anxiety r/t pressures of personal role
Pain r/t gastrointestinal disease, consumption of irritating foods

Dysphagia

Impaired swallowing r/t neuromuscular impairment
Risk for aspiration r/t loss of gag or cough reflex

Dysphasia

Impaired social interaction r/t difficulty in communicating
Impaired verbal communication r/t decrease in circulation to the brain

Dyspnea

Activity intolerance r/t imbalance between oxygen supply and demand
Fear r/t threat to state of well-being, potential death
Impaired gas exchange r/t alveolar-capillary damage
Ineffective airway clearance r/t decreased energy, fatigue
Ineffective breathing pattern r/t decreased lung expansion, neurological impairment affecting respiratory center, extreme anxiety
Sleep pattern disturbance r/t difficulty breathing, positioning required for effective breathing

Dysreflexia

Dysreflexia r/t bladder distention, bowel distention, noxious stimuli

Dysrhythmia

Activity intolerance r/t decreased cardiac output
Altered health maintenance r/t knowledge deficit regarding self-care with disease
Altered tissue perfusion: cerebral r/t interruption of cerebral arterial flow secondary to decreased cardiac output
Anxiety/fear r/t threat of death, change in health status
Decreased cardiac output r/t altered electrical conduction

Dysthymic Disorder

Altered health maintenance r/t inability to make good judgments regarding ways to obtain help
Altered sexual pattern r/t loss of sexual desire
Chronic low self-esteem r/t repeated unmet expectations
Ineffective individual coping r/t impaired social interaction
Sleep pattern disturbance r/t anxious thoughts
Social isolation r/t ineffective coping

Dystocia

Anxiety r/t difficult labor and knowledge deficit regarding normal labor pattern
Fatigue r/t prolonged labor
Grieving r/t loss of ideal labor experience
Ineffective individual coping r/t situational crisis
Pain r/t difficult labor and medical interventions
Powerlessness r/t perceived inability to control outcome of labor
Risk for fluid volume deficit r/t hemorrhage secondary to uterine atony
Risk for infection r/t prolonged rupture of membranes

Risk for injury (maternal and fetal) r/t difficult labor, medical interventions
Situational low self-esteem r/t perceived inability to have normal labor and delivery

Dysuria

Altered urinary elimination r/t urinary tract infection

E

Ear Surgery

Altered health maintenance r/t knowledge deficit regarding postoperative restrictions, expectations, and care
Pain r/t edema in ears from surgery
Risk for injury r/t dizziness from excessive stimuli to vestibular apparatus
Sensory/perceptual alteration: hearing r/t invasive surgery of ears, dressings
Refer to Hospitalized Child

Earache

Pain r/t trauma, edema
Sensory perceptual alteration: auditory r/t altered sensory reception, transmission, and/or integration

Eating Disorder

Refer to Anorexia Nervosa; Bulimia; Obesity

Eclampsia

Altered family processes r/t unmet expectations for pregnancy and childbirth
Fear r/t threat of well-being to self and fetus
Risk for altered fetal tissue perfusion r/t uteroplacental insufficiency
Risk for aspiration r/t seizure activity
Risk for fluid volume excess r/t decreased urine output secondary to renal dysfunction
Risk for injury (fetal) r/t hypoxia
Risk for injury (maternal) r/t seizure activity

ECT (Electroconvulsive Therapy)

Decisional conflict r/t lack of relevant information
Fear r/t real or imagined threat to well-being
Impaired memory r/t effects of treatment
Refer to Depression, Major

Ectopic Pregnancy

Altered role performance r/t loss of pregnancy
Body image disturbance r/t negative feelings about the body and reproductive functioning
Fear r/t threat to self, surgery, implications for future pregnancy
Fluid volume deficit r/t loss of blood
Pain r/t stretching or rupture of implantation site
Risk for altered family processes r/t situational crisis
Risk for ineffective individual coping r/t loss of pregnancy
Risk for infection r/t traumatized tissue and blood loss
Risk for spiritual distress r/t grief process
Situational low self-esteem r/t loss of pregnancy, inability to carry pregnancy to term

Eczema

Altered health maintenance r/t knowledge deficit regarding how to decrease inflammation and prevent further outbreaks
Body image disturbance r/t change in appearance from inflamed skin
Impaired skin integrity r/t side effect of medication, allergic reaction
Pain: pruritis r/t inflammation of skin

Edema

Altered health maintenance r/t knowledge deficit regarding treatment of edema
Fluid volume excess r/t excessive fluid intake, cardiac dysfunction, renal dysfunction, loss of plasma proteins
Risk for impaired skin integrity r/t impaired circulation, fragility of skin
Refer to cause of Edema

Elderly Abuse

Refer to Battered Person

Electroconvulsive Therapy

Refer to ECT

Emaciated Person

Altered nutrition: less than body requirements r/t inability to ingest food, digest food, or absorb nutrients due to biological, psychological, or economic factors

Embolectomy

Fear r/t threat of great body harm from embolus
Risk for fluid volume deficit: hemorrhage r/t postoperative complication, surgical area
Risk for peripheral neurovascular dysfunction r/t decreased circulation to extremity
Refer to Surgery—Postoperative Care

Emesis

Refer to Vomiting

Emotional Problems

Refer to Coping Problems

Emphysema

Refer to COPD

Encephalitis

Refer to Meningitis/Encephalitis

Endocardial Cushion Defect

Refer to Congenital Heart Disease/Cardiac Anomalies

Endocarditis

Activity intolerance r/t reduced cardiac reserve and prescribed bedrest
Altered health maintenance r/t knowledge deficit regarding treatment of disease, preventive measures against further incidence of disease
Altered tissue perfusion: cardiopulmonary/ peripheral r/t high risk for development of emboli
Decreased cardiac output r/t inflammation of lining of heart and change in structure in valve leaflets, increased myocardial workload
Pain r/t biological injury and inflammation
Risk for alteration in nutrition: less than body requirements r/t fever, hypermetabolic state associated with fever

Endometriosis

Altered health maintenance r/t knowledge deficit regarding disease condition, medications, and other treatments
Anticipatory grieving r/t possible infertility
Pain r/t onset of menses with distention of endometrial tissue
Sexual dysfunction r/t painful coitus

Endometritis

Anxiety r/t prolonged hospitalization, fear of the unknown
Hyperthermia r/t infectious process
Knowledge deficit r/t limited experience with condition, treatment, and antibiotic regimen
Pain r/t infectious process in reproductive tract

Energy Field Disturbance

Energy field disturbance r/t disruption in flow of energy as a result of pain, depression, fatigue, anxiety, or stress

Enuresis

Altered health maintenance r/t unachieved developmental task, neuromuscular immaturity, diseases of the urinary system, infections or illnesses such as diabetes mellitus or insipidus, regression in developmental stage secondary to hospitalization or stress, parental knowledge deficit regarding involuntary urination at night after age 6, fluid intake at bedtime, lack of control during sound sleep, male gender
Refer to Toilet Training

Environmental Interpretation Problems

Impaired environmental interpretation syndrome r/t dementia, Parkinson's disease, Huntington's disease, depression, alcoholism

Epididymitis

Altered health maintenance r/t knowledge deficit regarding treatment for pain and infection
Altered pattern of sexuality r/t edema of epididymis and testes
Anxiety r/t situational crisis, pain, threat to future fertility
Pain r/t inflammation in scrotal sac

Epiglottitis

Refer to Respiratory Infections, Acute Childhood

Epilepsy

Altered health maintenance r/t knowledge deficit regarding seizures and seizure control
Anxiety r/t threat to role functioning
Impaired memory r/t seizure activity
Risk for altered thought processes r/t excessive, uncontrolled neurological stimuli
Risk for aspiration r/t impaired swallowing, excessive secretions
Risk for injury r/t environmental factors during seizure
Refer to Seizure Disorders, Childhood

Episiotomy

Anxiety r/t fear of pain
Body image disturbance r/t fear of resuming sexual relations
Impaired physical mobility r/t pain, swelling, and tissue trauma
Impaired skin integrity r/t perineal incision
Pain r/t tissue trauma
Risk for infection r/t tissue trauma
Sexual dysfunction r/t altered body structure and tissue trauma

Epistaxis

Fear r/t large amount of blood loss
Risk for fluid volume deficit r/t excessive fluid loss

Epstein-Barr Virus

Refer to Mononucleosis

Esophageal Varices

Fear r/t threat of death
Fluid volume deficit: hemorrhage r/t portal hypertension, distended variceal vessels that can easily rupture
Refer to Cirrhosis

Esophagitis

Altered health maintenance r/t knowledge deficit regarding treatment of disease
Pain r/t inflammation of esophagus

ETOH Withdrawal

Refer to Alcohol Withdrawal

Evisceration

Refer to Dehiscence

Exposure to Hot or Cold Environment

Risk for altered body temperature r/t exposure

External Fixation

Body image disturbance r/t trauma and change to affected part
Risk for infection r/t pressure of pins on skin surface
Refer to Fractures

Eye Surgery

Altered health maintenance r/t knowledge deficit regarding postoperative activity, medications, and eyecare
Anxiety r/t possible loss of vision
Risk for injury r/t impaired vision
Self-care deficit r/t impaired vision
Sensory/perceptual alteration: visual r/t surgical procedure
Refer to Hospitalized Child

F

Failure to Thrive, Nonorganic

Altered growth and development r/t parental knowledge deficit, lack of stimulation, nutritional deficit, long-term hospitalization
Altered nutrition: less than body requirements r/t inadequate type/amounts of food for infant, inappropriate feeding techniques
Altered parenting r/t lack of parenting skills, inadequate role modeling
Chronic low self-esteem: parental r/t feelings in inadequacy, support system deficiencies, inadequate role model
Disorganized infant behavior r/t lack of boundaries
Risk for altered parent/infant attachment r/t inability of parents to meet infant's needs
Sleep pattern disturbance r/t inconsistency of caretaker, lack of quiet environment
Social isolation r/t limited support systems, self-imposed situation

Family Problems

Altered family process r/t situation transition and/or crises, developmental transition and/or crises
Family coping: potential for growth r/t needs sufficiently gratified and adaptive tasks effectively addressed to enable goals of self-actualization to surface
Ineffective family coping: compromised r/t inadequate or incorrect information or understanding by a primary person; temporary preoccupation by a significant person who is trying to manage emotional conflicts and personal suffering and is unable to perceive or act effectively in regard to client's needs; temporary family disorganization and role changes; other situational or developmental crises the significant person may be facing; little support provided by client, in turn, for primary person; prolonged disease or disability progression that exhausts supportive capacity of significant people
Ineffective family coping: disabling r/t significant person with chronically unexpressed feelings such as guilt, anxiety, hostility, despair; dissonant discrepancy of coping styles for dealing with adaptive tasks by the significant person and client or among significant people; highly ambivalent family relationships; arbitrary handling of family's resistance to treatment, which tends to solidify defensiveness as it fails to deal adequately with underlying anxiety
Ineffective management of therapeutic regimen: families r/t complexity of health care system, complexity of therapeutic regimen, decisional conflicts, economic difficulties, excessive demands made on individual or family, family conflict

Fatigue

Fatigue r/t decreased or increased metabolic energy production, overwhelming psychological or emotional demands, increased energy requirements to perform activities of daily living, excessive social and/or role demands, states of discomfort, altered body chemistry

Fear

Fear r/t identifiable physical or psychological threat to person

Febrile Seizures

Refer to Seizure Disorders, Childhood

Fecal Impaction

Refer to Impaction of Stool

Fecal Incontinence

Bowel incontinence r/t neurological impairment, gastrointestinal disorders, anorectal trauma

Feeding Problems—Newborn

Ineffective breast-feeding r/t prematurity, infant anomaly, maternal breast anomaly, previous breast surgery, previous history of breast-feeding failure, infant receiving supplemental feedings with artificial nipple, poor infant sucking reflex, nonsupportive partner and family, knowledge deficit, maternal anxiety or ambivalence

Ineffective infant feeding pattern r/t prematurity, neurological impairment or delay, oral hypersensitivity, prolonged NPO

Interrupted breast-feeding r/t maternal or infant illness, prematurity, maternal employment, contraindications to breast-feeding, need to abruptly wean infant

Femoral Popliteal Bypass

Anxiety r/t threat to or change in health status

Pain r/t surgical trauma and edema in surgical area

Risk for altered tissue perfusion: peripheral r/t impaired arterial circulation

Risk for fluid volume deficit: hemorrhage r/t abnormal blood loss

Risk for infection r/t invasive procedure

Risk for neurovascular dysfunction r/t vascular surgery, emboli

Fetal Alcohol Syndrome

Refer to Infant of Substance Abusing Mother

Fetal Distress/Nonreassuring Fetal Heart Rate Pattern

Altered tissue perfusion (fetal) r/t interruption of umbilical cord blood flow

Altered tissue perfusion (placental) r/t small or old placenta, interference with gas exchange transplacentally

Fear r/t threat to fetus

Fever

Hyperthermia r/t infectious process, damage to hypothalamus, exposure to hot environment, medications, anesthesia, inability or decreased ability to perspire

Fibrocystic Breast Disease

Refer to Breast Lumps

Filthy Home Environment

Impaired home maintenance management r/t individual or family member disease or injury, insufficient family organization or planning, impaired cognitive or emotional functioning, lack of knowledge, economic factors

Financial Crisis in the Home Environment

Impaired home maintenance management r/t insufficient finances

Fistulectomy

Refer to Hemorroidectomy (nursing care is the same)

Flashbacks

Post-trauma response r/t catastrophic event

Flat Affect

Hopelessness r/t prolonged activity restriction creating isolation, failing or deteriorating physiological condition, long-term stress, abandonment, lost belief in transcendent values or in God

Risk for loneliness r/t social isolation, lack of interest in surroundings

Fluid Volume Deficit

Fluid volume deficit r/t active fluid loss, failure of regulatory mechanisms

Fluid Volume Excess

Fluid volume excess r/t compromised regulatory mechanism, excess fluid intake, excess sodium intake

Foreign Body Aspiration

Altered health maintenance r/t parental knowledge deficit regarding small toys, pieces of toys, nuts, balloons
Impaired home maintenance management r/t insufficient family organization or planning, lack of resources or support systems, inability to maintain orderly and clean surroundings
Ineffective airway clearance r/t obstruction of airway
Risk for suffocation r/t inhalation of small object
Refer to Safety, Childhood

Formula Feeding

Altered health maintenance r/t maternal knowledge deficit regarding formula feeding
Decisional conflict (maternal) r/t multiple or divergent sources of information, values conflict, support system deficit
Grieving (maternal) r/t loss of desired breast-feeding experience
Risk for altered nutrition: more than body requirements r/t composition of formula and bottle feeding and overuse of food for reward or comfort measures
Risk for constipation (infant) r/t iron-fortified formula
Risk for infection (infant) r/t lack of passive maternal immunity and supine feeding position

Fractured Hip

Refer to Hip Fracture

Fractures

Altered health maintenance r/t knowledge deficit regarding care of the fracture
Diversional activity deficit r/t immobility
Impaired physical mobility r/t limb immobilization
Pain r/t muscle spasm, edema, and trauma
Risk for altered tissue perfusion r/t immobility, presence of cast
Risk for impaired skin integrity r/t immobility, presence of cast
Risk for peripheral neurovascular impairment r/t mechanical compression, treatment of fracture

Frequency of Urination

Altered urinary elimination r/t anatomical obstruction, sensory motor impairment, urinary tract infection
Stress incontinence r/t degenerative change in pelvic muscles and structural supports
Urge incontinence r/t decreased bladder capacity, irritation of bladder stretch receptors causing spasm, alcohol, caffeine, increased fluids, increased urine concentration, overdistended bladder
Urinary retention r/t high urethral pressure caused by weak detrusor, inhibition of reflex arc, strong sphincter, blockage

Frostbite

Impaired skin integrity r/t freezing of skin
Pain r/t decreased circulation from prolonged exposure to cold
Refer to Hypothermia

Frothy Sputum

Refer to Pulmonary Edema; CHF; Seizure Disorders

Fusion, Lumbar

Altered health maintenance r/t knowledge deficit regarding postoperative mobility restrictions, body mechanics
Anxiety r/t fear of surgical procedure and possible recurring problems
Impaired physical mobility r/t limitations related to the surgical procedure, presence of brace
Pain r/t discomfort at bone donor site
Risk for injury r/t improper body mechanics
Risk for perioperative positioning injury r/t immobilization

G

Gag Reflex, Depressed or Absent

Impaired swallowing r/t neuromuscular impairment
Risk for aspiration r/t depressed cough/gag reflex

Gallop Rhythm

Decreased cardiac output r/t decreased contractility of heart

Gallstones

Refer to Cholelithiasis

Gangrene

Altered tissue perfusion: peripheral r/t obstruction of arterial flow
Fear r/t possible loss of extremity

Gas Exchange, Impaired

Impaired gas exchange r/t ventilation perfusion imbalance

Gastric Surgery

Risk for injury r/t inadvertent insertion of nasogastric tube through gastric incision line

Refer to Abdominal Surgery

Gastric Ulcer

Refer to Ulcer, Peptic

Gastritis

Altered nutrition: less than body requirements r/t vomiting, inadequate intestinal absorption of nutrients, restricted dietary regimen

Pain r/t inflammation of gastric mucosa

Risk for fluid volume deficit r/t excessive loss from gastrointestinal tract secondary to vomiting, decreased intake

Gastroenteritis

Altered health maintenance r/t knowledge deficit regarding treatment of disease

Altered nutrition: less than body requirements r/t vomiting, inadequate intestinal absorption of nutrients, restricted dietary intake

Diarrhea r/t infectious process involving intestinal tract

Fluid volume deficit r/t excessive loss from gastrointestinal tract secondary to diarrhea, vomiting

Pain r/t increased peristalsis causing cramping

Refer to Gastroenteritis—Child

Gastroenteritis—Child

Altered health maintenance r/t lack of parental knowledge regarding fluid and dietary changes

Impaired skin integrity (diaper rash) r/t acidic excretions on perineal tissues

Refer to Gastroenteritis; Hospitalized Child

Gastroesophageal Reflux

Altered health maintenance r/t knowledge deficit regarding antireflux regimen (e.g., positioning, oral or enteral feeding techniques, medications), possible home apnea monitoring

Altered nutrition: less than body requirements r/t poor feeding, vomiting

Anxiety/fear (parental) r/t possible need for surgical intervention (Nissen fundoplication/gastrostomy tube)

Fluid volume deficit r/t persistent vomiting

Ineffective airway clearance r/t reflux of gastric contents into esophagus and tracheal or bronchial tree

Pain r/t irritation of esophagus from gastric acids

Risk for altered parenting r/t disruption in bonding secondary to irritable or inconsolable infant

Risk for aspiration r/t entry of gastric contents in tracheal or bronchial tree

Refer to Hospitalized Child; Child with Chronic Condition

Gastrointestinal Hemorrhage

Refer to GI Bleed

Gastroschisis/Omphalocele

Altered bowel elimination pattern r/t effects of congenital herniated abdominal contents

Anticipatory grieving r/t threatened loss of infant, loss of perfect birth or infant secondary to serious medical condition

Impaired gas exchange r/t effects of anesthesia and subsequent atelectasis

Ineffective airway clearance r/t complications of anesthetic effects

Risk for fluid volume deficit r/t inability to feed secondary to condition and subsequent electrolyte imbalance

Risk for infection r/t disrupted skin integrity with exposure of abdominal contents

Risk for injury r/t disrupted skin integrity and altered protection

Refer to Hospitalized Child; Premature Infant

Gastrostomy

Risk for impaired skin integrity r/t presence of gastric contents on skin

Refer to Tube Feedings

Gestational Diabetes (Diabetes in Pregnancy)

Altered fetal nutrition: more than body requirements r/t excessive glucose uptake

Altered health maintenance (maternal) r/t knowledge deficit regarding care of diabetic condition in pregnancy

Altered maternal nutrition: less than body requirements r/t decreased insulin production and glucose uptake into cells

Anxiety r/t threat to self and/or fetus

Powerlessness r/t lack of control over outcome of pregnancy

Risk for fetal injury r/t macrosomia, congenital defects, and maternal hypoglycemic or hyperglycemic incidents

Risk for maternal injury r/t delivery of large infant or hypoglycemic or hyperglycemic incidents

GI Bleed (Gastrointestinal Bleeding)

Altered nutrition: less than body requirements r/t nausea, vomiting
Fatigue r/t loss of circulating blood volume, decreased ability to transport oxygen
Fear r/t threat to well-being, potential death
Fluid volume deficit r/t gastrointestinal bleeding
Pain r/t irritated mucosa from acid secretion
Risk for ineffective individual coping r/t personal vulnerability in a crisis, bleeding, hospitalization

Gingivitis

Altered oral mucous membranes r/t ineffective oral hygiene

Glaucoma

Sensory/perceptual alteration: visual r/t increased intraocular pressure

Glomerulonephritis

Altered health maintenance r/t knowledge deficit regarding care of the disease
Altered nutrition: less than body requirements r/t anorexia, restrictive diet
Fluid volume excess r/t renal impairment
Pain r/t edema of kidney

Gonorrhea

Altered health maintenance r/t knowledge deficit regarding treatment and prevention of disease
Pain r/t inflammation of reproductive organs
Risk for infection r/t spread of organism throughout reproductive organs

Gout

Altered health maintenance r/t knowledge deficit regarding medications and home care
Impaired physical mobility r/t musculoskeletal impairment
Pain r/t inflammation of affected joint

Grand Mal Seizure

Refer to Seizure Disorder

Grandiosity

Defensive coping r/t inaccurate perception of self and abilities

Graves' Disease

Refer to Hyperthyroidism

Grieving

Anticipatory grieving r/t anticipated significant loss
Dysfunctional grieving r/t actual or perceived significant loss
Grieving r/t actual significant loss; change in life status, style, or function

Grooming, Inability to Groom Self

Dressing/grooming self-care deficit r/t intolerance to activity, decreased strength and endurance, pain, discomfort, perceptual or cognitive impairment, neuromuscular impairment, musculoskeletal impairment, depression, severe anxiety

Growth and Development Lag

Altered growth and development r/t inadequate caretaking, indifference, inconsistent responsiveness, multiple caretakers, separation from significant others, environmental and stimulation deficiencies, effects of physical disability, prescribed dependence

Guillain-Barre Syndrome

Inability to sustain spontaneous ventilation r/t weakness of muscles of respiration
Refer to Neurological Disorder

Guilt

Anticipatory grieving r/t potential loss of significant person, animal, or prized material possession
Dysfunctional grieving r/t actual loss of significant person, animal, or prized material possession
Potential for enhanced spiritual well-being r/t desire to be in harmony with self, others, and higher power/God
Self-esteem disturbance r/t unmet expectations of self

H

Hair Loss

Altered nutrition: less than body requirements r/t inability to ingest food due to biological, psychological, or economic factors
Body image disturbance r/t psychological reaction to loss of hair

Halitosis

Altered oral mucous membranes r/t ineffective oral hygiene

Hallucinations

Altered thought processes r/t inability to control bizarre thoughts
Anxiety r/t threat to self-concept
Risk for self-mutilation r/t command hallucinations
Risk for violence: self-directed or directed at others r/t catatonic excitement, manic excitement, rage/panic reactions, response to violent internal stimuli

Head Injury

Altered thought processes r/t pressure damage to brain
Altered tissue perfusion: cerebral r/t effects of increased intracranial pressure
Decreased adaptive capacity: intracranial r/t brain injury
Ineffective breathing patterns r/t pressure damage to breathing center in brain stem
Sensory/perceptual alteration r/t pressure damage to sensory centers in brain
Refer to Neurological Disorders

Headache

Pain: headache r/t lack of knowledge of pain control techniques or methods to prevent headaches

Health Maintenance Problems

Altered health maintenance r/t significant alteration in communication skills, lack of ability to make deliberate and thoughtful judgments, perceptual or cognitive impairment, ineffective individual coping, dysfunctional grieving, unachieved developmental tasks, ineffective family coping, disabling spiritual distress, lack of material resources

Health-Seeking Person

Health-seeking behavior r/t expressed desire for increased control of own personal health

Hearing Impairment

Impaired verbal communication r/t inability to hear own voice
Sensory/perceptual alteration: auditory r/t altered state of auditory system
Social isolation r/t difficulty with communication

Heartburn

Altered health maintenance r/t knowledge deficit regarding information about factors that cause esophageal reflex
Pain: heartburn r/t gastroesophageal reflux
Risk for altered nutrition: less than body requirements r/t pain after eating

Heart Failure

Refer to CHF

Heart Surgery

Refer to Coronary Artery Bypass Grafting

Heat Stroke

Altered thought processes r/t hyperthermia, increased oxygen needs
Fluid volume deficit r/t profuse diaphoresis
Hyperthermia r/t vigorous activity, hot environment

Helplessness

Hopelessness r/t prolonged activity restriction creating isolation, failing or deteriorating physiological condition, long-term stress, abandonment, lost belief in transcendent values or in God

Hematemesis

Refer to GI Bleed

Hematologic Disorder

Altered protection r/t abnormal blood profile
Refer to cause of Hematologic Disorder

Hematuria

Risk for fluid volume deficit r/t excessive loss of blood through urinary system

Hemianopsia

Anxiety r/t change in vision
Sensory/perceptual alteration r/t altered sensory reception, transmission, and/or integration
Unilateral neglect r/t effects of disturbed perceptual abilities

Hemiplegia

Anxiety r/t change in health status
Body image disturbance r/t functional loss of one side of the body
Impaired physical mobility r/t loss of neurological control of involved extremities
Risk for impaired skin integrity r/t alteration in sensation, immobility
Risk for injury r/t impaired mobility
Risk for unilateral neglect r/t neurological impairment; loss of sensation, vision, and/or movement
Self-care deficit: specify r/t neuromuscular impairment

Unilateral neglect r/t effects of disturbed perceptual abilities

Refer to CVA

Hemodialysis

Altered family processes r/t changes in role responsibilities due to therapy regimen

Altered health maintenance r/t knowledge deficit regarding hemodialysis procedure, restrictions, blood access care

Fluid volume excess r/t renal disease with minimal urine output

Ineffective individual coping r/t situational crisis

Noncompliance: dietary restrictions r/t denial of chronic illness

Powerlessness r/t treatment regimen

Risk for caregiver role strain r/t complexity of care receiver treatment

Risk for fluid volume deficit r/t excessive removal of fluid during dialysis

Risk for infection r/t exposure to blood products and risk for developing hepatitis B/C

Risk for injury: clotting of blood access r/t abnormal surface for blood flow

Refer to Renal Failure; Renal Failure Acute/Chronic, Child

Hemodynamic Monitoring

Risk for infection r/t invasive procedure

Risk for injury r/t inadvertent wedging of catheter; dislodgement of catheter; disconnection of catheter with embolism

Hemolytic Uremic Syndrome

Altered comfort: nausea/vomiting r/t effects of uremia

Fluid volume deficit r/t vomiting and diarrhea

Risk for impaired skin integrity r/t diarrhea

Risk for injury r/t decreased platelet count, seizure activity

Refer to Renal Failure, Acute/Chronic, Child; Hospitalized Child

Hemophilia

Altered health maintenance r/t knowledge and skill acquisition regarding home administration of intravenous clotting factors, protection from injury

Altered protection r/t deficient clotting factors

Fear r/t high risk for AIDS secondary to contaminated blood products

Impaired physical mobility r/t pain from acute bleeds and imposed activity restrictions

Pain r/t bleeding into body tissues

Risk for injury r/t deficient clotting factors and child's developmental level, age-appropriate play, inappropriate use of toys or sports equipment

Refer to Hospitalized Child; Child with Chronic Condition; Maturational Issues, Adolescent

Hemoptysis

Fear r/t serious threat to well-being

Risk for fluid volume deficit r/t excessive loss of blood

Risk for ineffective airway clearance r/t obstruction of airway with blood and mucus

Hemorrhage

Fear r/t threat to well-being

Fluid volume deficit r/t massive blood loss

Refer to cause of Hemorrhage; Hypovolemic Shock

Hemorrhoidectomy

Altered health maintenance r/t knowledge deficit regarding pain relief, use of stool softeners, dietary changes

Anxiety r/t embarrassment, need for privacy

Colonic constipation r/t fear of defecation

Pain r/t surgical procedure

Risk for fluid volume deficit: hemorrhage r/t inadequate clotting

Urinary retention r/t pain, anesthetic effect

Hemorrhoids

Altered health maintenance r/t knowledge deficit regarding care of condition

Constipation r/t painful defecation, poor bowel habits

Pain: pruritis r/t inflammation of hemorrhoids

Hemothorax

Fluid volume deficit r/t blood in pleural space

Refer to Pneumothorax

Hepatitis

Activity intolerance r/t weakness of fatigue secondary to infection

Altered health maintenance r/t knowledge deficit regarding disease process and home management

Altered nutrition: less than body requirements r/t anorexia, impaired use of proteins and carbohydrates

Diversional activity deficit r/t isolation

Fatigue r/t infectious process, altered body chemistry

Pain r/t edema of liver, bile irritating skin

Risk for fluid volume deficit r/t excessive loss of fluids via vomiting and diarrhea
Social isolation r/t treatment imposed isolation

Hernia

Refer to Inguinal Hernia Repair; Hiatus Hernia

Herniated Disk

Refer to Low Back Pain

Herniorrhapy

Refer to Inguinal Hernia Repair

Herpes in Pregnancy

Altered health maintenance r/t knowledge deficit regarding treatment of disease, protection of fetus
Altered urinary elimination r/t pain with urination
Fear r/t threat to fetus and impending surgery
Impaired tissue integrity r/t active herpes lesion
Pain r/t active herpes lesion
Risk for fetal injury r/t herpes virus
Situational low self-esteem r/t threat to fetus secondary to disease process

Herpes Simplex I

Altered oral mucous membranes r/t inflammatory changes in mouth

Herpes Simplex II

Altered health maintenance r/t knowledge deficit regarding treatment, prevention of spread of disease
Altered urinary elimination r/t pain with urination
Impaired tissue integrity r/t active herpes lesion
Pain r/t active herpes lesion
Situational low self-esteem r/t expressions of shame or guilt

Hiatus Hernia

Altered health maintenance r/t knowledge deficit regarding care of disease
Altered nutrition: less than body requirements r/t pain after eating
Pain: heartburn r/t gastroesophageal reflux

Hip Fracture

Acute confusion r/t sensory overload, sensory deprivation, medication side effects
Colonic constipation r/t immobility, narcotics, anesthesia
Fear r/t outcome of treatment, future mobility, and present helplessness
Impaired physical mobility r/t surgical incision and temporary absence of weight bearing
Pain r/t injury, surgical procedure
Powerlessness r/t health care environment
Risk for fluid volume deficit: hemorrhage r/t postoperative complication, surgical blood loss
Risk for impaired skin integrity r/t immobility
Risk for infection r/t invasive procedure
Risk for injury r/t dislodged prosthesis, unsteadiness when ambulating
Risk for perioperative positioning injury r/t immobilization, muscle weakness, emaciation
Self-care deficit: specify r/t musculoskeletal impairment

Hip Replacement

Refer to Total Joint Replacement

Hirshsprung's Disease

Altered health maintenance r/t parental knowledge deficit regarding temporary stoma care, dietary management, treatment for constipation or diarrhea
Altered nutrition: less than body requirements r/t anorexia, pain from distended colon
Constipation (bowel obstruction) r/t inhibited peristalsis secondary to congenital absence of parasympathetic ganglion cells in the distal colon
Grieving r/t loss of perfect child, birth of child with congenital defect, even though child expected to be normal within 2 years
Impaired skin integrity r/t stoma, potential skin care problems associated with stoma
Pain r/t distended colon, incisional postoperative pain
Refer to Hospitalized Child

Hirsutism

Body image disturbance r/t excessive hair

Hitting Behavior

Acute confusion r/t dementia, alcohol abuse, drug abuse, delirium
Risk for violence: directed at others r/t antisocial character, catatonic or manic excitement, organic brain syndrome, panic states, rage reactions, temporal lobe epilepsy, toxic reactions to drugs

HIV (Human Immunodeficiency Virus)

Altered protection r/t depressed immune system
Fear r/t possible death
Refer to AIDS

Hodgkin's Disease

Refer to Cancer; Anemia

Home Maintenance Problems

Impaired home maintenance management r/t individual or family member disease or injury, insufficient family organization or planning, insufficient finances, unfamiliarity with neighborhood resources, impaired cognitive or emotional functioning, lack of knowledge, lack of role modeling, inadequate support systems

Homelessness

Impaired home maintenance management r/t impaired cognitive or emotional functioning, inadequate support system, insufficient finances

Hopelessness

Hopelessness r/t prolonged activity restriction creating isolation, failing or deteriorating physiological condition, long-term stress, abandonment, lost belief in transcendent values or in God

Hospitalized Child

Activity intolerance r/t fatigue associated with acute illness

Altered family processes r/t situational crisis of illness or disease and hospitalization

Altered growth and development r/t regression or lack of progression toward developmental milestones secondary to frequent or prolonged hospitalization, inadequate or inappropriate stimulation, cerebral insult, chronic illness, effects of physical disability, prescribed dependence

Anxiety: separation (child) r/t familiar surroundings and separation from family and friends

Diversional activity deficit r/t immobility, monotonous environment, frequent or lengthy treatments, reluctance to participate, therapeutic isolation, separation from peers

Family coping: potential for growth r/t impact of crisis on family values, priorities, goals, or relationships in family

Fear r/t knowledge deficit or maturational level with fear of unknown, mutilation, painful procedures, surgery

Hopelessness (child) r/t prolonged activity restriction and/or uncertain prognosis

Ineffective family coping: compromised r/t possible prolonged hospitalization that exhausts supportive capacity of significant people

Ineffective individual coping (parent) r/t possible guilt regarding hospitalization of child, parental inadequacies

Risk for altered growth and development: regression r/t disruption of normal routine, unfamiliar environment or caregivers, developmental vulnerability of young children

Risk for altered nutrition: less than body requirements r/t anorexia, absence of familiar foods, cultural preferences

Risk for altered parent/child attachment r/t separation

Risk for injury r/t unfamiliar environment, developmental age, lack of parental knowledge regarding safety (e.g., side rails, IV site/pole)

Sleep pattern disturbance (child or parent) r/t 24-hour care needs of hospitalization

Pain r/t treatments, diagnostic or therapeutic procedures

Powerlessness (child) r/t health care environment, illness-related regimen

Hostile Behavior

Risk for violence: self-directed or directed at others r/t antisocial personality disorder

HTN (Hypertension)

Altered health maintenance r/t knowledge deficit regarding treatment and control of disease process

Altered nutrition: more than body requirements r/t lack of knowledge of relationship between diet and the disease process

Noncompliance r/t side effects of treatment, lack of understanding regarding importance of controling hypertension

Pain: headache r/t cerebral vascular changes

Hydrocele

Altered sexuality pattern r/t recent surgery on area of scrotum

Pain r/t severely enlarged hydrocele

Hydrocephalus

Altered family processes r/t situational crisis

Altered growth and development r/t sequelae of increased intracranial pressure

Altered nutrition: less than body requirements r/t inadequate intake secondary to anorexia, nausea, and/or vomiting; feeding difficulties

Altered tissue perfusion: cerebral r/t interrupted flow and/or hypervolemia of cerebral ventricles

Decisional conflict: parental r/t unclear or conflicting values regarding selection of treatment modality

Fluid volume excess: cerebral ventricles r/t compromised regulatory mechanism

Impaired skin (tissue) integrity r/t impaired physical mobility, mechanical irritation
Risk for infection r/t sequelae of invasive procedure (shunt placement)
Refer to Premature Infant; Child with Chronic Condition; Hospitalized Child; Mental Retardation, if appropriate

Hygiene, Inability to Provide Own Hygiene

Bathing/hygiene self-care deficit r/t intolerance to activity, decreased strength and endurance, pain, discomfort, perceptual or cognitive impairment, neuromuscular impairment, musculoskeletal impairment, depression, severe anxiety

Hyperactive Syndrome

Altered role performance (parent) r/t stressors associated with dealing with hyperactive child, perceived or projected blame for causes of child's behavior, unmet needs for support or care, lack of energy to provide for those needs
Decisional conflict r/t multiple or divergent sources of information regarding education, nutrition, and medication regimens, willingness to change own food habits, limited resources
Impaired social interaction r/t impulsive and overactive behaviors, concomitant emotional difficulties, distractibility and excitability
Ineffective family coping: compromised r/t unsuccessful strategies to control excessive activity, behaviors, frustration, and anger
Parental role conflict (when siblings present) r/t increased attention toward hyperactive child
Risk for altered parenting r/t disruptive or uncontrollable behaviors of child
Risk for violence (parent or child) r/t frustration with disruptive behavior, anger, unsuccessful relationship(s)
Self-esteem disturbance/chronic low self-esteem r/t inability to achieve socially acceptable behaviors, frustration; frequent reprimands, punishment, or scoldings secondary to uncontrolled activity and behaviors; mood fluctuations and restlessness; inability to succeed academically; lack of peer support

Hyperalimentation

Refer to TPN

Hyperbilirubinemia

Altered nutrition: less than body requirements (infant) r/t disinterest in feeding due to jaundice-related lethargy
Anxiety (parents) r/t threat to infant and unknown future
Parental role conflict r/t interruption of family life due to care regimen
Risk for altered body temperature (infant) r/t phototherapy
Risk for injury (infant) r/t kernicterus, phototherapy lights
Sensory/perceptual alteration: visual (infant) r/t use of eye patches for protection of eyes during phototherapy

Hypercalcemia

Altered nutrition: less than body requirements r/t gastrointestinal manifestations of hypercalcemia (nausea, anorexia, ileus)
Altered thought processes r/t elevated calcium levels that cause paranoia
Decreased cardiac output r/t bradydysrhythmias
Impaired physical mobility r/t decreased tone in smooth and striated muscle
Pain r/t activity
Risk for trauma r/t risk for fractures

Hypercapnea

Fear r/t difficulty breathing
Impaired gas exchange r/t ventilation perfusion imbalance

Hyperemesis Gravidarum

Altered comfort: nausea r/t hormonal changes of pregnancy
Altered nutrition: less than body requirements r/t vomiting
Anxiety r/t threat to self and infant, hospitalization
Fluid volume deficit r/t vomiting
Impaired home maintenance management r/t chronic nausea, inability to function
Powerlessness r/t illness-related regimen
Social isolation r/t hospitalization

Hyperglycemia

Ineffective management of therapeutic regimen r/t complexity of therapeutic regimen, decisional conflicts, economic difficulties, nonsupportive family, insufficient cues to action, knowledge deficits, mistrust, lack of acknowledgement of seriousness of condition
Refer to Diabetes Mellitus

Hyperkalemia

Risk for activity intolerance r/t muscle weakness
Risk for decreased cardiac output r/t possible dysrhythmias
Risk for fluid volume excess r/t untreated renal failure

Hypernatremia

Risk for fluid volume deficit r/t abnormal water loss, inadequate water intake

Hyperosmolar Nonketotic Coma

Altered thought processes r/t dehydration, electrolyte imbalance
Fluid volume deficit r/t polyuria, inadequate fluid intake
Risk for injury: seizures r/t hyperosmolar state, electrolyte imbalance
Refer to Diabetes

Hypersensitivity to Slight Criticism

Defensive coping r/t situational crisis, psychological impairment, substance abuse

Hypertension

Altered health maintenance r/t knowledge deficit regarding treatment and control of disease process
Altered nutrition: more than body requirements r/t lack of knowledge of relationship between diet and the disease process
Noncompliance r/t side effects of treatment
Pain: headache r/t cerebral vascular changes

Hyperthermia

Hyperthermia r/t exposure to hot environment, vigorous activity, medications, anesthesia, inappropriate clothing, increased metabolic rate, illness, trauma, dehydration, inability or decreased ability to perspire

Hyperthyroidism

Activity intolerance r/t increased oxygen demands from increased metabolic rate
Altered health maintenance r/t knowledge deficit regarding medications, methods of coping with stress
Altered nutrition: less than body requirements r/t increased metabolic rate, increased gastrointestinal activity
Anxiety r/t increased stimulation, loss of control
Diarrhea r/t increased gastric motility
Risk for injury: eye damage r/t exophthalmos
Sleep pattern disturbance r/t anxiety, excessive sympathetic discharge

Hyperventilation

Ineffective breathing pattern r/t anxiety, acid-base imbalance

Hypocalcemia

Activity intolerance r/t neuromuscular irritability
Altered nutrition: less than body requirements r/t effects of vitamin D deficiency, renal failure, malabsorption, laxative use
Ineffective breathing pattern r/t laryngospasm

Hypoglycemia

Altered health maintenance r/t knowledge deficit regarding disease process, self-care
Altered nutrition: less than body requirements r/t imbalance of glucose and insulin level
Altered thought processes r/t insufficient blood glucose to brain
Refer to Diabetes

Hypokalemia

Activity intolerance r/t muscle weakness
Decreased cardiac output r/t possible dysrhythmias from electrolyte imbalance

Hypomania

Sleep pattern disturbance r/t psychological stimulus
Refer to Manic Disorder

Hyponatremia

Altered thought processes r/t electrolyte imbalance
Fluid volume excess r/t excessive intake of hypotonic fluids

Hypoplastic Left Lung

Refer to Congenital Heart Disease/Cardiac Anomalies

Hypotension

Altered thought processes r/t decreased oxygen supply to brain
Altered tissue perfusion: cardiopulmonary/peripheral r/t hypovolemia, decreased contractility, decreased afterload
Decreased cardiac output r/t decreased preload, decreased contractility
Risk for fluid volume deficit r/t excessive fluid loss
Refer to cause of Hypotension

Hypothermia

Hypothermia r/t exposure to cold environment, illness, trauma, damage to hypothalamus, malnutrition, aging

Hypothyroidism

Activity intolerance r/t muscular stiffness, shortness of breath on exertion
Altered health maintenance r/t knowledge deficit regarding disease process and self-care

Altered nutrition: more than body requirements r/t decreased metabolic process
Altered thought processes r/t altered metabolic process
Colonic constipation r/t decreased gastric motility
Impaired gas exchange r/t possible respiratory depression
Impaired skin integrity r/t edema, dry or scaly skin

Hypovolemic Shock

Refer to Shock

Hypoxia

Altered thought processes r/t decreased oxygen supply to brain
Fear r/t breathlessness
Impaired gas exchange r/t altered oxygen supply, inability to transport oxygen
Impaired memory r/t hypoxia
Ineffective airway clearance r/t decreased energy and fatigue, increased secretions

Hysterectomy

Altered health maintenance r/t knowledge deficit regarding precautions and self-care following surgery
Anticipatory grieving r/t change in body image, loss of reproductive status
Constipation r/t narcotics, anesthesia, bowel manipulation during surgery
Ineffective individual coping r/t situational crisis of surgery
Pain r/t surgical injury
Risk for altered tissue perfusion r/t thromboembolism
Risk for fluid volume deficit r/t abnormal blood loss, hemorrhage
Risk for urinary retention r/t edema in area, anesthesia, narcotics, pain
Sexual dysfunction r/t disturbance in self-concept
Refer to Surgery

I

IBS (Irritable Bowel Syndrome)

Altered health maintenance r/t knowledge deficit regarding self-care with IBS
Constipation r/t low-residue diet, stress
Diarrhea r/t increased motility of intestines associated with stress
Ineffective management of therapeutic regimen r/t knowledge deficit, powerlessness
Pain r/t spasms and increased motility of bowel

ICD (Internal Cardioverter Defibrillator)

Preoperative

Anxiety r/t surgical procedure
Knowledge deficit r/t purpose and function of ICD

Postoperative

Altered health maintenance r/t knowledge deficit regarding self-care and care of internal cardiac defibrillator
Risk for decreased cardiac output r/t possible dysrhythmias
Risk for infection r/t invasive surgical procedure
Refer to Coronary Artery Bypass Grafting

IDDM (Insulin-Dependent Diabetes)

Refer to Diabetes Mellitus

Identity Disturbance

Personal identity disturbance r/t situational crisis, psychological impairment, chronic illness, pain

Idiopathic Thrombocytopenia Purpura

Refer to ITP

Ileal Conduit

Altered sexuality pattern r/t altered body function and structure
Body image disturbance r/t presence of stoma
Ineffective management of therapeutic regimen r/t new skills required to care for appliance and self
Knowledge deficit r/t care of stoma
Risk for impaired skin integrity r/t difficulty obtaining tight seal of appliance
Social isolation r/t alteration in physical appearance, fear of accidental spill of ostomy contents

Ileostomy

Altered sexuality pattern r/t altered body function and structure
Body image disturbance r/t presence of stoma
Constipation/diarrhea r/t dietary changes, change in intestinal motility
Ineffective management of therapeutic regimen r/t new skills required to care for appliance and self
Knowledge deficit r/t limited practice of stoma care, dietary modifications
Risk for impaired skin integrity r/t difficulty obtaining tight seal of appliance, caustic drainage
Social isolation r/t alteration in physical appearance, fear of accidental spill of ostomy contents

Ileus

Constipation r/t decreased gastric motility
Fluid volume deficit r/t loss of fluids from vomiting, fluids trapped in bowl
Pain r/t pressure, abdominal distention

Immobility

Altered thought process r/t sensory deprivation from immobility
Altered tissue perfusion: peripheral r/t interruption of venous flow
Constipation r/t immobility
Disuse syndrome r/t immobilization
Impaired physical mobility r/t medically imposed bedrest
Ineffective breathing pattern r/t inability to deep breathe in supine position
Powerlessness r/t forced immobility from health care environment
Risk for impaired skin integrity r/t pressure on immobile parts, shearing forces when moving

Immunosuppression

Altered protection r/t medications/treatments suppressing immune system function
Risk for infection r/t immunosuppression

Impaction of Stool

Colonic constipation r/t decreased fluid intake, less than adequate amounts of fiber and bulk-forming foods in diet, immobility

Imperforate Anus

Anxiety r/t ability to care for newborn
Knowledge deficit r/t home care for newborn
Risk for impaired skin integrity r/t presence of stool at surgical repair site

Impetigo

Altered health maintenance r/t parental knowledge deficit regarding care of impetigo
Impaired skin integrity r/t pruritis
Refer to Communicable Diseases, Childhood

Impotence

Self-esteem disturbance r/t physiological crisis, inability to practice usual sexual activity
Sexual dysfunction r/t altered body function

Inactivity

Impaired physical mobility r/t intolerance to activity, decreased strength and endurance, depression, severe anxiety, musculoskeletal impairment, perceptual or cognitive impairment, neuromuscular impairment, pain, discomfort

Incompetent Cervix

Refer to Premature Dilation of the Cervix

Incontinence of Stool

Bowel incontinence r/t decreased awareness of need to defecate, loss of sphincter control
Knowledge deficit r/t lack of information on normal bowel elimination
Risk for impaired skin integrity r/t incontinence of stool
Self-care deficit r/t toileting needs
Situational low self-esteem r/t inability to control the elimination of stool

Incontinence of Urine

Functional incontinence r/t altered environment; sensory, cognitive, or mobility deficits
Reflex incontinence r/t neurological impairment
Risk for impaired skin integrity r/t presence of urine
Self-care deficit: toileting r/t toileting needs
Situational low self-esteem r/t inability to control passage of urine
Stress incontinence r/t degenerative change in pelvic muscles and structural supports associated with increased age, high intra-abdominal pressure (e.g., obesity, gravid uterus), incompetent bladder outlet, overdistention between voidings, weak pelvic muscles and structural supports
Total incontinence r/t neuropathy preventing transmission of reflex indicating bladder fullness, neurological dysfunction causing triggering of micturation at unpredictable times, independent contraction of detrusor reflex due to surgery, trauma or disease affecting spinal cord nerves, anatomical fistula
Urge incontinence r/t decreased bladder capacity (e.g., history of pelvic inflammatory disease, abdominal surgeries, indwelling urinary catheter); irritation of bladder stretch receptors, causing spasm (e.g., bladder infection); alcohol; caffeine; increased fluids; increased urine concentration; overdistention of bladder

Indigestion

Altered comfort r/t unpleasant sensations experienced when eating, burning, bloating, heaviness
Altered nutrition: less than body requirements r/t discomfort when eating

Induction of Labor

Anxiety r/t medical interventions
Decisional conflict r/t perceived threat to idealized birth
Ineffective individual coping r/t situational crisis of medical intervention in birthing process
Risk for injury (maternal and fetal) r/t hypertonic uterus and potential prematurity of the newborn
Self-esteem disturbance r/t inability to carry out normal labor

Infant Apnea

Refer to Premature Infant; Respiratory Conditions of the Neonate; Sudden Infant Death Syndrome

Infant Feeding Pattern, Ineffective

Ineffective infant feeding pattern r/t prematurity, neurological impairment or delay, oral hypersensitivity, prolonged NPO

Infant of Diabetic Mother

Altered growth and development r/t prolonged and severe postnatal hypoglycemia
Altered nutrition: less than body requirements r/t hypotonia, lethargy, poor sucking, postnatal metabolic changes from hyperglycemia to hypoglycemia and hyperinsulinism
Fluid volume deficit r/t increased urinary excretion and osmotic diuresis
Risk for decreased cardiac output r/t increased incidence of cardiomegaly
Risk for impaired gas exchange r/t increased incidence of cardiomegaly, prematurity
Refer to Premature Infant; Respiratory Conditions of the Neonate

Infant Behavior

Disorganized infant behavior r/t pain, oral/motor problems, feeding intolerance, environmental overstimulation, lack of containment/boundries, prematurity, invasive/painful procedures
Potential for enhanced organized infant behavior r/t prematurity, pain
Risk for disorganized infant behavior r/t pain, oral/motor problems, environmental overstimulation, lack of containment/boundaries

Infant of Substance-Abusing Mother (Fetal Alcohol Syndrome, Crack Baby, Other Drug Withdrawal Infants)

Altered growth and development r/t effects of maternal use of drugs, effects of neurological impairment, decreased attentiveness to environmental stimuli or inadequate stimuli
Altered nutrition: less than body requirements r/t feeding problems; uncoordinated or ineffective suck and swallow; effects of diarrhea, vomiting, or colic associated with maternal substance abuse
Altered parenting r/t impaired or absent attachment behaviors, inadequate support systems
Altered protection r/t effects of maternal substance abuse
Diarrhea r/t effects of withdrawal, increased peristalsis secondary to hyperirritability
Ineffective airway clearance r/t pooling of secretions secondary to lack of adequate cough reflex, effects of viral or bacterial lower airway infection secondary to altered protective state
Ineffective infant feeding pattern r/t uncoordinated or ineffective sucking reflex
Interrupted breast-feeding r/t use of drugs or alcohol by mother
Risk for infection: skin, meningeal, respiratory r/t effects of withdrawal
Sensory-perceptual alteration r/t hypersensitivity to environmental stimuli
Sleep pattern disturbance r/t hyperirritability or hypersensitivity to environmental stimuli
Refer to Failure to Thrive; Sudden Infant Death Syndrome; Hospitalized Child; Cerebral Palsy; Hyperactive Syndrome

Infantile Spasms

Refer to Seizure Disorders, Childhood

Infection

Altered protection r/t inadequate nutrition, abnormal blood profiles, drug therapies, treatments
Hyperthermia r/t increased metabolic rate

Infection, Potential for

Risk for infection r/t inadequate primary defenses, (e.g., broken skin, traumatized tissue, decrease in ciliary action, stasis of body fluids, change in pH secretions, altered peristalsis), inadequate secondary defenses (e.g., decreased hemoglobin, leukopenia, suppressed inflammatory response), immunosuppression, inadequate acquired immunity, tissue destruction and increased environmental exposure, chronic disease, invasive procedures, malnutrition, pharmaceutical agents, trauma, rupture of amniotic membranes, or insufficient knowledge to avoid exposure to pathogens

Inflammatory Bowel Disease, Child and Adult

Altered nutrition: less than body requirements r/t anorexia, decreased absorption of nutrients from gastrointestinal tract
Diarrhea r/t effects of inflammatory changes of the bowel
Fluid volume deficit r/t frequent and loose stools
Impaired skin integrity r/t frequent stools and development of anal fissures
Ineffective individual coping r/t repeated episodes of diarrhea
Pain r/t abdominal cramping and anal irritation
Social isolation r/t diarrhea
Refer to Crohn's Disease; Hospitalized Child; Child with Chronic Condition; Maturational Issues, Adolescent

Influenza

Altered health maintenance r/t knowledge deficit regarding self-care with influenza
Fluid volume deficit r/t inadequate fluid intake
Hyperthermia r/t infectious process
Ineffective management of therapeutic regimen r/t lack of knowledge regarding preventive immunizations
Pain r/t inflammatory changes in joints

Inguinal Hernia Repair

Impaired physical mobility r/t pain at surgical site and fear of causing hernia to "break open"
Pain r/t surgical procedure
Risk for infection r/t surgical procedure
Urinary retention r/t possible edema at surgical site

Injury

Risk for injury r/t environmental conditions interacting with the client's adaptive and defensive resources

Insomnia

Anxiety r/t actual or perceived loss of sleep
Sleep pattern disturbance r/t sensory alterations, internal factors, external factors

Insulin Shock

Refer to Hypoglycemia

Intermittent Claudication

Altered tissue perfusion: peripheral r/t interruption of arterial flow
Knowledge deficit r/t lack of knowledge of cause and treatment of peripheral vascular diseases
Pain r/t decreased circulation to extremities with activity
Risk for injury r/t tissue hypoxia
Risk for peripheral neurovascular dysfunction r/t disruption in arterial flow
Refer to Peripheral Vascular Disease

Internal Cardioverter Defibrillator

Refer to ICD

Internal Fixation

Risk for infection r/t traumatized tissue, broken skin
Refer to Fracture

Interstitial Cystitis

Altered urinary elimination r/t inflammation of the bladder
Pain r/t inflammatory process
Risk for infection r/t suppressed inflammatory response

Intervertebral Disk Excision

Refer to Laminectomy

Intestinal Obstruction

Refer to Ileus

Intoxication

Acute confusion r/t alcohol abuse
Altered thought process r/t effect of substance on central nervous system
Anxiety r/t loss of control of actions
Ineffective individual coping r/t use of mind-altering substances as a means of coping
Risk for violence r/t inability to control thoughts and actions
Sensory/perceptual alterations: visual, auditory, kinesthetic, tactile, olfactory r/t neurochemical imbalance in the brain

Intra-aortic Balloon Counterpulsation

Anxiety r/t device providing cardiovascular assistance
Decreased cardiac output r/t failing heart needing counterpulsation
Impaired physical mobility r/t restriction of movement because of mechanical device
Risk for peripheral neurovascular dysfunction r/t vascular obstruction of balloon catheter, thrombus formation, emboli, edema

Intracranial Pressure, Increased

Acute confusion r/t increased intracranial pressure
Altered thought processes r/t pressure damage to brain

Altered tissue perfusion: cerebral r/t the effects of increased intracranial pressure
Decreased adaptive capacity: intracranial r/t sustained increase in intracranial pressure (≥ 10 to 15 mm Hg)
Ineffective breathing patterns r/t pressure damage to breathing center in brain stem
Sensory/perceptual alteration r/t pressure damage to sensory centers in brain
Refer to cause of Increased Intracranial Pressure

Intrauterine Growth Retardation

Altered growth and development r/t insufficient supply of oxygen and nutrients
Altered nutrition: less than body requirements r/t insufficient placenta
Anxiety (maternal) r/t threat to fetus
Impaired gas exchange r/t insufficient placental perfusion
Ineffective individual coping (maternal) r/t situational crisis and threat to fetus
Risk for injury r/t insufficient supply of oxygen and nutrients
Situational low self-esteem (maternal) r/t guilt over threat to fetus

Intubation—Endotracheal or Nasogastric

Altered nutrition: less than body requirements r/t inability to ingest food due to presence of tubes
Altered oral mucous membrane r/t presence of tubes
Body image disturbance r/t altered appearance with mechanical devices
Impaired verbal communication r/t endotracheal tube

Irregular Pulse

Refer to Dysrhythmia

Irritable Bowel Syndrome

Refer to IBS

Isolation

Risk for loneliness r/t lack of affection, physical isolation, cathectic deprivation, social isolation
Social isolation r/t factors contributing to the absence of satisfying personal relationships, such as delay in accomplishing developmental tasks, immature interests, alterations in mental status, unacceptable social behavior, unaccepted social values, altered state of wellness, inadequate personal resources, inability to engage in satisfying personal relationships

Itching

Altered comfort r/t irritation of the skin
Risk for infection r/t potential break in skin

ITP (Idiopathic Thrombocytopenia Purpura)

Altered protection r/t decreased platelet count
Diversional activity deficit r/t activity restrictions and safety precautions
Impaired home health maintenance r/t parental lack of ability to follow through with safety precautions secondary to child's developmental stage (active toddler)
Risk for injury r/t decreased platelet count and developmental level, age-appropriate play
Refer to Hospitalized Child

J

Jaundice

Altered comfort: pruritis r/t toxic metabolites excreted in the skin
Altered thought processes r/t toxic blood metabolites
Risk for impaired skin integrity r/t pruritis, itching
Refer to Cirrhosis

Jaw Surgery

Altered nutrition: less than body requirements r/t jaws wired closed
Impaired swallowing r/t edema from surgery
Knowledge deficit r/t emergency care for wired jaw (cutting bands and wires), oral care
Pain r/t surgical procedure
Risk for aspiration r/t wired jaws

Jittery

Anxiety r/t unconscious conflict about essential values and goals, threat to or change in health status

Joint Replacement

Risk for peripheral neurovascular dysfunction r/t orthopedic surgery
Refer to Total Joint Replacement

JRA (Juvenile Rheumatoid Arthritis)

Refer to Rheumatoid Arthritis

K

Kaposi's Sarcoma

Refer to AIDS

Kawasaki Disease (Formerly Called Mucocutaneous Lymph Node Syndrome)

Altered nutrition: less than body requirements r/t altered oral mucous membranes
Altered oral mucous membranes r/t inflamed mouth and pharynx; swollen lips that progress to dry, cracked, and fissured
Anxiety (parental) r/t progression of disease, complications of arthritis and cardiac involvement
Hyperthermia r/t inflammatory disease process
Impaired skin integrity r/t inflammatory skin changes
Pain r/t enlarged lymph nodes; erythematous skin rash that progresses to desquamation, peeling, and denuding of skin
Refer to Hospitalized Child

Kegel's Exercise

Health-seeking behavior r/t desire for information to relieve incontinence
Stress incontinence r/t degenerative change in pelvic muscles
Urge-incontinence r/t decreased bladder capacity

Ketoacidosis

Altered nutrition: less than body requirements r/t body's inability to use nutrients
Fluid volume deficit r/t excess excretion of urine, nausea, vomiting, increased respiration
Impaired memory r/t fluid and electrolyte imbalance
Ineffective management of therapeutic regimen r/t denial of illness, lack of understanding of preventive measures and adequate blood sugar control
Noncompliance (with diabetic regimen) r/t ineffective coping with chronic disease
Refer to Diabetes

Kidney Failure

Refer to Renal Failure

Kidney Stones

Altered patterns of urinary elimination: frequency, urgency r/t anatomical obstruction, irritation caused by stone
Knowledge deficit r/t fluid requirements and dietary restrictions
Pain r/t obstruction from renal calculi
Risk for fluid volume deficit r/t nausea, vomiting
Risk for infection r/t obstruction of urinary tract with stasis of urine

Knee Replacement

Refer to Total Joint Replacement

Knowledge Deficit

Altered health maintenance r/t lack of or significant alteration in communication skills (written, verbal, and/or gestural)
Knowledge deficit r/t lack of exposure, lack of recall, information misinterpretation, cognitive limitation, lack of interest in learning, unfamiliarity with information resources

Kock Pouch

Refer to Continent Ileostomy

Korsakoff's Syndrome

Acute confusion r/t alcohol abuse
Impaired memory r/t neurological changes
Risk for altered nutrition r/t lack of adequate balanced intake
Risk for injury r/t sensory dysfunction, lack of coordination when ambulating

L

Labor, Induction of

Refer to Induction of Labor

Labor—Normal

Anxiety r/t fear of the unknown, situational crisis
Fatigue r/t childbirth
Health-seeking behaviors r/t healthy outcome of pregnancy, prenatal care, and childbirth eduction
Knowledge deficit r/t lack of preparation for labor
Impaired tissue integrity r/t passage of infant through birth canal, episiotomy
Pain r/t uterine contractions, stretching of cervix and birth canal
Risk for fluid volume deficit r/t excessive loss of blood
Risk for infection r/t multiple vaginal examinations, tissue trauma, and prolonged rupture of membranes
Risk for injury (fetal) r/t hypoxia

Laminectomy

Anxiety r/t change in health status, surgical procedure
Impaired physical mobility r/t neuromuscular impairment
Knowledge deficit r/t appropriate postoperative and postdischarge activities
Pain r/t localized inflammation and edema
Risk for impaired tissue perfusion r/t edema, hemorrhage, or embolism
Risk for perioperative positioning injury r/t prone position
Sensory/perceptual alteration: tactile r/t possible edema or nerve injury
Urinary retention r/t competing sensory impulses, effects of narcotics/anesthesia
Refer to Surgery; Scoliosis

Laparotomy

Refer to Abdominal Surgery

Laproscopic Laser Cholecystectomy

Refer to Cholecystectomy; Laser Surgery

Laryngectomy

Altered health maintenance r/t knowledge deficit regarding self-care with laryngectomy
Alteration in family process r/t surgery, serious condition of family member, difficulty communicating
Alteration in nutrition: less than body requirements r/t absence of oral feeding, difficulty swallowing, increased need for fluids
Alteration in oral mucous membranes r/t absence of oral feeding
Anticipatory grieving r/t loss of voice, fear of death
Body image disturbance r/t change in body structure and function
Impaired swallowing r/t edema, laryngectomy tube
Impaired verbal communication r/t removal of the larynx
Ineffective airway clearance r/t surgical removal of the glottis, decreased humidification of air
Risk for infection r/t invasive procedure, surgery

Laser Surgery

Constipation r/t laser intervention in vulva and perianal areas
Knowledge deficit r/t preoperative and postoperative care associated with laser procedure
Pain r/t heat from action of the laser
Risk for infection r/t delayed heating reaction of tissue exposed to laser
Risk for injury r/t accidental exposure to laser beam

Laxative Abuse

Perceived constipation r/t health belief, faulty appraisal, impaired thought processes

Lens Implant

Refer to Cataract Extraction

Lethargy/Listlessness

Altered tissue perfusion: cerebral r/t lack of oxygen supply to brain
Fatigue r/t decreased metabolic energy production
Sleep pattern disturbance r/t internal or external stressors
Refer to cause of Lethargy

Leukemia

Altered protection r/t abnormal blood profile
Risk for fluid volume deficit r/t side effects of treatment, nausea, vomiting, bleeding
Risk for infection r/t ineffective immune system
Refer to Chemotherapy; Cancer

Leukopenia

Risk for infection r/t low white blood count

Level of Consciousness, Decreased

Refer to Confusion

Lice

Refer to Communicable Diseases, Childhood

Limb Reattachment Procedures

Anticipatory grieving r/t unknown outcome of reattachment procedure
Anxiety r/t unknown outcome of reattachment procedure, use and appearance of limb
Body image disturbance r/t unpredictability of function and appearance of reattached body part
Risk for fluid volume deficit: hemorrhage r/t severed vessels
Risk for perioperative positioning injury r/t immobilization
Risk for peripheral neurovascular dysfunction r/t trauma, orthopedic and neurovascular surgery, compression of nerves and blood vessels
Refer to Surgery, Postoperative Care

Liver Biopsy

Anxiety r/t procedure and results
Risk for fluid volume deficit r/t hemorrhage from biopsy site

Liver Disease

Refer to Cirrhosis; Hepatitis

Lobectomy

Refer to Thoracotomy

Loneliness

Risk for loneliness r/t lack of affection, physical isolation, cathectic deprivation, social isolation

Loose Stools

Diarrhea r/t increased gastric motility (refer to underlying disease)

Low Back Pain

Altered health maintenance r/t knowledge deficit regarding self-care with back pain
Chronic pain r/t degenerative processes, musculotendinous strain, injury, inflammation, congenital deformities
Impaired physical mobility r/t back pain
Urinary retention r/t possible spinal cord compression

Lumbar Puncture

Anxiety r/t invasive procedure and unknown results
Knowledge deficit r/t information about the procedure
Pain: headache r/t possible loss of cerebral spinal fluid
Risk for infection r/t invasive procedure

Lung Cancer

Refer to Cancer; Thoracotomy

Lupus Erythematosus

Altered health maintenance r/t knowledge deficit regarding medication, diet, and activity
Body image disturbance r/t change in skin, rash, lesions, ulcers, mottled erythema
Fatigue r/t increased metabolic requirements
Pain r/t inflammatory process
Powerlessness r/t unpredictability of course of the disease
Risk for impaired skin integrity r/t chronic inflammation, edema, altered circulation
Spiritual distress r/t chronicity of disease, unknown etiology

Lyme Disease

Fatigue r/t increased energy requirements
Knowledge deficit r/t lack of information concerning the disease, prevention, and treatment
Pain r/t inflammation of joints, urticaria, rash
Risk for decreased cardiac output r/t dysrhythmias

Lymphedema

Fluid volume excess r/t compromised regulatory system; inflammation, obstruction, or removal of lymph glands
Knowledge deficit r/t management of condition

Lymphoma

Refer to Cancer

M

Magnetic Resonance Imaging

Refer to MRI

Major Depressive Disorder

Refer to Depression

Malabsorption Syndrome

Alteration in nutrition: less than body requirements r/t inability of body to absorb nutrients because of biological factors
Diarrhea r/t lactose intolerance; gluten sensitivity; resection of small bowel
Knowledge deficit r/t lack of information about diet and nutrition
Risk for fluid volume deficit r/t diarrhea

Maladaptive Behavior

Refer to Crisis; Suicide Attempt

Malnutrition

Altered nutrition: less than body requirements r/t inability to ingest food, digest food, or absorb nutrients due to biological, psychological, or economic factors; institutionalization (i.e., lack of menu choices)
Altered protection r/t inadequate nutrition
Ineffective management of therapeutic regimen r/t economic difficulties
Knowledge deficit r/t misinformation about normal nutrition, social isolation, lack of food preparation facilities

Manic Disorder, Bipolar I

Altered family processes r/t family member's illness
Altered nutrition: less than body requirements r/t lack of time and motivation to eat, constant movement
Altered role performance r/t impaired social interactions

Altered thought processes r/t mania
Anxiety r/t change in role function
Fluid volume deficit r/t decreased intake
Impaired home maintenance management r/t altered psychological state, inability to concentrate
Ineffective denial r/t fear of inability to control behavior
Ineffective individual coping r/t situational crisis
Ineffective management of therapeutic regimen r/t lack of social supports
Ineffective management of therapeutic regimen: families r/t unpredictability of client, excessive demands on family, chronicity of condition
Noncompliance r/t denial of illness
Risk for caregiver role strain r/t unpredictability of the condition, mood swings
Risk for violence: self-directed or directed at others r/t bizarre hallucinations, delusions
Sleep pattern disturbance r/t constant anxious thoughts

Manipulative Behavior

Defensive coping r/t superior attitude toward others
Impaired social interaction r/t self-concept disturbance
Ineffective individual coping r/t inappropriate use of defense mechanisms
Risk for loneliness r/t inability to interact appropriately with others
Risk for self-mutilation r/t inability to cope with increased psychological or physiological tension in a healthy manner

Marasmus

Refer to Failure to Thrive (FTT)

Marshall-Marchetti-Krantz Operation

Preoperative

Stress incontinence r/t weak pelvic muscles and pelvic supports

Postoperative

Knowledge deficit r/t lack of exposure to information regarding care after surgery and at home
Pain r/t manipulation of organs and surgical incision
Risk for infection r/t presence of urinary catheter
Urinary retention r/t swelling of urinary meatus

Mastectomy

Body image disturbance r/t loss of sexually significant body part
Fear r/t change in body image and prognosis
Knowledge deficit r/t self-care activities
Pain r/t surgical procedure
Risk for impaired physical mobility r/t nerve or muscle damage, pain
Sexual dysfunction r/t change in body image, fear of loss of feminism

Refer to Cancer; Surgery

Mastitis

Altered role performance r/t change in capacity to function in expected role
Anxiety r/t threat to self and concern over safety of milk for infant
Ineffective breast-feeding r/t breast pain, conflicting advice from health care providers
Knowledge deficit r/t antibiotic regimen and comfort measures
Pain r/t infectious disease process and swelling of breast tissue

Maternal Infection

Altered protection r/t invasive procedures, traumatized tissue, stress of recent childbirth

Refer to Post Partum, Normal Care

Maturational Issues, Adolescent

Altered family processes r/t developmental crises of adolescence secondary to challenge of parental authority and values, situational crises secondary to change in parental marital status
Impaired social interaction r/t ineffective, unsuccessful, or dysfunctional interaction with peers
Ineffective individual coping r/t maturational crises
Knowledge deficit: potential for enhanced health maintenance r/t information misinterpretation, lack of education regarding age-related factors
Risk for injury/trauma r/t thrill-seeking behaviors
Social isolation r/t perceived alteration in physical appearance, social values not accepted by dominant peer group

Refer to Sexuality—Adolescent; Substance Abuse (if relevant)

Measles (Rubeola)

Refer to Communicable Diseases, Childhood

Meconium Aspiration

Refer to Respiratory Conditions of the Neonate

Melanoma

Altered health maintenance r/t knowledge deficit regarding self-care and treatment of melanoma
Body image disturbance r/t altered pigmentation, surgical incision

Fear r/t threat to well-being
Pain r/t surgical incision
Refer to Cancer

Melena

Fear r/t presence of blood in feces
Risk for fluid volume deficit r/t hemorrhage
Refer to GI Bleed

Memory Deficit

Impaired memory r/t acute or chronic hypoxia, anemia, decreased cardiac output, fluid and electrolyte imbalance, neurological disturbance, excessive environmental disturbances

Meningitis/Encephalitis

Altered comfort: nausea and vomiting r/t central nervous system (CNS) inflammation
Altered comfort: photophobia r/t increased sensitivity to external stimuli secondary to CNS inflammation
Altered growth and development r/t brain damage secondary to infectious process, increased intracranial pressure
Altered thought processes r/t inflammation of brain, fever
Altered tissue perfusion: cerebral r/t inflamed cerebral tissues and meninges, increased intracranial pressure
Decreased adaptive capacity: intracranial r/t sustained increase in intracranial pressure (≥ 10 to 15 mm Hg)
Fluid volume excess r/t increased intracranial pressure, syndrome of inappropriate secretion of antidiuretic hormone (SIADH)
Impaired mobility r/t neuromuscular or CNS insult
Ineffective airway clearance r/t seizure activity
Pain r/t neck (nuchal) rigidity, inflammation of meninges, headache, kinesthetic sensory-perceptual alteration (skin is painful to touch), fever, earache
Risk for aspiration r/t seizure activity
Risk for injury r/t seizure activity
Sensory-perceptual alteration: hearing r/t CNS infection, ear infection
Sensory-perceptual alteration: kinesthetic r/t CNS infection
Sensory-perceptual alteration: visual r/t photophobia secondary to CNS infection
Refer to Hospitalized Child

Meningocele

Refer to Neurotube Defects

Menopause

Altered sexuality patterns r/t altered body structure, lack of physiological lubrication, lack of knowledge of artificial lubrication
Effective management of therapeutic regimen r/t verbalized desire to manage menopause
Health-seeking behavior r/t menopause and therapies associated with change in hormonal levels
Ineffective thermoregulation r/t changes in hormonal levels
Risk for altered nutrition: more than body requirements r/t change in metabolic rate caused by fluctuating hormone levels

Menorrhagia

Fear r/t loss of large amounts of blood
Risk for fluid volume deficit r/t excessive loss of menstrual blood

Mental Illness

Altered thought process r/t factors to consider: head injury, mental disorder, personality disorder, organic mental disorder, substance abuse, severe interpersonal conflict, sleep deprivation, sensory deprivation or overload, impaired cerebral perfusion
Defensive coping r/t psychological impairment, substance abuse
Ineffective denial r/t refusal to acknowledge abuse problem, fear of the social stigma of disease
Ineffective family coping: compromised r/t lack of available support from client
Ineffective family coping: disabling r/t chronically unexpressed feelings of guilt, anxiety, hostility, or despair
Ineffective individual coping r/t situational crisis, coping with mental illness
Ineffective management of therapeutic regimen: community r/t inadequate services to care for mentally ill clients, lack of information regarding how to access services
Ineffective management of therapeutic regimen: families r/t chronicity of condition, unpredictability of client, unknown prognosis
Risk for loneliness r/t social isolation

Mental Retardation

Altered family processes r/t crisis of diagnosis and situational transition
Altered growth and development r/t cognitive or perceptual impairment, developmental delay
Chronic low self-esteem r/t perceived differences

Family coping: potential for growth r/t adaptation and acceptance of child's condition and needs
Grieving r/t loss of perfect child; birth of child with congenital defect or subsequent head injury
Impaired home maintenance management r/t insufficient support systems
Impaired social interaction r/t developmental lag or delay, perceived differences
Impaired swallowing r/t neuromuscular impairment
Impaired verbal communication r/t developmental delay
Parental role conflict r/t home care of child with special needs
Risk for self-mutilation r/t separation anxiety, depersonalization
Self-care deficit: bathing/hygiene; dressing/grooming; feeding; toileting r/t perceptual or cognitive impairment
Refer to Safety—Childhood; Child with Chronic Condition

Metabolic Acidosis

Refer to Ketoacidosis

Metabolic Alkalosis

Fluid volume deficit r/t fluid volume loss, vomiting, gastric suctioning, failure of regulatory mechanisms

MI (Myocardial Infarction)

Altered family processes r/t crisis, role change
Altered health maintenance r/t knowledge deficit regarding self-care and treatment of MI
Altered sexuality pattern r/t fear of chest pain, possibility of heart damage
Anxiety r/t threat of death, possible change in role status
Colonic constipation r/t decreased peristalsis from decreased physical activity, medication effect, change in diet
Decreased cardiac output r/t ventricular damage, ischemia, dysrhythmias
Fear r/t threat to well-being
Ineffective denial r/t fear or knowledge deficit about heart disease
Ineffective family coping r/t spouse or significant other's fear of partner loss
Pain r/t myocardial tissue damage from inadequate blood supply
Situational low self-esteem r/t crisis of MI

Midlife Crisis

Ineffective individual coping r/t inability to deal with changes associated with aging
Potential for enhanced spiritual well-being r/t desire to find purpose and meaning to life
Powerlessness r/t lack of control over life situation
Spiritual distress r/t questioning belief/value system

Migraine Headache

Altered health maintenance r/t knowledge deficit regarding prevention and treatment of headaches
Pain: headache r/t vasodilation of cerebral and extracerebral vessels

Miscarriage

Refer to Pregnancy Loss

Mitral Stenosis

Activity intolerance r/t imbalance between oxygen supply and demand
Altered health maintenance r/t knowledge deficit regarding self-care with disorder
Anxiety r/t possible worsening of symptoms, activity intolerance, fatigue
Decreased cardiac output r/t incompetent heart valves, abnormal forward or backward blood flow, flow into a dilated chamber, flow through an abnormal passage between chambers
Fatigue r/t reduced cardiac output

Mitral Valve Prolapse

Altered health maintenance r/t knowledge deficit regarding methods to relieve pain and treat dysrhythmias and shortness of breath, need for prophylactic antibiotics before invasive procedures
Altered tissue perfusion: cerebral r/t postural hypotension
Anxiety r/t symptoms of condition: palpitations, chest pain
Fatigue r/t abnormal catecholamine regulation, decreased intravascular volume
Fear r/t lack of knowledge about mitral valve prolapse, feelings of having a heart attack
Pain r/t mitral valve regurgitation
Risk for infection r/t invasive procedures

Mobility, Impaired Physical

Impaired physical mobility r/t intolerance to activity, decreased strength and endurance, pain, discomfort, perceptual or cognitive impairment, neuromuscular impairment, musculoskeletal impairment, depression, severe anxiety

Modified Radical Mastectomy

Decisional conflict r/t treatment of choice for Breast Cancer
Refer to Mastectomy

Mononucleosis

Activity intolerance r/t generalized weakness
Altered health maintenance r/t knowledge deficit concerning transmission and treatment of disease
Hyperthermia r/t infectious process
Impaired swallowing r/t irritation of oropharyngeal cavity
Pain r/t enlargement of lymph nodes, irritation of oropharyngeal cavity
Risk for injury r/t possible rupture of spleen

Mood Disorders

Caregiver role strain r/t symptoms associated with disorder of care receiver
Impaired adjustment r/t hopelessness, altered locus of control
Social isolation r/t alterations in mental status
Refer to specific disorder: Depression; Dysthymic Disorder; Manic Disorder; Hypomania

Moon Face

Body image disturbance r/t change in appearance from disease or medication
Refer to Cushing's Syndrome

Mottling of Peripheral Skin

Altered tissue perfusion: peripheral r/t interruption of arterial flow, decreased circulating blood volume

Mouth Lesions

Refer to Mucous Membranes, Altered Oral

MRI (Magnetic Resonance Imaging)

Anxiety r/t fear of being in closed spaces
Knowledge deficit r/t preparation for examination, presence of any metal in body contraindication for test

Mucocutaneous Lymph Node Syndrome

Refer to Kawasaki Disease

Mucous Membranes, Altered Oral

Altered oral mucous membranes r/t pathological conditions—oral cavity (radiation to head or neck), dehydration, chemical trauma (e.g., acidic foods, drugs, noxious agents, alcohol), mechanical trauma (e.g., ill-fitting dentures, braces, endotracheal or nasogastric tubes, surgery in oral cavity), NPO for more than 24 hours, ineffective oral hygiene, mouth breathing, malnutrition, infection, lack of or decreased salivation, medication

Multi-infarct Dementia

Refer to Dementia

Multiple Gestation

Altered nutrition: less than body requirements r/t physiological demands of a multifetal pregnancy
Anxiety r/t uncertain outcome of pregnancy
Fatigue r/t physiological demands of a multifetal pregnancy and/or care of more than one infant
Impaired home maintenance management r/t fatigue
Impaired physical mobility r/t increased uterine size
Knowledge deficit r/t caring for more than one infant
Risk for ineffective breast-feeding r/t lack of support, physical demands of feeding more than one infant
Sleep pattern disturbance r/t discomforts of multiple gestation or care of infants
Stress incontinence r/t increased pelvic pressure

Multiple Personality Disorder (Dissociative Identity Disorder)

Anxiety r/t loss of control of behavior and feelings
Body image disturbance r/t feelings of powerlessness with personality changes
Chronic low self-esteem r/t inability to deal with life events, history of abuse
Defensive coping r/t unresolved past traumatic events, severe anxiety
Hopelessness r/t long-term stress
Ineffective individual coping r/t history of abuse
Personal identity disturbance r/t severe child abuse
Risk for self-mutilation r/t need to act out to relieve stress
Refer to Dissociative Disorder

Multiple Sclerosis (MS)

Anticipatory grieving r/t risk for loss of normal body functioning
Disuse syndrome r/t physical immobility
Energy field disturbance r/t disruption in energy flow resulting from disharmony between mind and body
Impaired physical mobility r/t neuromuscular impairment
Ineffective airway clearance r/t decreased energy/fatigue
Potential for enhanced spiritual well-being r/t struggling with chronic debilitating condition
Powerlessness r/t progressive nature of disease
Risk for altered nutrition: less than body requirements r/t impaired swallowing, depression
Risk for injury r/t altered mobility, sensory dysfunction

Self-care deficit: specify r/t neuromuscular impairment
Sensory/perceptual alteration: specify r/t pathology in sensory tracts
Sexual dysfunction r/t biopsychosocial alteration of sexuality
Spiritual distress r/t perceived hopelessness of diagnosis
Urinary retention r/t inhibition of the reflex arc
Refer to Neurological Disorders

Mumps

Refer to Communicable Diseases, Childhood

Murmurs

Decreased cardiac output r/t incompetent heart valves, abnormal forward or backward blood flow, flow into a dilated chamber, flow through an abnormal passage between chambers

Muscular Atrophy/Weakness

Risk for disuse syndrome r/t impaired physical mobility

Muscular Dystrophy (MD)

Activity intolerance r/t fatigue
Altered nutrition: less than body requirements r/t impaired swallowing or chewing
Altered nutrition: more than body requirements r/t inactivity
Constipation r/t immobility
Decreased cardiac output r/t effects of congestive heart failure
Disuse syndrome r/t complications of immobility
Fatigue r/t increased energy requirements to perform activities of daily living
Impaired mobility r/t muscle weakness and development of contractures
Ineffective airway clearance r/t muscle weakness and decreased cough
Risk for aspiration r/t impaired swallowing
Risk for impaired gas exchange r/t ineffective airway clearance and ineffective breathing patterns secondary to muscle weakness
Risk for impaired skin integrity r/t immobility, braces or adaptive devices
Risk for ineffective breathing patterns r/t muscle weakness
Risk for infection r/t pooling of pulmonary secretions secondary to immobility and muscle weakness
Risk for injury r/t muscle weakness and unsteady gait
Self-care deficits: feeding, bathing, dressing, toileting r/t muscle weakness and fatigue
Refer to Hospitalized Child; Child with Chronic Condition; Terminally Ill Child/Death of Child

MVA (Motor Vehicle Accident)

Refer to Injury; Head Injury; Fracture; Pneumothorax

Myasthenia Gravis

Altered family process r/t crisis of dealing with diagnosis
Altered nutrition: less than body requirements r/t difficulty eating and swallowing
Fatigue r/t paresthesia, aching muscles
Impaired physical mobility r/t defective transmission of nerve impulses at the neuromuscular junction
Impaired swallowing r/t neuromuscular impairment
Ineffective airway clearance r/t decreased ability to cough and swallow
Ineffective management of therapeutic regimen r/t lack of knowledge of treatment, uncertainty of outcome
Risk for caregiver role strain r/t severity of illness of client
Refer to Neurological Disorders

Mycoplasma Pneumonia

Refer to Pneumonia

Myelocele

Refer to Neurotube Defects

Myelogram, Contrast

Pain r/t irritation of nerve roots
Risk for altered tissue perfusion: cerebral r/t hypotension, loss of cerebral spinal fluid
Risk for fluid volume deficit r/t possible dehydration, loss of cerebral spinal fluid
Urinary retention r/t pressure on spinal nerve roots

Myelomeningocele

Refer to Neurotube Defects

Myocardial Infarction

Refer to MI

Myocarditis

Activity intolerance r/t reduced cardiac reserve and prescribed bedrest
Decreased cardiac output r/t impaired contractility of ventricles
Knowledge deficit r/t treatment of disease
Refer to CHF if appropriate

Myringotomy

Altered health maintenance r/t knowledge deficit regarding self-care following surgery
Fear r/t hospitalization, surgical procedure
Risk for infection r/t invasive procedure
Pain r/t surgical procedure
Sensory/perceptual alteration r/t possible hearing impairment

Myxedema

Refer to Hypothyroidism

N

Narcissistic Personality Disorder

Decisional conflict r/t lack of realistic problem-solving skills
Defensive coping r/t grandiose sense of self
Impaired social interaction r/t self-concept disturbance
Risk for loneliness r/t inability to interact appropriately with others

Narcolepsy

Anxiety r/t fear of lack of control over falling asleep
Risk for trauma r/t falling asleep during potentially dangerous activity
Sleep pattern disturbance r/t uncontrollable desire to sleep

Nasogastric Suction

Altered comfort r/t presence of nasogastric tube
Altered oral mucous membranes r/t presence of nasogastric tube
Risk for fluid volume deficit r/t loss of gastro-intestinal fluids without adequate replacement

Nausea

Altered comfort: nausea r/t alteration in gastrointestinal function
Risk for altered nutrition: less than body requirements r/t nausea (specify cause)
Risk for fluid volume deficit r/t inadequate fluid intake secondary to nausea

Near-Drowning

Altered health maintenance r/t parental knowledge deficit regarding safety measures appropriate for age
Anticipatory/dysfunctional grieving r/t potential death of child, unknown sequelae, guilt over accident
Aspiration r/t aspiration of fluid into the lungs
Fear (parental) r/t possible death of child, possible permanent and debilitating sequelae
Hypothermia r/t CNS injury, prolonged submersion in cold water
Impaired gas exchange r/t laryngospasm, breath holding, aspiration
Ineffective airway clearance/ineffective breathing pattern r/t aspiration, impaired gas exchange
Potential for enhanced spiritual well-being r/t struggle with survival of life-threatening situation
Risk for altered growth and development r/t hypoxemia, cerebral anoxia
Risk for infection r/t aspiration, invasive monitoring
Refer to Safety—Childhood; Hospitalized Child; Child with Chronic Condition; Terminally Ill Child/Death of Child

Neck Vein Distention

Decreased cardiac output r/t decreased contractility of heart and the resulting increased payload
Fluid volume excess r/t excess fluid intake, compromised regulatory mechanisms
Refer to Congestive Heart Failure

Necrotizing Enterocolitis (NEC)

Altered nutrition: less than body requirements r/t decreased ability to absorb nutrients, decreased perfusion to gastrointestinal tract
Altered tissue perfusion: gastrointestinal r/t shunting of blood away from mesenteric circulation and toward vital organs secondary to perinatal stress, hypoxia
Fluid volume deficit r/t vomiting, gastrointestinal bleeding
Ineffective breathing pattern r/t abdominal distention, hypoxia
Risk for infection r/t bacterial invasion of gastrointestinal tract, invasive procedures
Refer to Premature Infant; Hospitalized Child

Negative Feelings About Self

Chronic low self-esteem r/t long standing negative self-evaluation
Self-esteem disturbance r/t inappropriate learned negative feelings about self

Neglectful Care of Family Member

Altered family processes r/t situational transition or crisis
Caregiver role strain r/t care demands of family member and lack of social or financial support
Ineffective family coping: disabling r/t highly ambivalent family relationships, lack of respite care

Ineffective management of therapeutic regimen: community r/t deficits in community for support of caregivers and detection of client neglect
Knowledge deficit r/t care needs

Neglect, Unilateral

Refer to Unilateral Neglect of One Side of Body

Neoplasm

Fear r/t possible malignancy
Refer to Cancer

Nephrectomy

Alteration in urinary elimination r/t loss of kidney
Anxiety r/t surgical recovery, prognosis
Constipation r/t lack of return of peristalsis
Ineffective breathing pattern r/t location of surgical incision
Pain r/t incisional discomfort
Risk for fluid volume deficit r/t vascular losses, decreased intake
Risk for infection r/t invasive procedure, lack of deep breathing due to location of surgical incision

Nephrostomy, Percutaneous

Altered urinary elimination r/t nephrostomy tube
Pain r/t invasive procedure
Risk for infection r/t invasive procedure

Nephrotic Syndrome

Activity intolerance r/t generalized edema
Altered comfort r/t edema
Altered nutrition: less than body requirements r/t anorexia, protein loss
Altered nutrition: more than body requirements r/t increased appetite secondary to steroid therapy
Body image disturbance r/t edematous appearance and side effects of steroid therapy
Fluid volume excess r/t edema secondary to oncotic fluid shift resulting from serum protein loss and renal retention of salt and water
Risk for impaired skin integrity r/t edema
Risk for infection r/t altered immune mechanisms secondary to disease itself and effects of steroids
Risk for noncompliance r/t side effects encountered with home steroid therapy
Social isolation r/t edematous appearance
Refer to Hospitalized Child; Child with Chronic Condition

Nerve Entrapment

Refer to Carpal Tunnel Syndrome

Neuritis

Activity intolerance r/t pain with movement
Altered health maintenance r/t knowledge deficit regarding self-care with neuritis
Pain r/t stimulation of affected nerve endings, inflammation of sensory nerves

Neurogenic Bladder

Reflex incontinence r/t neurological impairment
Urinary retention r/t interruption in the lateral spinal tracts

Neurological Disorders

Acute confusion r/t dementia, alcohol abuse, drug abuse, delirium
Altered family process r/t situational crisis, illness or disability of family member
Altered nutrition: less than body requirements r/t impaired swallowing, depression, difficulty feeding self
Anticipatory grieving r/t loss of usual body functioning
Impaired home maintenance management r/t client or family member's disease
Impaired memory r/t neurological disturbance
Impaired physical mobility r/t neuromuscular impairment
Impaired swallowing r/t neuromuscular dysfunction
Ineffective airway clearance r/t perceptual or cognitive impairment, decreased energy, fatigue
Ineffective individual coping r/t disability requiring change in life-style
Powerlessness r/t progressive nature of disease
Risk for disuse syndrome r/t physical immobility, neuromuscular dysfunction
Risk for impaired skin integrity r/t altered sensation, altered mental status, paralysis
Risk for injury r/t altered mobility, sensory dysfunction, cognitive impairment
Self-care deficit: specify r/t neuromuscular dysfunction
Sexual dysfunction r/t biopsychosocial alteration of sexuality
Social isolation r/t altered state of wellness

Neurotube Defects (Meningocele, Myelomeningocele, Spina Bifida, Anencephaly)

Altered growth and development r/t physical impairments, possible cognitive impairment
Chronic low self-esteem r/t perceived differences, decreased ability to participate in physical and social activities at school

Colonic constipation r/t immobility or less than adequate mobility
Family coping: potential for growth r/t effective adaptive response by family members
Grieving r/t loss of perfect child, birth of child with congenital defect
Impaired mobility r/t neuromuscular impairment
Impaired skin integrity r/t incontinence
Reflex incontinence r/t neurogenic impairment
Risk for altered nutrition: more than body requirements r/t diminished, limited, or impaired physical activity
Risk for impaired skin integrity (lower extremities) r/t decreased sensory perception
Sensory/perceptual alteration: visual r/t altered reception secondary to strabismus
Total incontinence r/t neurogenic impairment
Urge incontinence r/t neurogenic impairment
Refer to Premature Infant; Child with Chronic Condition

Newborn, Normal

Altered protection r/t immature immune system
Effective breast-feeding r/t normal oral structure and gestational age greater than 34 weeks
Ineffective thermoregulation r/t immaturity of neuroendocrine system
Potential for enhanced organized infant behavior r/t appropriate environmental stimuli
Risk for infection r/t open umbilical stump
Risk for injury r/t immaturity and need for caretaking

Newborn, Postmature

Hypothermia r/t depleted stores of subcutaneous fat
Impaired skin integrity r/t cracked and peeling skin secondary to decreased vernix
Risk for ineffective airway clearance r/t meconium aspiration
Risk for injury r/t hypoglycemia secondary to depleted glycogen stores

Newborn, Small for Gestational Age (SGA)

Altered nutrition: less than body requirements r/t history of placental insufficiency
Ineffective thermoregulation r/t decreased brown fat, subcutaneous fat
Risk for injury r/t hypoglycemia, perinatal asphyxia, meconium aspiration

Nicotine Addiction

Altered health maintenance r/t lack of ability to make a judgment about smoking cessation
Powerlessness r/t perceived lack of control over ability to give up nicotine

NIDDM (Noninsulin-Dependent Diabetes Mellitus)

Health-seeking behaviors r/t desiring information on exercise and diet to manage diabetes
Refer to Diabetes Mellitus

Nightmares

Energy field disturbance r/t disharmony of body and mind
Post-trauma response r/t disasters, wars, epidemics, rape, assault, torture, catastrophic illness or accident
Rape-trauma syndrome, rape-trauma syndrome: compound reaction, rape-trauma syndrome: silent reaction r/t forced violent sexual penetration against the victim's will and consent

Nipple Soreness

Pain r/t injury to nipples
Refer to Painful Breasts—Sore Nipples

Nocturia

Altered urinary elimination r/t sensory motor impairment, urinary tract infection
Total incontinence r/t neuropathy preventing transmission of reflex indicating bladder fullness, neurological dysfunction causing triggering of micturition at unpredictable times, independent contraction of detrusor reflex due to surgery, trauma or disease affecting spinal cord nerves, anatomical fistula
Urge incontinence r/t decreased bladder capacity, irritation of bladder stretch receptors causing spasm, alcohol, caffeine, increased fluids, increased urine concentration, overdistention of bladder

Nocturnal Paroxysmal Dyspnea

Refer to PND

Noncompliance

Noncompliance r/t client value system, health beliefs, cultural influences, spiritual values, client-provider relationships, knowledge deficit

Noninsulin-Dependent Diabetes Mellitus (NIDDM)

Refer to Diabetes Mellitus

Nutrition, Altered

Altered nutrition: less than body requirements r/t inability to ingest or digest food or absorb nutrients due to biological, psychological, or economic factors

Altered nutrition: more than body requirements r/t excessive intake in relation to metabolic need

Nutrition, altered: high risk for more than body requirements r/t obesity in parents, use of food as reward or comfort measure, dysfunctional eating pattern, eating in response to cues other than hunger

Obesity

Altered nutrition: more than body requirements r/t caloric intake exceeding energy expenditure

Body image disturbance r/t eating disorder, excess weight

Chronic low self-esteem r/t ineffective individual coping, overeating

Obsessive-Compulsive Disorder

Altered thought process r/t persistent thoughts, ideas, and impulses that seem irrelevant and will not relent

Anxiety r/t threat to self-concept, unmet needs

Decisional conflict r/t inability to make a decision for fear of reprisal

Ineffective family coping: disabling r/t family process being disrupted by client's ritualistic activities

Ineffective individual coping r/t expression of feelings in an unacceptable way, ritualistic behavior

Powerlessness r/t unrelenting repetitive thoughts to perform irrational activities

Obstruction, Bowel

Refer to Bowel Obstruction

Oligohydramnios

Anxiety (maternal) r/t fear of unknown and threat to fetus

Risk for injury (fetal) r/t decreased umbilical cord blood flow secondary to compression

Oliguria

Fluid volume deficit r/t active fluid loss, failure of regulatory mechanism

Refer to Renal Failure; Shock; Cardiac Output Decrease

Omphalocele

Refer to Gastroschisis

Oophorectomy

Risk for altered sexuality patterns r/t altered body function

Refer to Surgery

Open Reduction of Fracture with Internal Fixation (Femur)

Anxiety r/t outcome of corrective procedure

Impaired physical mobility r/t position required postoperatively, abduction of leg, avoidance of acute flexion

Powerlessness r/t loss of control, unanticipated change in life-style

Risk for perioperative positioning injury r/t immobilization

Risk for peripheral neurovascular dysfunction r/t mechanical compression, orthopedic surgery, immobilization

Refer to Surgery, Postoperative Care

Opportunistic Infection

Altered infection r/t abnormal blood profiles

Refer to AIDS

Oral Mucous Membrane, Altered

Altered oral mucous membrane r/t pathological conditions—oral cavity (radiation to head or neck); dehydration; chemical trauma (e.g., acidic foods, drugs, noxious agents, alcohol); mechanical trauma (e.g., ill-fitting dentures, braces, endotracheal and nasogastric tubes, surgery in oral cavity); NPO for more than 24 hours; ineffective oral hygiene; mouth breathing; malnutrition; infection; lack of or decreased salivating; medication

Organic Mental Disorders

Impaired social interaction r/t altered thought processes

Risk for injury r/t disorientation to time, place, and person

Refer to Dementia

Orthopedic Traction

Altered role performance r/t limited physical mobility

Impaired social interaction r/t limited physical mobility

Refer to Traction and Casts

Orthopnea

Decreased cardiac output r/t inability of heart to meet demands of body

Ineffective breathing pattern r/t inability to breathe with the head of the bed flat

Orthostatic Hypotension

Refer to Dizziness

Osteoarthritis

Activity intolerance r/t pain after exercise or use of joint
Pain r/t movement
Refer to Arthritis

Osteomylitis

Altered health maintenance r/t continued immobility at home, possible extensive casts, continued antibiotics
Diversional activity deficit r/t prolonged immobilization and hospitalization
Fear: parental r/t concern regarding possible growth plate damage secondary to infection, concern that infection may become chronic
Hyperthermia r/t infectious process
Impaired physical mobility r/t imposed immobility secondary to infected area
Pain r/t inflammation in affected extremity
Risk for colonic constipation r/t immobility
Risk for impaired skin integrity r/t irritation from splint/cast
Risk for spread of infection r/t inadequate primary and secondary defenses
Refer to Hospitalized Child

Osteoporosis

Altered nutrition: less than body requirements r/t inadequate intake of calcium and vitamin D
Effective management of therapeutic regimen: individual r/t appropriate choices for diet and exercise to prevent and manage condition
Impaired physical mobility r/t pain, skeletal changes
Knowledge deficit r/t diet, exercise, need to abstain from alcohol and nicotine
Pain r/t fracture, muscle spasms
Risk for injury: fractures r/t lack of activity; risk of falling resulting from environmental hazards, neuromuscular disorders, diminished senses, cardiovascular responses, and responses to drugs

Ostomy

Refer to Colostomy; Ileostomy; Ileal Conduit; Child with Chronic Condition

Otitis Media

Pain r/t inflammation, infectious process
Risk for infection r/t eustachian tube obstruction, traumatic eardrum perforation, infectious disease process
Sensory/perceptual alteration: auditory r/t incomplete resolution of otitis media, presence of excess drainage in the middle ear

Ovarian Carcinoma

Altered health maintenance r/t knowledge deficit regarding self-care and treatment of condition
Fear r/t unknown outcome, possible poor prognosis
Refer to Hysterectomy; Chemotherapy; Radiation Therapy

P

Pacemaker

Anxiety r/t change in health status, presence of pacemaker
Knowledge deficit r/t self-care program, when to seek medical attention
Pain r/t surgical procedure
Risk for decreased cardiac output r/t malfunction of pacemaker
Risk for infection r/t invasive procedure, presence of foreign body (catheter and generator)

Paget's Disease

Body image disturbance r/t possible enlarged head, bowed tibias, kyphosis
Knowledge deficit r/t appropriate diet of high protein and high calcium, mild exercise
Risk for trauma: fracture r/t excessive bone destruction

Pain

Pain r/t injury agents (biological, chemical, physical, psychological)

Pain, Chronic

Chronic pain r/t chronic physical or psychosocial disability

Painful Breasts—Engorgement

Altered role performance r/t change in physical capacity to assume the role of breast-feeding mother
Impaired tissue integrity r/t excessive fluid in breast tissues
Pain r/t distention of breast tissue
Risk for ineffective breast-feeding r/t pain and infant's inability to latch on to engorged breast
Risk for infection r/t milk stasis

Painful Breasts—Sore Nipples

Altered role performance r/t change in physical capacity to assume the role of breast-feeding mother
Impaired skin integrity r/t mechanical factors involved in suckling and breast-feeding management
Ineffective breast-feeding r/t pain
Pain r/t cracked nipples
Risk for infection r/t break in skin

Pallor of Extremities

Altered tissue perfusion: peripheral r/t interruption of vascular flow

Pancreatic Cancer

Anticipatory grieving r/t shortened life span
Fear r/t poor prognosis of the disease
Ineffective family coping r/t poor prognosis
Knowledge deficit r/t disease-induced diabetes, home management
Spiritual distress r/t poor prognosis
Refer to Cancer; Radiation Therapy; Surgery

Pancreatitis

Altered health maintenance r/t knowledge deficit concerning diet, alcohol use, and medication
Altered nutrition: less than body requirements r/t inadequate dietary intake, increased nutritional needs secondary to acute illness, increased metabolic needs caused by increased body temperature
Diarrhea r/t decrease in pancreatic secretions resulting in steatorrhea
Fluid volume deficit r/t vomiting, decreased fluid intake, fever, diaphoresis, fluid shifts
Ineffective breathing pattern r/t splinting from severe pain
Ineffective denial r/t ineffective coping, alcohol use
Pain r/t irritation and edema of the inflamed pancreas

Panic Disorder

Anxiety r/t situational crisis
Ineffective individual coping r/t personal vulnerability
Post-trauma response r/t previous catastrophic event
Risk for loneliness r/t inability to socially interact because of fear of losing control
Social isolation r/t fear of lack of control

Paralysis

Altered health maintenance r/t knowledge deficit regarding self-care with paralysis
Body image disturbance r/t biophysical changes, loss of movement, immobility
Colonic constipation r/t effects of spinal cord disruption, diet inadequate in fiber
Disuse syndrome r/t paralysis
Impaired home maintenance management r/t physical disability
Impaired physical mobility r/t neuromuscular impairment
Pain r/t prolonged immobility
Powerlessness r/t illness-related regimen
Reflex incontinence r/t neurological impairment
Risk for impaired skin integrity r/t altered circulation, altered sensation, and immobility
Risk for injury r/t altered mobility, sensory dysfunction
Self-care deficit: specify r/t neuromuscular impairment
Sexual dysfunction r/t loss of sensation, biopsychosocial alteration
Refer to Child with Chronic Condition; Hospitalized Child; Neurotube Defects; Hemiplegia; Spinal Cord Injury

Paralytic Ileus

Altered oral mucous membranes r/t presence of nasogastric tube
Constipation r/t decreased gastric motility
Fluid volume deficit r/t loss of fluids from vomiting, retention of fluid in the bowels
Pain r/t pressure, abdominal distention

Paranoid Personality Disorder

Altered thought processes r/t psychological conflicts
Anxiety r/t uncontrollable intrusive, suspicious thoughts
Chronic low self-esteem r/t inability to trust others
Risk for loneliness r/t social isolation
Risk for violence: directed at others r/t suspicious of others and others' actions
Sensory/perceptual alteration: specify r/t psychological dysfunction; suspicious thoughts
Social isolation r/t inappropriate social skills

Paraplegia

Refer to Spinal Cord Injury

Parathyroidectomy

Anxiety r/t surgery
Risk for impaired verbal communication r/t possible laryngeal damage, edema

Risk for ineffective airway clearance r/t edema or hematoma formation, airway obstruction
Risk for infection r/t surgical procedure
Refer to Hypocalcemia

Parental Role Conflict

Parental role conflict r/t separation from child due to chronic illness; intimidation with invasive or restrictive modalities (e.g., isolation, intubation); specialized care center policies; home care of a child with special needs (e.g., apnea monitoring, postural drainage, hyperalimentation); change in marital status; interruptions of family life due to home care regimen (e.g., treatments, caregivers, lack of respite)

Parenting, Altered

Altered parenting r/t lack of available role model; ineffective role model; physical and psychosocial abuse of nurturing figure; lack of support between and from significant other(s); unmet social, emotional, or maturational needs of parenting figures; interruption in bonding process, (e.g., maternal, paternal, other); unrealistic expectations for self, infant, partner; physical illness; presence of stress (e.g., financial, legal, recent crisis, cultural move); lack of knowledge; limited cognitive functioning; lack of role identity; lack or inappropriate response of child to relationship; multiple pregnancies

Parent Attachment

Risk for altered parent/infant/child attachment r/t inability of parents to meet personal needs; anxiety associated with the parental role; substance abuse; premature infant; ill infant/child who is unable to effectively initiate parental contact as a result of altered behavioral organization, separation, physical barriers, or lack of privacy

Parenting, Risk for Altered

Risk for altered parenting r/t lack of available role model; ineffective role model; physical and psychosocial abuse of nurturing figure; lack of support between or from significant other(s); unmet social, emotional, or maturational needs of parenting figures; interruption in bonding process (e.g., maternal, paternal, other); unrealistic expectations for self, infant, partner; physical illness; presence of stress (e.g., financial, legal, recent crisis, cultural move); lack of knowledge; limited cognitive functioning; lack of role identity; lack or inappropriate response of child to relationship; multiple pregnancies

Paresthesia

Sensory/perceptual alteration: tactile r/t altered sensory reception, transmission, or integration

Parkinson's Disease

Alteration in nutrition: less than body requirements r/t tremor, slowness in eating, difficulty in chewing and swallowing
Constipation r/t weakness of defecation muscles, lack of exercise, inadequate fluid intake, decreased autonomic nervous system activity
Impaired verbal communication r/t decreased speech volume, slowness of speech, impaired facial muscles
Risk for injury r/t tremors, slow reactions, altered gait
Refer to Neurological Disorders

Paroxysmal Nocturnal Dyspnea

Refer to PND

Patent Ductus Arteriosus (PDA)

Refer to Congenital Heart Disease/Cardiac Anomalies

Patient-Controlled Analgesia

Refer to PCA

Patient Education

Effective management of therapeutic regimen r/t verbalized desire to manage illness and prevent complications
Health-seeking behaviors r/t expressed or observed desire to seek a higher level of wellness or control of health practices
Knowledge deficit r/t lack of exposure to information, information misinterpretation, unfamiliarity with information resources
Potential for enhanced spiritual well-being r/t desire to reach harmony with self, others, and higher power/God

PCA (Patient-Controlled Analgesia)

Altered comfort: pruritis, nausea, vomiting r/t side effects of medication
Effective management of therapeutic regimen r/t ability to manage pain with appropriate use of patient-controlled analgesia
Knowledge deficit r/t self-care of pain control
Risk for injury r/t possible complications associated with PCA

Pelvic Inflammatory Disease

Refer to PID

Penile Prosthesis

Altered sexuality pattern r/t use of penile prosthesis
Health-seeking behavior r/t information regarding use and care of prosthesis
Risk for infection r/t invasive surgical procedure
Risk for situational low self-esteem r/t altered sexuality pattern

Peptic Ulcer

Refer to Ulcer

Percutaneous Transluminal Coronary Angioplasty (PTCA)

Refer to Angioplasty

Pericardial Friction Rub

Decreased cardiac output r/t inflammation in pericardial sac, fluid accumulation compressing heart
Pain r/t inflammation, effusion

Pericarditis

Activity intolerance r/t reduced cardiac reserve and prescribed bedrest
Altered tissue perfusion: cardiopulmonary/ peripheral r/t risk for development of emboli
Knowledge deficit r/t unfamiliarity with information sources
Pain r/t biological injury, inflammation
Risk for alteration in nutrition: less than body requirements r/t fever, hypermetabolic state associated with fever
Risk for decreased cardiac output r/t inflammation in pericardial sac, fluid accumulation compressing heart function

P

Perioperative Positioning

Risk for perioperative positioning injury r/t disorientation, immobilization, muscle weakness, sensory/perceptual disturbances resulting from anesthesia, obesity, emaciation, edema

Peripheral Neurovascular Dysfunction, Risk for

Risk for peripheral neurovascular dysfunction r/t fractures, mechanical compression, orthopedic surgery, trauma, immobilization, burns, vascular obstruction

Peripheral Vascular Disease

Activity intolerance r/t imbalance between peripheral oxygen supply and demand
Altered health maintenance r/t knowledge deficit regarding self-care and treatment of disease
Altered tissue perfusion: peripheral r/t interruption of vascular flow
Chronic pain: intermittent claudication r/t ischemia
Risk for impaired skin integrity r/t altered circulation or sensation
Risk for injury r/t tissue hypoxia, altered mobility, altered sensation
Risk for peripheral neurovascular dysfunction r/t possible vascular obstruction

Peritoneal Dialysis

Impaired home maintenance management r/t complex home treatment of client
Knowledge deficit r/t treatment procedure, self-care with peritoneal dialysis
Pain r/t instillation of dialysate, temperature of dialysate
Risk for fluid volume excess r/t retention of dialysate
Risk for ineffective breathing pattern r/t pressure from the dialysate
Risk for ineffective individual coping r/t disability requiring change in life-style
Risk for infection: peritoneal r/t invasive procedure, presence of catheter, dialysate

Refer to Renal Failure, Oliguric; Renal Failure, Acute/Chronic, Child; Hospitalized Child; Child with Chronic Condition

Peritonitis

Altered nutrition: less than body requirements r/t nausea, vomiting
Constipation r/t decreased oral intake, decrease of peristalsis
Fluid volume deficit r/t retention of fluid in bowel with loss of circulating blood volume
Ineffective breathing pattern r/t pain, increased abdominal pressure
Pain r/t inflammation and stimulation of somatic nerves

Persistent Fetal Circulation

Refer to Congenital Heart Disease/Cardiac Anomalies

Personal Identity Problems

Personal identity disturbance r/t situational crisis, psychological impairment, chronic illness, pain

Personality Disorder

Chronic low self-esteem r/t inability to set and achieve goals
Decisional conflict r/t low self-esteem, feelings that choices will always be wrong
Impaired adjustment r/t ambivalent behavior toward others, testing of others' loyalty
Impaired social interaction r/t knowledge or skill deficit regarding ways to interact effectively with others, self-concept disturbances
Ineffective family coping: compromised r/t inability of client to provide positive feedback to family, chronicity exhausting family
Personal identity disturbance r/t lack of consistent positive self-image
Risk for loneliness r/t inability to interact appropriately with others
Spiritual distress r/t lack of identifiable values, no meaning to life
Refer to Antisocial Personality Disorder; Borderline Personality Disorder

Pertussis (Whooping Cough)

Refer to Respiratory Infections, Acute Childhood

Petechiae

Refer to Clotting Disorder

Pharyngitis

Refer to Sore Throat

Pheochromocytoma

Altered health maintenance r/t knowledge deficit regarding treatment and self-care
Anxiety r/t symptoms from increased catecholamines: headache, palpitations, sweating, nervousness, nausea, vomiting, syncope
Risk for altered tissue perfusion: cardiopulmonary and renal r/t episodes of hypertension
Sleep pattern disturbance r/t high levels of catecholamines
Refer to Surgery

Phobia (Specific)

Anxiety r/t inability to control emotions when dreaded object or situation is encountered
Fear r/t presence or anticipation of specific object or situation
Ineffective individual coping r/t transfer of fears from self to dreaded object situation
Powerlessness r/t anxiety over encountering unknown or known entity
Refer to Anxiety; Panic Disorder

Photosensitivity

Altered health maintenance r/t knowledge deficit regarding medications inducing photosensitivity
Risk for impaired skin integrity r/t exposure to sun

Physical Abuse

Refer to Abuse

PID (Pelvic Inflammatory Disease)

Altered health maintenance r/t knowledge deficit regarding self-care and treatment of disease
Altered sexuality patterns r/t medically imposed abstinence from sexual activities until the acute infection subsides, change in reproductive potential
Risk for infection r/t insufficient knowledge to avoid exposure to pathogens; proper hygiene, nutrition, and other health habits
Pain r/t biological injury; inflammation, edema, and congestion of pelvic tissues
Refer to Maturational Issues, Adolescent

PIH (Pregnancy-Induced Hypertension/Preeclampsia)

Altered family processes r/t situational crisis
Altered parenting r/t bedrest
Altered role performance r/t change in physical capacity to assume role of pregnant woman or resume other roles
Anxiety r/t fear of the unknown, threat to self and infant, change in role functioning
Diversional activity deficit r/t bedrest
Fluid volume excess r/t decreased renal function
Impaired home maintenance management r/t bedrest
Impaired physical mobility r/t medically prescribed limitations
Impaired social interaction r/t imposed bedrest
Knowledge deficit r/t lack of experience with situation
Powerlessness r/t complication threatening pregnancy and medically prescribed limitations
Risk for injury (fetal) r/t decreased uteroplacental perfusion, seizures
Risk for injury (maternal) r/t vasospasm, high blood pressure
Situational low self-esteem r/t loss of idealized pregnancy

Piloerection

Hypothermia r/t exposure to cool environment

Placenta Previa

Altered family processes r/t maternal bedrest or hospitalization
Altered role performance r/t maternal bedrest or hospitalization
Altered tissue perfusion: placental r/t dilation of cervix, loss of placental implantation site
Body image disturbance r/t negative feelings about body and reproductive ability, feelings of helplessness
Diversional activity deficit r/t long-term hospitalization
Fear r/t threat to self and fetus, unknown future
Impaired home maintenance management r/t maternal bedrest or hospitalization
Impaired physical mobility r/t medical protocol, maternal bedrest
Ineffective individual coping r/t threat to self and fetus
Risk for altered parenting r/t maternal bedrest or hospitalization
Risk for fluid volume deficit r/t maternal blood loss
Risk for injury (fetal and maternal) r/t threat to uteroplacental perfusion and hemorrhage
Situational low self-esteem r/t situational crisis
Spiritual distress r/t inability to participate in usual religious rituals, situational crisis

Pleural Effusion

Fluid volume excess r/t compromised regulatory mechanisms; heart, liver. or kidney failure
Hyperthermia r/t increased metabolic rate secondary to infection
Ineffective breathing pattern r/t pain
Pain r/t inflammation, fluid accumulation

Pleural Friction Rub

Ineffective breathing pattern r/t pain
Pain r/t inflammation, fluid accumulation
Refer to cause of Pleural Friction Rub

Pleurisy

Ineffective breathing pattern r/t pain
Pain r/t pressure on pleural nerve endings associated with fluid accumulation or inflammation
Risk for impaired gas exchange r/t ventilation perfusion imbalance
Risk for impaired physical mobility r/t activity intolerance, inability to "catch breath"
Risk for ineffective airway clearance r/t increased secretions, ineffective cough because of pain

PMS (Premenstrual Tension Syndrome)

Effective management of therapeutic regimen: individual r/t desire for information to manage and prevent symptoms
Fatigue r/t hormonal changes
Fluid volume excess r/t alterations of hormonal levels inducing fluid retention
Knowledge deficit r/t methods to deal with and prevent syndrome
Pain r/t hormonal stimulation of gastrointestinal structures

PND (Paroxysmal Nocturnal Dyspnea)

Anxiety r/t inability to breathe during sleep
Decreased cardiac output r/t failure of the left ventricle
Ineffective breathing pattern r/t increase in carbon dioxide levels, decrease in oxygen levels
Sleep pattern disturbance r/t suffocating feeling from fluid in lungs awakening from sleep

Pneumonia

Activity intolerance r/t imbalance between oxygen supply and demand
Altered health maintenance r/t knowledge deficit regarding self-care and treatment of disease
Altered nutrition: less than body requirements r/t loss of appetite
Altered oral mucous membranes r/t dry mouth from mouth breathing, decreased fluid intake
Hyperthermia r/t dehydration, increased metabolic rate, illness
Impaired gas exchange r/t decreased functional lung tissue
Ineffective airway clearance r/t inflammation and presence of secretions
Knowledge deficit r/t risk factors predisposing person to pneumonia, treatment
Risk for fluid volume deficit r/t inadequate intake of fluids
For child with Pneumonia, refer to Respiratory Infections, Acute Childhood

Pneumothorax

Fear r/t threat to own well-being, difficulty breathing
Impaired gas exchange r/t ventilation perfusion imbalance
Pain r/t recent injury, coughing, deep breathing
Risk for injury r/t possible complications associated with closed chest drainage system

Poisoning, Risk for

Risk for poisoning r/t internal: reduced vision, verbalization of occupational settings without adequate safeguards, lack of safety or drug education, lack of proper precaution, cognitive or emotional difficulties, insufficient finances; external: large supplies of drugs in house, medicines stored in unlocked cabinets accessible to children or confused persons, dangerous products placed or stored within the reach of children or confused persons, availability of illicit drugs potentially contaminated by poisonous additives, flaking or peeling paint or plaster in presence of young children, chemical contamination of food and water, unprotected contact with heavy metals or chemicals, paint or lacquer used in poorly ventilated areas or without effective protection, presence of poisonous vegetation, presence of atmospheric pollutants

Polydipsia

Refer to Diabetes Mellitus

Polyphagia

Refer to Diabetes Mellitus

Polyuria

Refer to Diabetes Mellitus

Postoperative Care

Refer to Surgery, Postoperative

Postpartum Blues

Altered parenting r/t hormone-induced depression
Altered role performance r/t new responsibilities of parenting
Anxiety r/t new responsibilities of parenting
Body image disturbance r/t normal postpartum recovery
Fatigue r/t childbirth and postpartum
Impaired adjustment r/t lack of support systems
Impaired home maintenance management r/t fatigue, care of the newborn
Impaired social interaction r/t change in role functioning
Ineffective individual coping r/t hormonal changes, maturational crisis
Knowledge deficit r/t life-style changes
Sexual dysfunction r/t fears of another pregnancy, postpartum pain and lochia flow
Sleep pattern disturbance r/t new responsibilities of parenting

Postpartum Hemorrhage

Activity intolerance r/t anemia from loss of blood
Altered tissue perfusion r/t hypovolemia
Body image disturbance r/t loss of ideal childbirth
Decreased cardiac output r/t hypovolemia
Fear r/t threat to self and unknown future
Fluid volume deficit r/t uterine atony, loss of blood
Impaired home maintenance management r/t lack of stamina
Interrupted breast-feeding r/t separation from infant for medical treatment
Knowledge deficit r/t lack of exposure to situation
Pain r/t nursing and medical interventions to control bleeding
Risk for altered parenting r/t weakened maternal condition
Risk for infection r/t loss of blood, depressed immunity

Postpartum, Normal Care

Altered role performance r/t new responsibilities of parenting
Altered urinary elimination r/t effects of anesthesia or tissue trauma
Anxiety r/t change in role functioning and parenting
Constipation r/t hormonal effects on smooth muscles, fear of straining with defecation, effects of anesthesia
Effective breast-feeding r/t basic breast-feeding knowledge, support of partner and health care provider
Family coping: potential for growth r/t adaptation to new family member
Fatigue r/t childbirth, new responsibilities of parenting, body changes
Health-seeking behaviors r/t postpartum recovery and adaptation
Impaired skin integrity r/t episiotomy, lacerations
Ineffective breast-feeding r/t lack of knowledge, lack of support, lack of motivation
Knowledge deficit (infant care) r/t lack of preparation for parenting
Pain r/t episiotomy, lacerations, bruising, breast engorgement, headache, sore nipples, epidural or IV site, hemorrhoids
Risk for altered parenting r/t lack of role models and knowledge deficit
Risk for infection r/t tissue trauma, blood loss
Sexual dysfunction r/t fear of pain or pregnancy
Sleep pattern disturbance r/t care of infant

Post-Trauma Response

Post-trauma response r/t disaster, wars, epidemics, rape, assault, torture, catastrophic illness or accident

Post-Traumatic Stress Disorder

Altered thought process r/t sense of reliving the experience (flashbacks)
Anxiety r/t exposure to internal or external cues that symbolize or resemble an aspect of the traumatic event
Energy field disturbance r/t disharmony of mind, body, and spirit
Ineffective breathing pattern r/t hyperventilation associated with anxiety
Ineffective individual coping r/t extreme anxiety
Post-trauma response r/t exposure to a traumatic event
Potential for enhanced spiritual well-being r/t desire for harmony after stressful event
Risk for violence r/t fear of self or others
Sensory/perceptual alteration r/t psychological stress
Sleep pattern disturbance r/t recurring nightmares
Spiritual distress r/t feelings of detachment or estrangement from others

Potassium, Increase or Decrease

Refer to Hyperkalemia or Hypokalemia

Powerlessness

Powerlessness r/t prolonged activity restriction creating isolation, failing or deteriorating physiological condition, long-term stress, abandonment, lost belief in transcendent values or in God

Preeclampsia

Refer to PIH

Pregnancy—Cardiac Disorders

Refer to Cardiac Disorders in Pregnancy

Pregnancy-Induced Hypertension/Preeclampsia

Refer to PIH

Pregnancy Loss

Altered role performance r/t inability to take on parenting role
Altered sexuality patterns r/t self-esteem disturbance due to pregnancy loss and anxiety about future pregnancies
Anxiety r/t threat to role functioning, health status, and situational crisis
Ineffective family coping: compromised r/t lack of support by significant other due to personal suffering
Ineffective individual coping r/t situational crisis
Pain r/t surgical intervention
Potential for enhanced spiritual well-being r/t desire for acceptance of loss
Risk for altered sexuality patterns r/t self-esteem disturbance, anxiety, grief
Risk for dysfunctional grieving r/t loss of pregnancy
Risk for fluid volume deficit r/t blood loss
Risk for infection r/t retained products of conception
Spiritual distress r/t intense suffering

Pregnancy—Normal

Altered family process r/t developmental transition of pregnancy
Altered nutrition: less than body requirements r/t growing fetus, nausea
Altered nutrition: more than body requirements r/t knowledge deficit regarding nutritional needs of pregnancy
Body image disturbance r/t altered body function and appearance
Family coping: potential for growth r/t satisfying partner relationship, attention to gratification of needs, effective adaptation to developmental tasks of pregnancy
Fear r/t labor and delivery
Health-seeking behaviors r/t desire to promote optimal fetal and maternal health
Ineffective individual coping r/t personal vulnerability, situational crisis
Knowledge deficit r/t primiparity
Sexual dysfunction r/t altered body function, self-concept, and body image with pregnancy
Sleep pattern disturbance r/t sleep deprivation secondary to discomfort of pregnant state
Refer to Discomforts of Pregnancy

Premature Dilation of the Cervix (Incompetent Cervix)

Altered role performance r/t inability to continue usual patterns of responsibility
Anticipatory grieving r/t potential loss of infant
Diversional activity deficit r/t bedrest
Fear r/t potential loss of infant
Impaired physical mobility r/t imposed bedrest to prevent preterm birth
Impaired social interaction r/t bedrest
Ineffective individual coping r/t bedrest, threat to fetus

Knowledge deficit r/t treatment regimen, prognosis for pregnancy
Powerlessness r/t inability to control outcome of pregnancy
Risk for infection r/t invasive procedures to prevent preterm birth
Risk for injury (fetal) r/t preterm birth, use of anesthetics
Risk for injury (maternal) r/t surgical procedures to prevent preterm birth (e.g., cerclage)
Sexual dysfunction r/t fear of harm to fetus
Situational low self-esteem r/t inability to complete normal pregnancy

Premature Infant (Child)

Altered growth and development: developmental lag r/t prematurity, environmental and stimulation deficiencies, multiple caretakers
Altered nutrition: less than body requirements r/t delayed or understimulated rooting reflex and easy fatigue during feeding, diminished endurance
Disorganized infant behavior r/t prematurity
Impaired gas exchange r/t effects of cardiopulmonary insufficiency
Impaired swallowing r/t decreased or absent gag reflex, fatigue
Ineffective thermoregulation r/t large body surface/weight ratio, immaturity of thermal regulation, state of prematurity
Potential for enhanced organized infant behavior r/t prematurity
Risk for infection r/t inadequate, immature, or undeveloped acquired immune response
Risk for injury r/t prolonged mechanical ventilation, retrolental fibroplasia (RLF) secondary to 100% oxygen environment
Sensory/perceptual alterations r/t noxious stimuli, noisy environment
Sleep pattern disturbance r/t noisy and noxious intensive care environment

Premature Infant (Parent)

Anticipatory grieving r/t loss of "perfect child," may lead to dysfunctional grieving
Dysfunctional grieving (prolonged) r/t unresolved conflicts
Decisional conflict r/t support system deficit, multiple sources of information
Ineffective breast-feeding r/t disrupted establishment of effective pattern secondary to prematurity or insufficient opportunities
Ineffective family coping: compromised r/t disrupted family roles and disorganization, prolonged condition exhausting supportive capacity of significant people
Parental role conflict r/t expressed concerns, expressed inability to care for child's physical, emotional, or developmental needs
Risk for altered parent/infant/child attachment r/t separation, physical barriers, lack of privacy
Spiritual distress r/t challenged belief or value systems regarding moral or ethical implications of treatment plans
Refer to Hospitalized Child; Child with Chronic Condition

Premature Rupture of Membranes

Anticipatory grieving r/t potential loss of infant
Anxiety r/t threat to infant's health status
Body image disturbance r/t inability to carry pregnancy to term
Ineffective individual coping r/t situational crisis
Risk for infection r/t rupture of membranes
Risk for injury (fetal) r/t risk of premature birth
Situational low self-esteem r/t inability to carry pregnancy to term

Premenstrual Tension Syndrome

Refer to PMS

Prenatal Care—Normal

Altered family processes r/t developmental transition
Altered nutrition: less than body requirements r/t nausea from normal hormonal changes
Altered urinary elimination r/t frequency caused by increased pelvic pressure and hormonal stimulation
Anxiety r/t unknown future and threat to self secondary to pain of labor
Constipation r/t decreased gastrointestinal motility secondary to hormonal stimulation
Fatigue r/t increased energy demands
Health-seeking behaviors r/t consistent prenatal care and education
Ineffective breathing pattern r/t increased intrathoracic pressure and decreased energy secondary to enlarged uterus
Knowledge deficit r/t lack of experience with pregnancy and care
Risk for activity intolerance r/t enlarged abdomen and increased cardiac workload
Risk for injury (maternal) r/t change in balance and center of gravity secondary to enlarged abdomen
Risk for sexual dysfunction r/t enlarged abdomen and fear of harm to infant
Sleep pattern disturbance r/t discomforts of pregnancy and fetal activity

Prenatal Testing

Anxiety r/t unknown outcome and delayed test results
Pain r/t invasive procedures
Risk for infection r/t invasive procedures during amniocentesis or chorionic villi sampling
Risk for injury (fetal) r/t invasive procedures

Preoperative Teaching

Knowledge deficit r/t preoperative regimens, postoperative precautions, expectations of role of client during preoperative or postoperative time
Refer to Surgery, Preoperative Care

Pressure Ulcer

Altered nutrition: less than body requirements r/t limited access to food, inability to absorb nutrients due to biological factors, anorexia
Impaired skin integrity (stage I or II pressure ulcer) r/t physical immobility, mechanical factors, altered circulation, skin irritants
Impaired tissue integrity (stage III or IV pressure ulcer) r/t altered circulation, impaired physical mobility
Pain r/t tissue destruction, exposure of nerves
Risk for infection r/t physical immobility; mechanical factors (shearing forces, pressure, restraint); altered circulation; skin irritants
Total incontinence r/t neurological dysfunction

Preterm Labor

Altered role performance r/t inability to carry out normal roles secondary to bedrest or hospitalization, change in expected course of pregnancy
Anticipatory grieving r/t loss of idealized pregnancy, potential loss of fetus
Anxiety r/t threat to fetus, change in role functioning, change in environment and interaction patterns, use of tocolytic drugs
Diversional activity deficit r/t long-term hospitalization
Impaired home maintenance management r/t medical restrictions
Impaired physical mobility r/t medically imposed restrictions
Impaired social interaction r/t prolonged bedrest or hospitalization
Ineffective individual coping r/t situational crisis, preterm labor
Risk for injury (fetal) r/t premature birth and immature body systems
Risk for maternal injury r/t use of tocolytic drugs
Sexual dysfunction r/t actual or perceived limitation imposed by preterm labor and/or prescribed treatment, separation from partner due to hospitalization
Situational low self-esteem r/t threatened ability to carry pregnancy to term
Sleep pattern disturbance r/t change in usual pattern secondary to contractions, hospitalization, or treatment regimen

Problem-Solving Ability

Defensive coping r/t situational crisis
Impaired adjustment r/t altered locus of control
Ineffective individual coping r/t situational crisis
Potential for enhanced spiritual well-being r/t desire to draw on inner strength and find meaning and purpose to life

Projection

Anxiety r/t threat to self-concept
Chronic low self-esteem r/t failure at life events
Defensive coping r/t inability to acknowledge that own behavior may be a problem and blames others
Impaired social interaction r/t self-concept disturbance, confrontive communication style
Risk for loneliness r/t blaming others for problems

Prolapsed Umbilical Cord

Altered tissue perfusion (fetal) r/t interruption in umbilical blood flow
Fear r/t threat to fetus, impending surgery
Risk for injury (fetal) r/t cord compression, altered tissue perfusion
Risk for injury (maternal) r/t emergency surgery

Prolonged Gestation

Altered nutrition: less than body requirements (fetal) r/t aging of placenta
Anxiety r/t potential change in birthing plans, need for increased medical intervention, unknown outcome for fetus
Defensive coping r/t underlying feeling of inadequacy regarding ability to give birth normally
Powerlessness r/t perceived lack of control over outcome of pregnancy
Situational low self-esteem r/t perceived inadequacy of body functioning

Prostatectomy

Refer to TURP (Transurethral Prostatectomy)

Prostatic Hypertrophy

Altered health maintenance r/t knowledge deficit regarding self-care and prevention of complications
Risk for infection r/t urinary residual postvoiding, bacterial invasion of bladder
Sleep pattern disturbance r/t nocturia
Urinary retention r/t obstruction

Prostatitis

Altered health maintenance r/t knowledge deficit regarding treatment
Altered protection r/t depressed immune system
Risk for urge incontinence r/t irritation of bladder

Protection, Altered

Altered protection r/t extremes of age, inadequate nutrition, alcohol abuse, abnormal blood profiles (leukopenia, thrombocytopenia, anemia, coagulation), drug therapies (antineoplastic, corticosteroid, immune, anticoagulant, thrombolytic), treatments (surgery, radiation), diseases (e.g., cancer, immune disorders)

Pruritis

Altered comfort: pruritis r/t inflammation in tissues
Knowledge deficit r/t methods to treat and prevent itching
Risk for impaired skin integrity r/t scratching from pruritis

Psoriasis

Altered health maintenance r/t knowledge deficit regarding treatment modalities
Body image disturbance r/t lesions on body
Impaired skin integrity r/t lesions on body
Powerlessness r/t lack of control over condition with frequent exacerbations and remissions

Psychosis

Alteration in family process r/t inability to express feelings, impaired communication
Alteration in nutrition: less than body requirements r/t lack of awareness of hunger, disinterest toward food
Alteration in thought process r/t inaccurate interpretations of environment
Altered health maintenance r/t cognitive impairment, ineffective individual and family coping
Anxiety r/t unconscious conflict with reality
Impaired home maintenance management r/t impaired cognitive or emotional functioning, inadequate support systems
Impaired social interaction r/t impaired communication patterns, self-concept disturbance, altered thought process
Impaired verbal communication r/t psychosis, inaccurate perceptions, hallucinations, delusions
Ineffective individual coping r/t inadequate support systems, unrealistic perceptions, altered thought processes, impaired communication
Fear r/t altered contact with reality
Risk for violence: self-directed or directed at others r/t lack of trust, panic, hallucinations, delusional thinking
Self-care deficit r/t loss of contact with reality, impairment in perception
Self-esteem disturbance r/t excessive use of defense mechanisms, (e.g., projection, denial, rationalization)
Sleep pattern disturbance r/t sensory alterations contributing to fear and anxiety
Social isolation r/t lack of trust, regression, delusional thinking, repressed fears
Refer to Schizophrenia

PTCA (Percutaneous Transluminal Coronary Angioplasty)

Refer to Angioplasty

Pulmonary Edema

Altered health maintenance r/t knowledge deficit regarding treatment regimen
Anxiety r/t fear of suffocation
Impaired gas exchange r/t ambulation of extravascular fluid in lung tissues and alveoli
Ineffective breathing pattern r/t presence of tracheobronchial secretions
Refer to CHF

Pulmonary Embolism

Altered tissue perfusion: pulmonary r/t interruption of pulmonary blood flow secondary to lodged embolus
Fear r/t severe pain, possible death
Impaired gas exchange r/t altered blood flow to alveoli secondary to lodged embolus
Knowledge deficit r/t activities to prevent embolism, self-care after diagnosis of embolism
Pain r/t biological injury, lack of oxygen to cells
Risk for altered cardiac output r/t right ventricular failure secondary to obstructed pulmonary artery
Refer to Anticoagulant Therapy

Pulmonary Stenosis

Refer to Congenital Heart Disease/Cardiac Anomalies

Pulse Deficit

Decreased cardiac output r/t dysrthymias
Refer to Dysrhythmia

Pulse Oximetry

Knowledge deficit r/t use of oxygen-monitoring equipment
Refer to Hypoxia

Pulse Pressure, Increased

Refer to Intracranial Pressure, Increased

Pulse Pressure, Narrowed

Refer to Shock

Pulses, Absent or Diminished Peripheral

Altered tissue perfusion: peripheral r/t interruption of arterial flow
Risk for peripheral neurovascular dysfunction r/t fractures, mechanical compression, orthopedic surgery trauma, immobilization, burns, vascular obstruction
Refer to cause of Absent or Diminished Peripheral Pulses

Purpura

Refer to Clotting Disorder

Pyelonephritis

Altered comfort r/t chills and fever
Altered health maintenance r/t knowledge deficit regarding self-care, treatment of disease, and prevention of further urinary tract infections
Altered urinary elimination r/t irritation of urinary tract
Pain r/t inflammation and irritation of urinary tract
Sleep pattern disturbance r/t urinary frequency

Pyloric Stenosis

Altered health maintenance r/t parental knowledge deficit regarding home care feeding regimen, wound care
Altered nutrition: less than body requirements r/t vomiting secondary to pyloric sphincter obstruction
Fluid volume deficit r/t vomiting, dehydration
Pain r/t surgical incision
Refer to Hospitalized Child

Q

Quadriplegia

Anticipatory grieving r/t loss of normal life-style, severity of disability
Ineffective breathing pattern r/t inability to use intercostal muscles
Risk for dysreflexia r/t bladder distention, bowel distention, skin irritation, lack of client and caregiver knowledge
Refer to Spinal Cord Injury

R

Rabies

Altered health maintenance r/t knowledge deficit regarding care of wound, isolation and observation of infected animal
Health-seeking behaviors r/t prophylactic immunization of domestic animals, avoidance of contact with wild animals
Hopelessness r/t poor prognosis
Pain r/t multiple immunization injections

Radiation Therapy

Activity intolerance r/t fatigue from possible anemia
Alteration in nutrition: less than body requirements r/t anorexia, nausea, vomiting, irradiation of areas of pharynx and esophagus
Alteration in oral mucous membranes r/t irradiation effects
Altered protection r/t suppression of bone marrow
Body image disturbance r/t change in appearance, hair loss
Diarrhea r/t irradiation effects
Knowledge deficit r/t what to expect with radiation therapy
Risk for impaired skin integrity r/t irradiation effects
Social isolation r/t possible limitations of time exposure of caregivers and significant others to client

Radical Neck Dissection

Refer to Laryngectomy

Rage

Risk for violence: directed at others r/t panic state, manic excitement, organic brain syndrome
Risk for self-mutilation r/t command hallucinations

Rape-Trauma Syndrome

Rape-trauma syndrome r/t forced, violent sexual penetration against the victim's will and consent
Rape-trauma syndrome: compound reaction r/t forced and violent sexual penetration against the victim's will and consent; activation of previous health disruptions (e.g., physical illness, psychiatric illness, substance abuse)
Rape-trauma syndrome: silent reaction r/t forced and violent sexual penetration against the victim's will and consent, demonstration of repression of the incident

Rash

Altered comfort: pruritis r/t inflammation in skin
Impaired skin integrity r/t mechanical trauma
Risk for infection r/t traumatized tissue, broken skin

Rationalization

Defensive coping r/t situational crisis, inability to accept blame for consequences of own behavior
Ineffective denial r/t fear of consequences, actual or perceived loss
Potential for enhanced spiritual well-being r/t possibility of seeking harmony with self, others, and higher power/God

Rats, Rodents in the Home

Impaired home maintenance management r/t lack of knowledge or insufficient finances

Raynaud's Disease

Altered tissue perfusion: peripheral r/t transient reduction of blood flow
Knowledge deficit r/t lack of information about disease process, possible complications, self-care needs regarding disease process and medication

RDS (Respiratory Distress Syndrome)

Refer to Respiratory Conditions of the Neonate

Rectal Fullness

Constipation r/t decreased activity level, decreased fluid intake, inadequate fiber in diet, decreased peristalsis, side effects from antidepressant or antipsychotic therapy

Rectal Pain/Bleeding

Constipation r/t pain on defecation
Knowledge deficit r/t possible causes of rectal bleeding, pain, treatment modalities
Pain r/t pressure of defecation
Risk for fluid volume deficit: bleeding r/t untreated rectal bleeding

Rectal Surgery

Refer to Hemorrhoidectomy

Rectocele Repair

Altered health maintenance r/t knowledge deficit of postoperative care of surgical site, dietary measures, and exercise to prevent constipation
Colonic constipation r/t painful defecation
Pain r/t surgical procedure
Risk for infection r/t surgical procedure and possible contamination of site with feces
Urinary retention r/t edema related to surgery

Reflex Incontinence

Reflex incontinence r/t neurological impairment

Regression

Altered role performance r/t powerlessness over health status
Anxiety r/t threat to or change in health status
Defensive coping r/t denial of obvious problems or weaknesses
Powerlessness r/t health care environment
Refer to Hospitalized Child; Separation Anxiety

Regretful

Anxiety r/t situational or maturational crises

Rehabilitation

Altered comfort r/t difficulty in performing rehabilitation tasks
Impaired physical mobility r/t injury, surgery, or psychosocial condition warranting rehabilitation
Ineffective individual coping r/t loss of normal function
Self-care deficit r/t impaired physical mobility

Relaxation Techniques

Energy field disturbance r/t use of imagery, relaxation and therapeutic touch to relieve stress
Health-seeking behaviors r/t requesting knowledge on ways to relieve stress

Religious Concern

Potential for enhanced spiritual well-being r/t desire for increased spirituality
Spiritual distress r/t separation from religious or cultural ties

Relocation Stress Syndrome

Relocation stress syndrome r/t past, concurrent, and recent losses; losses involved with decision to move; feeling of powerlessness; lack of adequate support system; little or no preparation for the impending move; moderate-to-high degree of environmental change; history and types of previous transfers; impaired psychosocial health status; decreased physical health status; advanced age

Renal Failure

Activity intolerance r/t effects of anemia and congestive heart failure
Altered comfort: pruritis r/t effects of uremia
Altered nutrition: less than body requirements r/t anorexia, nausea, vomiting, altered taste sensation, dietary restrictions
Altered oral mucous membranes r/t irritation from nitrogenous waste products
Altered urinary elimination r/t effects of disease, need for dialysis
Decreased cardiac output r/t effects of congestive heart failure, elevated potassium levels interfering with conduction system
Fatigue r/t effects of chronic uremia and anemia
Fluid volume excess r/t decreased urine output, sodium retention, inappropriate fluid intake
Ineffective individual coping r/t depression secondary to chronic disease
Risk for altered oral mucous membranes r/t dehydration, effects of uremia
Risk for infection r/t altered immune functioning
Risk for injury r/t bone changes, neuropathy, muscle weakness
Risk for noncompliance r/t complex medical therapy
Spiritual distress r/t dealing with chronic illness

Renal Failure, Acute/Chronic, Child

Body image disturbance r/t growth retardation; bone changes; visibility of dialysis access devices (shunt, fistula); edema
Diversional activity deficit r/t immobility during dialysis

Refer to Renal Failure; Hospitalized Child; Child with Chronic Illness

Renal Failure, Nonoliguric

Anxiety r/t change in health status
Risk for fluid volume deficit r/t loss of large volumes of urine

Refer to Renal Failure

Renal Transplantation, Donor

Decisional conflict r/t harvesting of kidney from traumatized donor
Family coping: potential for growth r/t decision to allow organ donation
Potential for enhanced spirituality r/t inner peace resulting from allowance of organ donation
Spiritual distress r/t anticipatory grieving from loss of significant person

Refer to Nephrectomy

Renal Transplantation Recipient

Altered protection r/t immunosupression therapy
Alteration in urinary elimination r/t possible impaired renal function
Anxiety r/t possible rejection, procedure
Impaired health maintenance r/t long-term home treatment after transplantation, diet, signs of rejection, use of medications
Knowledge deficit r/t specific nutritional needs, possible paralytic ileus, fluid or sodium restrictions
Risk for infection r/t use of immunosuppressive therapy to control rejection
Spiritual distress r/t obtaining transplanted kidney from someone's traumatic loss

Respiratory Acidosis

Refer to Acidosis, Respiratory

Respiratory Conditions of the Neonate (Respiratory Distress Syndrome—RDS, Meconium Aspiration, Diaphragmatic Hernia)

Fatigue r/t increased energy requirements and metabolic demands
Impaired gas exchange r/t decreased surfactant, immature lung tissue
Ineffective airway clearance r/t sequelae of attempts to breathe in utero, resulting in meconium aspiration
Ineffective breathing patterns r/t prolonged ventilator dependence
Risk for infection r/t tissue destruction or irritation secondary to aspiration of meconium fluid

Refer to Hospitalized Child; Premature Infant; Bronchopulmonary Dysplasia

Respiratory Distress

Refer to Dyspnea

Respiratory Distress Syndrome (RDS)

Refer to Respiratory Conditions of the Neonate

Respiratory Infections, Acute Childhood (Croup, Epiglotitis, Pertussis, Pneumonia, Respiratory Syncytial Virus)

Activity intolerance r/t generalized weakness, dyspnea, fatigue, poor oxygenation

Altered nutrition: less than body requirements r/t anorexia, fatigue, generalized weakness, poor sucking and breathing coordination, dyspnea
Anxiety/fear r/t oxygen deprivation, difficulty breathing
Fluid volume deficit r/t insensible losses (fever, diaphoresis), inadequate oral fluid intake
Hyperthermia r/t infectious process
Impaired gas exchange r/t insufficient oxygenation secondary to inflammation or edema of epiglottis, larynx, or bronchial passages
Ineffective airway clearance r/t excess tracheobronchial secretions
Ineffective breathing patterns r/t inflamed bronchial passages, coughing
Risk for aspiration r/t inability to coordinate breathing, coughing, and sucking
Risk for infection: transmission to others r/t virulent infectious organisms
Risk for injury (to pregnant others) r/t exposure to aerosolized medications (e.g., ribavirin, pentamidine), and resultant potential fetal toxicity
Risk for suffocation r/t inflammation of larynx or epiglottis
Refer to Hospitalized Child

Respiratory Syncytial Virus

Refer to Respiratory Infections, Acute Childhood

Retching

Altered comfort r/t visceral disorders
Altered nutrition: less than body requirements r/t inability to ingest food

Retinal Detachment

Anxiety r/t change in vision, threat of loss of vision
Knowledge deficit r/t symptoms, need for early intervention to prevent permanent damage
Risk for impaired home maintenance management r/t postoperative care, activity limitations, care of affected eye
Sensory perceptual alteration: visual r/t changes in vision, sudden flashes of light, floating spots, blurring of vision

Reye's Syndrome

Altered health maintenance r/t knowledge deficit regarding use of salicylates during viral illness of child
Altered nutrition: less than body requirements r/t effects of liver dysfunction, vomiting
Altered thought processes r/t degenerative changes in fatty brain tissue
Anticipatory grieving r/t uncertain prognosis and sequelae
Fluid volume deficit r/t vomiting, hyperventilation
Fluid volume excess (cerebral) r/t cerebral edema
Impaired gas exchange r/t hyperventilation, sequelae of increased intracranial pressure
Impaired skin integrity r/t effects of decorticate or decerebrate posturing, seizure activity
Ineffective breathing patterns r/t neuromuscular impairment
Ineffective family coping: compromised r/t acute situational crisis
Risk for injury r/t combative behavior, seizure activity
Sensory-perceptual alterations r/t cerebral edema
Situational low self-esteem (family) r/t negative perceptions of self, perceived inability to manage family situation, expressions of guilt
Refer to Hospitalized Child

Rh Incompatibility

Anxiety r/t unknown outcome of pregnancy
Health-seeking behaviors r/t prenatal care, compliance with diagnostic and treatment regimen
Knowledge deficit r/t treatment regimen from lack of experience with situation
Powerlessness r/t perceived lack of control over outcome of pregnancy
Risk for fetal injury r/t intrauterine destruction of red blood cells, transfusions

Rheumatic Fever

Refer to Endocarditis

Rheumatoid Arthritis, Juvenile (JRA)

Altered growth and development r/t effects of physical disability, chronic illness
Fatigue r/t chronic inflammatory disease
Impaired physical mobility r/t pain, restricted joint movement
Pain r/t swollen or inflamed joints, restricted movement, physical therapy
Risk for impaired skin integrity r/t splints, adaptive devices
Risk for injury r/t impaired physical mobility, splints, adaptive devices, increased bleeding potential secondary to anti-inflammatory medications
Self-care deficits: feeding, bathing/hygiene, dressing/grooming, toileting r/t restricted joint movement, pain
Refer to Child with Chronic Condition; Hospitalized Child

Rib Fracture

Ineffective breathing pattern r/t fractured ribs
Pain r/t movement, deep breathing
Refer to Ventilator Client, if relevant

Ridicule of Others

Defensive coping r/t situational crisis, psychological impairment; substance abuse

Roaches, Invasion of Home with

Impaired home maintenance management r/t lack of knowledge, insufficient finances

Role Performance, Altered

Altered role performance r/t inability to perform role as anticipated

RSV (Respiratory Synctical Virus)

Refer to Respiratory Infection, Acute Childhood

Rubella

Refer to Communicable Diseases, Childhood

Rubor of Extremities

Altered tissue perfusion: peripheral r/t interruption of arterial flow
Refer to Peripheral Vascular Disease

S

Sadness

Dysfunctional grieving r/t actual or perceived loss
Potential for enhanced spiritual well-being r/t desire for harmony following actual or perceived loss
Spiritual distress r/t intense suffering

Safety, Childhood

Health-seeking behaviors: enhanced parenting r/t adequate support systems, appropriate requests for help, desire and request for safety information, requests for information or assistance regarding parenting skills
Knowledge deficit: potential for enhanced health maintenance r/t parental knowledge and skill acquisition regarding appropriate safety measures
Risk for altered health maintenance r/t parental knowledge deficit regarding appropriate safety needs per developmental stage, childproofing house, infant and child car restraints, water safety, teaching child how to avoid molestation
Risk for altered parenting r/t lack of available and effective role model, lack of knowledge, misinformation from other family members ("old wives' tales")
Risk for aspiration and/or suffocation r/t pillow or propped bottle placed in infant's crib; sides of playpen/crib wide enough that child can get head through; child left in car with engine running; enclosed areas; plastic bags or small objects used as toys; toys with small, breakaway parts; refrigerators or freezers with doors not removed left accessible as play areas for children; children left unattended in or near bathtubs, pools, or spas; low-slung clotheslines; electric garage doors without automatic stop/reopen; pacifier hung around infant's neck; food not cut into small, bite-size, and age-appropriate pieces; balloons, hot dogs, nuts, or popcorn given to infants or young children (especially under 1 year of age); use of baby powder
Risk for injury/trauma r/t developmental age; altered home maintenance management (house not "childproofed"); altered parenting; hot liquids within child's reach; nonuse of infant and child car restraints; no gates at top of stairs; lack of immunizations for age; no fences or pool or spa covers; leaving child in car unattended with windows up or in hot weather; firearms loaded and within child's reach
Risk for poisoning r/t use of lead-based paint; presence of asbestos or radon gas; licit and illicit drugs not locked in cabinet; household products left in accessible area (bleach, detergent, drain cleaners, household cleaners); alcohol and perfume within reach of child; presence of poisonous plants; atmospheric pollutants

Salmonella

Refer to Gastroenteritis

Salpingectomy

Anticipatory grieving r/t possible loss due to tubal pregnancy
Decisional conflict r/t sterilization procedure
Risk for altered urinary elimination r/t trauma to ureter during surgery
Refer to Hysterectomy; Surgery

Sarcoidosis

Altered health maintenance r/t knowledge deficit regarding home care and medication regimen
Anxiety r/t change in health status
Impaired gas exchange r/t ventilation perfusion imbalance

Pain r/t possible disease affecting the joints
Risk for decreased cardiac output r/t dysrthymias

SBE (Self-Breast Examination)

Health-seeking behaviors r/t desire to have information about self-breast examination

Scabies

Refer to Communicable Diseases, Childhood

Scared

Anxiety r/t threat of death, threat to or change in health status
Fear r/t hospitalization, real or imagined threat to own well-being

Schizophrenia

Alteration in family process r/t inability to express feelings, impaired communication
Alteration in nutrition: less than body requirements r/t fear of eating, unaware of hunger, disinterest toward food
Alteration in thought process r/t inaccurate interpretations of environment
Altered health maintenance r/t cognitive impairment, ineffective individual and family coping, lack of material resources
Anxiety r/t unconscious conflict with reality
Diversional activity deficit r/t social isolation, possible regression
Fear r/t altered contact with reality
Impaired home maintenance management r/t impaired cognitive or emotional functioning, insufficient finances, inadequate support systems
Impaired social interaction r/t impaired communication patterns, self-concept disturbance, altered thought process
Impaired verbal communication r/t psychosis, disorientation, inaccurate perception, hallucinations, delusions
Ineffective individual coping r/t inadequate support systems, unrealistic perceptions, inadequate coping skills, altered thought processes, impaired communication
Ineffective management of therapeutic regimen: families r/t chronicity and unpredictability of condition
Risk for caregiver role strain r/t bizarre behavior of client, chronicity of condition
Risk for loneliness r/t inability to interact socially
Risk for violence: self-directed or directed at others r/t lack of trust, panic, hallucinations, delusional thinking
Self-care deficit r/t loss of contact with reality, impairment in perception
Self-esteem disturbance r/t excessive use of defense mechanisms (e.g., projection, denial, rationalization)
Sleep pattern disturbance r/t sensory alterations contributing to fear and anxiety
Social isolation r/t lack of trust, regression, delusional thinking, repressed fears

Scoliosis

Altered health maintenance r/t knowledge deficit regarding treatment modalities, restrictions, home care, postoperative activities
Body image disturbance r/t use of therapeutic braces, postsurgery scars, restricted physical activity
Impaired adjustment r/t lack of developmental maturity to comprehend long-term consequences of noncompliance with treatment procedures
Impaired gas exchange r/t restricted lung expansion secondary to severe presurgery curvature of spine; immobilization
Impaired physical mobility r/t restricted movement, dyspnea secondary to severe curvature of spine
Impaired skin integrity r/t braces, casts, surgical correction
Ineffective breathing patterns r/t restricted lung expansion secondary to severe curvature of spine
Pain r/t musculoskeletal restrictions, surgery, reambulation with cast or spinal rod
Risk for infection r/t surgical incision
Risk for perioperative positioning injury r/t prone position

Refer to Hospitalized Child; Maturational Issues, Adolescent

Sedentary Life-style

Activity intolerance r/t sedentary life-style

Seizure Disorders, Adult

Acute confusion r/t postseizure state
Altered health maintenance r/t lack of knowledge regarding anticonvulsive therapy
Impaired memory r/t seizure activity
Risk for altered thought processes r/t effects of anticonvulsant medications
Risk for ineffective airway clearance r/t accumulation of secretions during seizure
Risk for injury r/t uncontrolled movements during seizure, falls, drowsiness secondary to anticonvulsants

Social isolation r/t unpredictability of seizures, community-imposed stigma

Refer to Epilepsy

Seizure Disorders, Childhood (Epilepsy, Febrile Seizure, Infantile Spasms)

Altered health maintenance r/t lack of knowledge regarding anticonvulsive therapy, fever reduction (febrile seizures)

Risk for altered growth and development r/t effects of seizure disorder, parental overprotection

Risk for altered thought processes r/t effects of anticonvulsant medications

Risk for ineffective airway clearance r/t accumulation of secretions during seizure

Risk for injury r/t uncontrolled movements during seizure, falls, drowsiness secondary to anticonvulsants

Social isolation r/t unpredictability of seizures, community-imposed stigma

Refer to Epilepsy

Self-Breast Examination

Refer to SBE

Self-Care Deficit, Bathing/Hygiene

Self-care deficit: dressing/grooming r/t intolerance to activity, decreased strength and endurance, pain, discomfort, perceptual or cognitive impairment, neuromuscular impairment, musculoskeletal impairment, depression, severe anxiety

Self-Care Deficit, Dressing/Grooming

Self-care deficit: dressing/grooming r/t intolerance to activity, decreased strength and endurance, pain, discomfort, perceptual or cognitive impairment, neuromuscular impairment, musculoskeletal impairment, depression, severe anxiety

Self-Care Deficit, Feeding

Self-care deficit: feeding r/t intolerance to activity, decreased strength and endurance, pain, discomfort, perceptual or cognitive impairment, neuromuscular impairment, musculoskeletal impairment, depression, severe anxiety

Self-Care Deficit, Toileting

Self-care deficit: toileting r/t impaired transfer ability, impaired mobility status, intolerance to activity, decreased strength and endurance, pain, discomfort, perceptual or cognitive impairment, neuromuscular impairment, musculoskeletal impairment, depression, severe anxiety

Self-Destructive Behavior

Post-trauma response r/t unresolved feelings related to traumatic event

Risk for self-mutilation r/t feelings of depression, rejection, self-hatred, or depersonalization; command hallucinations

Risk for violence: self-directed r/t panic state, history of child abuse, toxic reaction to medication

Self-Esteem, Chronic Low

Chronic low self-esteem r/t long-standing negative self-evaluation

Self-Esteem Disturbance

Self-esteem disturbance r/t inappropriate and learned negative feelings about self

Self-Esteem, Situational Low

Situational low self-esteem r/t situational crisis

Self-Mutilation, Risk for

Risk for self-mutilation r/t inability to cope with increased psychological or physiological tension in a healthy manner; feelings of depression, rejection, self-hatred, separation anxiety, guilt, and depersonalization; fluctuating emotions; command hallucinations; need for sensory stimuli; parental emotional deprivation; dysfunctional family

Senile Dementia

Refer to Dementia

Sensory/Perceptual Alterations

Sensory/perceptual alterations: visual, auditory, kinesthetic, gustatory, tactile, olfactory r/t altered, excessive, or insufficient environmental stimuli; altered sensory reception, transmission, and/or integration; endogenous (electrolyte) or exogenous (e.g., drugs) chemical alterations; psychological stress

Separation Anxiety

Ineffective individual coping r/t maturational and situational crises, vulnerability secondary to developmental age, hospitalization, separation from family and familiar surroundings, multiple caregivers

Refer to Hospitalized Child

Sepsis—Child

Altered comfort: increased sensitivity to environmental stimuli r/t sensory-perceptual alterations: visual, auditory, kinesthetic
Altered nutrition: less than body requirements r/t anorexia, generalized weakness, poor sucking reflex
Altered tissue perfusion: cardiopulmonary, peripheral r/t arterial or venous blood flow exchange problems, septic shock
Ineffective thermal regulation r/t infectious process; septic shock
Risk for impaired skin integrity r/t desquamation secondary to disseminated intravascular coagulation (DIC)
Refer to Hospitalized Child; Premature Infant

Septicemia

Altered nutrition: less than body requirements r/t anorexia, generalized weakness
Altered tissue perfusion r/t decreased systemic vascular resistance
Fluid volume deficit r/t vasodilation of peripheral vessels, leaking of capillaries
Refer to Sepsis—Child; Shock; Shock, Septic

Sexual Dysfunction

Sexual dysfunction r/t biopsychosocial alteration of sexuality; ineffectual or absent role models; physical abuse or harmful relationships; vulnerability; conflicting values; lack of privacy; lack of significant other; altered body structure or function (pregnancy, recent childbirth, drugs, surgery, anomalies, disease process, trauma, radiation); misinformation or lack of knowledge

Sexuality, Adolescent

Body image disturbance r/t anxiety secondary to unachieved developmental milestone (puberty) or knowledge deficit regarding reproductive maturation as manifested by amenorrhea or expressed concerns regarding lack of growth of secondary sex characteristics
Decisional conflict: sexual activity r/t undefined personal values or beliefs, multiple or divergent sources of information, lack of relevant information
Knowledge deficit: potential for enhanced health maintenance r/t multiple or divergent sources of information or lack of relevant information regarding sexual transmission of disease, contraception, and prevention of toxic shock syndrome
Risk for rape-trauma syndrome r/t secondary to date rape, campus rape, insufficient knowledge regarding self-protection mechanisms
Refer to Maturational Issues, Adolescent

Sexuality Patterns, Alteration in

Altered sexuality patterns r/t knowledge or skill deficit regarding alternative responses to health-related transitions, altered body function or structure, illness or medical problems, lack of privacy, lack of significant other, ineffective or absent role models, fear of pregnancy or of acquiring a sexually transmitted disease, impaired relationship with a significant other

Sexually Transmitted Disease

Refer to STD

Shakiness

Anxiety r/t situational or maturational crisis, threat of death

Shame

Self-esteem disturbance r/t inability to deal with past traumatic events, blames self for events not responsible for

Shivering

Hypothermia r/t exposure to cool environment

Shock

Altered tissue perfusion: cardiopulmonary, peripheral r/t arterial/venous blood flow exchange problems
Fear r/t serious threat to health status
Risk for injury r/t prolonged shock resulting in multiple organ failure, death
Refer to Shock, Cardiogenic; Shock, Hypovolemic; Shock, Septic

Shock, Cardiogenic

Decreased cardiac output r/t decreased myocardial contractility, dysrhythmias
Refer to Shock

Shock, Hypovolemic

Fluid volume deficit r/t abnormal loss of fluid
Refer to Shock

Shock, Septic

Altered protection r/t inadequately functioning immune system
Fluid volume deficit r/t abnormal loss of fluid through capillaries, pooling of blood in peripheral circulation
Refer to Shock; Sepsis, Child; Septicemia

Shoulder Repair

Risk for perioperative positioning injury r/t immobility

Self-care deficit: bathing/hygiene, dressing/grooming, feeding r/t immobilization of affected shoulder

Refer to Surgery; Total Joint Replacement

Sickle Cell Anemia/Crisis

Activity intolerance r/t fatigue, effects of chronic anemia

Fluid volume deficit r/t decreased intake, increased fluid requirements during sickle cell crisis, decreased ability of kidneys to concentrate urine

Impaired physical mobility r/t pain, fatigue

Pain r/t viscous blood, tissue hypoxia

Risk for altered tissue perfusion (renal, cerebral, cardiac, gastrointestinal, peripheral) r/t effects of red cell sickling, infarction of tissues

Risk for infection r/t alterations in splenic function

Refer to Hospitalized Child; Child with Chronic Condition

SIDS

Altered family processes r/t stress secondary to special care needs of infant with apnea

Anticipatory grieving r/t potential loss of infant

Anxiety/fear (parental) r/t life-threatening event

Knowledge deficit: potential for enhanced health maintenance r/t knowledge or skill acquisition of CPR and home apnea monitoring

Sleep pattern disturbance (parental, infant) r/t home apnea monitoring

Refer to Terminally Ill Child/Death of Child

Situational Crisis

Altered family processes r/t situational crisis

Ineffective individual coping r/t situational crisis

Potential for enhanced spiritual well-being r/t desire for harmony following crisis

Skin Cancer

Altered health maintenance r/t knowledge deficit regarding self-care with skin cancer

Impaired skin integrity r/t abnormal cell growth in skin, treatment of skin cancer

Skin Disorders

Impaired skin integrity r/t External: hyperthermia, hypothermia, chemical substances, mechanical factors (shearing forces, pressure, restraint), radiation, physical immobilization, humidity; Internal: medication, altered nutritional state (obesity, emaciation), altered metabolic state, altered circulation, altered sensation, altered pigmentation, skeletal prominence, developmental factors, immunological deficit, alterations in turgor (change in elasticity)

Skin Integrity, Risk for Impaired

Risk for impaired skin integrity r/t internal or external factors that are potentially harmful to skin

Skin Turgor, Change in Elasticity

Fluid volume deficit r/t active fluid loss

Note: decreased skin turgor can be normal finding in the elderly.

Sleep Apnea

Refer to PND

Sleep Deprivation

Altered sensory perception r/t lack of sleep

Fatigue r/t lack of sleep

Sleep Pattern Disorders

Sleep pattern disorders r/t sensory alterations; internal factors (illness, psychological stress); external factors (environmental changes, social cues)

Sleep Pattern Disturbance, Parent/Child

Sleep pattern disturbance (child) r/t anxiety or apprehension secondary to parental deprivation (Refer to Suspected Child Abuse and Neglect), fear, night terrors, enuresis, inconsistent parental responses to child's requests to alter bedtime rules, frequent nighttime awakening, inability to wean from parents' bed, hypervigilance

Sleep pattern disturbance (parental) r/t time-intensive home treatments, increased caretaker demands

Slurring of Speech

Impaired verbal communication r/t decrease in circulation to brain, brain tumor, anatomical defect, cleft palate

Situational low self-esteem r/t speech impairment

Small Bowel Resection

Refer to Abdominal Surgery

Smell, Loss of

Sensory/perceptual alteration: olfactory r/t altered sensory reception, transmission, or integration

Smoking Behavior

Altered health maintenance r/t denial of effects of smoking, lack of effective support for smoking withdrawal

Social Interaction, Impaired

Social interaction: impaired r/t knowledge or skill deficit about ways to enhance mutuality, communication barriers, self-concept disturbance, absence of available significant others or peers, limited physical mobility, therapeutic isolation, sociocultural dissonance, environmental barriers, altered thought processes

Social Isolation

Social isolation r/t factors contributing to the absence of satisfying personal relationships, such as delay in accomplishing developmental tasks, immature interests, alterations in physical appearance, alterations in mental status, unaccepted social behavior, unaccepted social values, altered state of wellness, inadequate personal resources, inability to engage in satisfying personal relationships, fear

Sociopath

Refer to Antisocial Personality Disorder

Sodium, Decrease/Increase

Refer to Hyponatremia, Hypernatremia

Somatoform Disorder

Anxiety r/t unresolved conflicts being channeled into physical complaints or conditions
Chronic pain r/t unexpressed anger, multiple physical disorders, depression
Ineffective individual coping r/t lack of insight into underlying conflicts

Sore Nipples: Breast-feeding

Ineffective breast-feeding r/t knowledge deficit regarding correct feeding procedure
Refer to Painful Breasts—Sore Nipples

Sore Throat

Altered oral mucous membranes r/t inflammation or infection of oral cavity
Impaired swallowing r/t irritation of oropharyngeal cavity
Knowledge deficit r/t treatment to relieve cause and discomfort
Pain r/t inflammation, irritation, dryness

Sorrow

Anticipatory grieving r/t impending loss of significant person or object
Grieving r/t loss of significant person, object, or role
Potential for enhanced spiritual well-being r/t desire to find purpose and meaning of loss

Speech Disorders

Anxiety r/t difficulty with communication
Impaired verbal communication r/t anatomical defect, cleft palate, psychological barriers, decrease in circulation to brain

Spina Bifida

Refer to Neurotube Defects

Spinal Cord Injury

Altered health maintenance r/t knowledge deficit regarding self-care with spinal cord injury
Body image disturbance r/t change in body function
Constipation r/t immobility, loss of sensation
Diversional activity deficit r/t long-term hospitalization, frequent lengthy treatments
Dysfunctional grieving r/t loss of usual body function
Fear r/t powerlessness over loss of body function
Impaired home maintenance r/t change in health status, insufficient family planning or finances, knowledge deficit, inadequate support systems
Impaired physical mobility r/t neuromuscular impairment
Reflex incontinence r/t spinal cord lesion interfering with conduction of cerebral messages
Risk for disuse syndrome r/t paralysis
Risk for dysreflexia r/t bladder or bowel distention, skin irritation, knowledge deficits of patient and caregiver
Risk for impaired skin integrity r/t immobility, paralysis
Risk for ineffective breathing pattern r/t neuromuscular impairment
Risk for infection r/t chronic disease, stasis of body fluids
Risk for loneliness r/t physical immobility
Self-care deficit r/t neuromuscular impairment
Sexual dysfunction r/t altered body function
Urinary retention r/t inhibition of reflex arc
Refer to Hospitalized Child; Child with Chronic Condition; Neurotube Defects

Spiritual Distress

Spiritual distress r/t separation from religious or cultural ties; challenged belief and value system resulting from moral or ethical implications of therapy or from intense suffering

Spiritual Well-Being

Potential for enhanced spiritual well-being r/t desire for harmonious interconnectedness, desire to find purpose and meaning to life

Splenectomy

Refer to Abdominal Surgery

Stapedectomy

Altered sensory perception: auditory r/t hearing loss related to edema from surgery
Pain r/t headache
Risk for infection r/t invasive procedure
Risk for injury: falling r/t dizziness

Stasis Ulcer

Impaired tissue integrity r/t chronic venous congestion
Refer to Varicose Veins

STD (Sexually Transmitted Disease)

Altered health maintenance r/t knowledge deficit regarding transmission, symptoms, and treatment of sexually transmitted disease
Altered sexuality patterns r/t illness, altered body function
Fear r/t altered body function, risk for social isolation, fear of incurable illness
Pain r/t biological or psychological injury
Risk for infection (spread of infection) r/t lack of knowledge concerning transmission of disease
Social isolation r/t fear of contracting or spreading the disease
Refer to Maturational Issues, Adolescent

Stertorous Respirations

Ineffective airway clearance r/t pharyngeal obstruction

Stillbirth

Refer to Pregnancy Loss

Stoma

Refer to Ostomy

Stomatitis

Altered oral mucous membranes r/t pathological conditions of oral cavity

Stone, Kidney

Refer to Kidney Stone

Stool, Hard, Dry

Colonic constipation r/t inadequate fluid intake, inadequate fiber intake, decreased activity level, decreased gastric motility

Straining with Defecation

Colonic constipation r/t less than adequate fluid intake, less than adequate dietary intake
Risk for decreased cardiac output r/t vagal stimulation with dysrhythmias secondary to Valsalva's maneuver

Stress

Anxiety r/t feelings of helplessness, feelings of being threatened
Energy field disturbance r/t low energy level, feelings of hopelessness
Fear r/t powerlessness over feelings
Ineffective individual coping r/t ineffective use of problem-solving process, feelings of apprehension or helplessness
Potential for enhanced spiritual well-being r/t desire for harmony and peace in stressful situation
Self-esteem disturbance r/t inability to deal with life events

Stress Incontinence

Stress incontinence r/t degenerative change in pelvic muscles
Refer to Incontinence of Urine

Stridor

Ineffective airway clearance r/t obstruction, tracheobronchial infection, trauma

Stroke

Refer to CVA

Stuttering

Impaired verbal communication r/t anxiety, psychological problems

Subarachnoid Hemorrhage

Altered tissue perfusion: cerebral r/t bleeding from cerebral vessel
Pain: headache r/t irritation of meninges from blood, increased intracranial pressure
Refer to Intracranial Pressure, Increased

Substance Abuse

Altered family process: alcohol r/t inadequate coping skills
Altered nutrition: less than body requirements r/t anorexia

Altered protection r/t malnutrition, sleep deprivation
Anxiety r/t loss of control
Compromised/dysfunctional family coping r/t co-dependency issues
Ineffective individual coping r/t use of substances to cope with life events
Powerlessness r/t substance addiction
Risk for altered parent/infant/child attachment r/t substance abuse
Risk for injury r/t alteration in sensory-perception
Risk for violence r/t reactions to substances used, impulsive behavior, disorientation, impaired judgment
Self-esteem disturbance r/t failure at life events
Sleep pattern disturbance r/t irritability, nightmares, tremors
Social isolation r/t unacceptable social behavior or values
Refer to Maturational Issues, Adolescent

Substance Abuse, Adolescent

Refer to Alcohol Withdrawal; Substance Abuse; Maturational Issues, Adolescent

Substance Abuse in Pregnancy

Altered health maintenance r/t addiction
Defensive coping r/t denial of situation, differing value system
Knowledge deficit r/t lack of exposure to information about effects of substance abuse in pregnancy
Noncompliance r/t differing value system, cultural influences, addiction
Risk for altered parenting r/t lack of ability to meet infant's needs
Risk for fetal injury r/t effects of drugs on fetal growth and development
Risk for infection r/t intravenous drug use, life-style
Risk for maternal injury r/t drug use
Refer to Substance Abuse

Sucking Reflex

Effective breast-feeding r/t regular and sustained suckling and swallowing at the breast

Sudden Infant Death Syndrome, Near Miss (Infant Apnea)

Refer to SIDS

Suffocation, Risk for

Risk for suffocation r/t internal: reduced olfactory sensation, reduced motor abilities, lack of safety education, lack of safety precautions, cognitive or emotional difficulties, disease or injury process; external: pillow placed in infant's crib, propped bottle placed in infant's crib, vehicle warming in closed garage, children playing with plastic bags, children inserting small objects into their mouths or noses, discarded or unused refrigerators or freezers with doors, children left unattended in or near bathtubs/pools/hot tubs, low-strung clothesline, pacifier hung around infant's neck, eating large mouthfuls of food

Suicide Attempt

Hopelessness r/t perceived or actual loss, substance abuse, low self-concept, inadequate support systems
Ineffective individual coping r/t anger, dysfunctional grieving
Post-trauma response r/t history of traumatic events, abuse, rape, incest, war, torture
Potential for enhanced spiritual well-being r/t desire for harmony and inner strength to help redefine purpose for life
Risk for violence: self-directed r/t suicidal ideation, feelings of hopelessness or worthlessness, lack of impulse control, feelings of anger or hostility (self-directed)
Self-esteem disturbance r/t guilt, inability to trust, feelings of worthlessness or rejection
Social isolation r/t inability to engage in satisfying personal relationships
Spiritual distress r/t hopelessness, despair

Support System

Family coping: potential for growth r/t ability to adapt to tasks related to care and support of significant other during health crisis

Suppression of Labor

Refer to Preterm Labor; Tocolytic Therapy

Surgery, Postoperative Care

Activity intolerance r/t pain, surgical procedure
Altered nutrition: less than body requirements r/t anorexia, nausea, vomiting, decreased peristalsis
Anxiety r/t change in health status, hospital environment
Knowledge deficit r/t postoperative expectations, life-style changes
Pain r/t inflammation or injury in surgical area
Risk for altered tissue perfusion: peripheral r/t hypovolemia, circulatory stasis, obesity, prolonged immobility, decreased coughing, decreased deep breathing

Risk for colonic constipation r/t decreased activity, decreased food or fluid intake, anesthesia, pain medication
Risk for fluid volume deficit r/t hypermetabolic state, fluid loss during surgery, presence of indwelling tubes
Risk for ineffective breathing pattern r/t pain, location of incision, effects of anesthesia/narcotics
Risk for infection r/t invasive procedure, pain, anesthesia, location of incision, weakened cough due to aging
Urinary retention r/t anesthesia, pain, fear, unfamiliar surroundings, client's position

Surgery, Preoperative Care

Anxiety r/t threat to or change in health status, situational crisis, fear of unknown
Knowledge deficit r/t preoperative procedures, postoperative expectations
Sleep pattern disturbance r/t anxiety about upcoming surgery

Suspected Child Abuse and Neglect (SCAN)—Child

Altered growth and development: regression vs delayed r/t diminished or absent environmental stimuli, inadequate caretaking, inconsistent responsiveness by caretaker
Altered nutrition: less than body requirements r/t inadequate caretaking
Anxiety/fear (child) r/t threat of punishment for perceived wrongdoing
Chronic low self-esteem r/t lack of positive feedback, excessive negative feedback
Diversional activity deficit r/t diminished or absent environmental or personal stimuli
Impaired skin integrity r/t altered nutritional state, physical abuse
Pain r/t physical injuries
Post-trauma response r/t physical abuse, incest, rape, molestation
Potential for enhanced community coping r/t obtaining resources to prevent child abuse and neglect
Rape-trauma syndrome: compound/silent reaction r/t altered life-style secondary to abuse and changes in residence
Risk for poisoning r/t inadequate safeguards, lack of proper safety precautions, accessibility of illicit substances secondary to impaired home maintenance management
Risk for suffocation (secondary to aspiration) r/t propped bottle, unattended child
Risk for trauma r/t inadequate precautions, cognitive or emotional difficulties
Sleep pattern disturbance r/t hypervigilance, anxiety
Social isolation: family imposed r/t fear of disclosure of family dysfunction and abuse

Refer to Hospitalized Child; Maturational Issues, Adolescent

Suspected Child Abuse and Neglect (SCAN)—Parent

Altered family process: alcoholism r/t inadequate coping skills
Altered health maintenance r/t knowledge deficit of parenting skills secondary to unachieved developmental tasks
Altered parenting r/t unrealistic expectations of child; lack of effective role model; unmet social, emotional, or maturational needs of parents, interruption in bonding process
Chronic low self-esteem r/t lack of successful parenting experiences
Impaired home maintenance management r/t disorganization, parental dysfunction, neglect of safe and nurturing environment
Ineffective family coping: disabling r/t dysfunctional family, underdeveloped nurturing parental role, lack of parental support systems or role models
Powerlessness r/t inability to perform parental role responsibilities
Risk for violence towards child r/t inadequate coping mechanisms, unresolved stressors, unachieved maturational level by parent

Suspicion

Impaired social interaction r/t altered thought process, paranoid delusions, hallucinations
Powerlessness r/t repetitive paranoid thinking
Risk for violence: directed at self or others r/t inability to trust

Swallowing Difficulties

Impaired swallowing r/t neuromuscular impairment (e.g., decreased or absent gag reflex, decreased strength or excursion of muscles involved in mastication), perceptual impairment, facial paralysis, mechanical obstruction (e.g., edema, tracheostomy tube, tumor), fatigue, limited awareness, reddened or irritated oropharyngeal cavity, improper feeding or positioning

Syncope

Altered tissue perfusion: cerebral r/t interruption of blood flow
Anxiety r/t fear of falling
Decreased cardiac output r/t dysrhythmias
Impaired physical mobility r/t fear of falling
Risk for injury r/t altered sensory-perception, transient loss of consciousness, risk for falls
Social isolation r/t fear of falling

Syphilis

Refer to STD

Systemic Lupus Erythematosus

Refer to Lupus Erythematosus

T

T&A (Tonsil & Adenoidectomy)

Altered comfort r/t effects of anesthesia (nausea and vomiting)
Ineffective airway clearance r/t hesitation or reluctance to cough secondary to pain
Knowledge deficit: potential for enhanced health maintenance r/t insufficient knowledge regarding postoperative nutritional and rest requirements, signs and symptoms of complications, positioning
Pain r/t surgical incision
Risk for altered nutrition: less than body requirements r/t hesitation or reluctance to swallow
Risk for aspiration/suffocation r/t postoperative drainage and impaired swallowing
Risk for fluid volume deficit r/t decreased intake secondary to painful swallowing, effects of anesthesia (nausea and vomiting), hemorrhage

Tachycardia

Refer to Dysrhythmia

Tachypnea

Ineffective breathing pattern r/t pain, anxiety
Refer to cause of Tachypnea

Taste Abnormality

Sensory/perceptual alteration: gustatory r/t medication side effects; altered sensory reception, transmission, and/or integration; aging changes

TBI (Traumatic Brain Injury)

Acute confusion r/t brain injury
Altered family process r/t traumatic injury to family member
Altered thought processes r/t pressure damage to brain
Altered tissue perfusion: cerebral r/t the effects of increased intracranial pressure
Decreased adaptive capacity: intracranial r/t brain injury
Ineffective breathing patterns r/t pressure damage to breathing center in brain stem
Sensory/perceptual alteration: specify r/t pressure damage to sensory centers in brain

Temperature, Decreased

Hypothermia r/t exposure to cool environment

Temperature, Increased

Hyperthermia r/t dehydration, illness, trauma

Temperature Regulation, Impaired

Ineffective thermoregulation r/t trauma, illness

Tension

Anxiety r/t threat to or change in health status, situational crisis
Energy field disturbance r/t change in health status, discouragement, pain

Terminally Ill Adult

Anticipatory grieving r/t loss of self or significant other
Decisional conflict r/t planning for Advance Directives
Ineffective family coping r/t inability to discuss impending death
Spiritual distress r/t suffering before death

Terminally Ill Child/Death of Child—Parental

Altered family processes r/t situational crisis
Altered parenting r/t risk for overprotection of surviving siblings
Anticipatory grieving r/t possible, expected, or imminent death of child
Decisional conflict r/t continuation or discontinuation of treatment, Do Not Resuscitate status, ethical issues regarding organ donation
Family coping: potential for growth r/t impact of crisis on family values, priorities, goals, or relationships; expressed interest or desire to attach meaning to child's life and death

Grieving r/t death of child
Hopelessness r/t overwhelming stresses secondary to terminal illness
Impaired social interaction r/t dysfunctional grieving
Ineffective denial r/t dysfunctional grieving
Ineffective family coping: compromised r/t inability or unwillingness to discuss impending death and feelings with child or to support child through terminal stages of illness
Powerlessness r/t inability to alter course of events
Risk for dysfunctional grieving r/t prolonged, unresolved, or obstructed progression through stages of grief and mourning
Sleep pattern disturbance r/t grieving process
Social isolation: imposed by others r/t feelings of inadequacy in providing support to grieving parents
Social isolation: self-imposed r/t unresolved grief, perceived inadequate parenting skills
Spiritual distress r/t sudden and unexpected death, prolonged suffering before death, questioning the death of youth, questioning meaning of own existence

Terminally Ill Child—Infant/Toddler

Ineffective individual coping r/t separation from parents and familiar environment secondary to inability to grasp external meaning of death

Terminally Ill Child—Preschool Child

Fear r/t perceived punishment, bodily harm, feelings of guilt secondary to magical thinking (thoughts cause events)

Terminally Ill Child—School-Age Child/Preadolescent

Fear r/t perceived punishment, body mutilation, feelings of guilt

Terminally Ill Child—Adolescent

Altered body image r/t effects of terminal disease, already critical feelings of group identity and self-image
Impaired social interaction/social isolation r/t forced separation from peers
Ineffective individual coping r/t inability to establish personal and peer identity secondary to threat of being different or "not being," inability to achieve maturational tasks

Refer to Hospitalized Child; Child with Chronic Condition

Tetralogy of Fallot

Refer to Congenital Heart Disease/Cardiac Anomalies

Therapeutic Regimen, Effective Management of: Individual

Effective management of therapeutic regimen: individual r/t adequate ability to manage needed health care

Therapeutic Regimen, Ineffective Management of

Ineffective management of therapeutic regimen r/t complexity of health care system; complexity of therapeutic regimen; decisional conflicts; economic difficulties; excessive demands made on individual or family; family conflict; family patterns of health care; inadequate number and types of cues to action; knowledge deficits; mistrust of regimen or health care personnel; perceived seriousness, susceptibility, barriers, or benefits; powerlessness; social support deficits

Therapeutic Regimen, Ineffective Management of: Families

Ineffective management of therapeutic regimen: families r/t complexity of health care system, complexity of therapeutic regimen, decisional conflicts, economic difficulties, excessive demands on individual or family, family conflict

Therapeutic Touch

Energy field disturbance r/t low energy levels, disturbance in energy fields, pain, depression, fatigue

Thermoregulation, Ineffective

Ineffective thermoregulation r/t trauma, illness, immaturity, aging, fluctuating environmental temperature

Thoracotomy

Activity intolerance r/t pain, imbalance between oxygen supply and demand, presence of chest tubes
Ineffective airway clearance r/t drowsiness, pain with breathing and coughing
Ineffective breathing pattern r/t decreased energy, fatigue, pain
Knowledge deficit r/t self-care, effective breathing exercises, pain relief
Pain r/t surgical procedure, coughing, deep breathing
Risk for infection r/t invasive procedure

Risk for injury r/t disruption of closed-chest drainage system
Risk for perioperative positioning injury r/t lateral positioning and immobility

Thought Disorders

Altered thought processes r/t disruption in cognitive thinking, processing

Thought Processes, Altered

Altered thought processes r/t head injury, mental disorder, personality disorder, organic mental disorder, substance abuse, severe interpersonal conflict, sleep deprivation, sensory deprivation or overload, impaired cerebral perfusion

Thrombocytopenic Purpura

Refer to ITP

Thrombophlebitis

Altered tissue perfusion: peripheral r/t interruption of venous blood flow
Colonic constipation r/t inactivity, bedrest
Diversional activity deficit r/t bedrest
Impaired physical mobility r/t pain in extremity, forced bedrest
Knowledge deficit r/t pathophysiology of condition, self-care needs, treatment regimen and outcome
Pain r/t vascular inflammation, edema
Risk for injury r/t possible embolus
Refer to Anticoagulant Therapy

Thyroidectomy

Risk for altered verbal communication r/t edema, pain, vocal cord of laryngeal nerve damage
Risk for ineffective airway clearance r/t edema or hematoma formation, airway obstruction
Risk for injury r/t possible parathyroid damage or removal
Refer to Surgery

TIA (Transient Ischemic Attack)

Acute confusion r/t hypoxia
Altered tissue perfusion: cerebral r/t lack of adequate oxygen supply to the brain
Health-seeking behaviors r/t obtaining knowledge regarding treatment and prevention of inadequate oxygenation
Risk for decreased cardiac output r/t dysrhythmias contributing to inadequate oxygen supply to brain
Risk for injury r/t possible syncope
Refer to Syncope

Tinnitus

Altered health maintenance r/t knowledge deficit regarding self-care with tinnitus
Sensory/perceptual alteration: auditory r/t altered sensory reception, transmission, and/or integration

Tissue Damage—Corneal, Integumentary, or Subcutaneous

Impaired tissue integrity r/t altered circulation, nutritional deficit or excess, fluid deficit or excess, knowledge deficit, impaired physical mobility, chemical irritants (including body excretions, secretions, medications), thermal irritants (temperature extremes), mechanical irritants (pressure, shear, friction), radiation irritants (including therapeutic radiation)

Tissue Perfusion, Decreased

Altered tissue perfusion r/t arterial or venous interruption of flow, exchange problems, hypovolemia, hypervolemia

Tocolytic Therapy

Altered health maintenance r/t knowledge deficit regarding management of preterm labor and treatment regimen
Risk for fluid volume excess r/t effects of tocolytic drugs
Refer to Preterm Labor

Toileting Problems

Self-care deficit: toileting r/t impaired transfer ability, impaired mobility status, intolerance of activity, neuromuscular impairment, cognitive impairment

Toilet Training

Health-seeking behaviors: bladder/bowel training r/t achievement of developmental milestone secondary to enhanced parenting skills

Tonsillectomy and Adenoidectomy

Refer to T&A

Total Anomalous Pulmonary Venous Return

Refer to Congenital Heart Disease/Cardiac Anomalies

Total Incontinence

Total incontinence r/t neuropathy, neurological dysfunction, compromised contraction of detrusor reflex, anatomical incontinence (fistula)

Total Joint Replacement—Total Hip/ Total Knee

Body image disturbance r/t large scar, presence of prosthesis
Impaired physical mobility r/t musculoskeletal impairment, surgery, prosthesis
Knowledge deficit r/t self-care, treatment regimen, outcomes
Pain r/t possible edema, physical injury, surgery
Risk for infection r/t invasive procedure, anesthesia, immobility
Risk for injury: neurovascular r/t altered peripheral tissue perfusion, altered mobility, prosthesis

Total Parenteral Nutrition

Refer to TPN

Toxemia

Refer to PIH

TPN (Total Parenteral Nutrition)

Altered nutrition: less than body requirements r/t inability to ingest or digest food or absorb nutrients due to biological or psychological factors
Risk for fluid volume excess r/t rapid administration of TPN
Risk for infection r/t concentrated glucose solution, invasive administration of fluids

Tracheoesophageal Fistula

Altered nutrition: less than body requirements r/t difficulties in swallowing
Ineffective airway clearance r/t aspiration of feeding secondary to inability to swallow
Risk for aspiration r/t common passage of air and food
Refer to Respiratory Conditions of the Neonate; Hospitalized Child

Tracheostomy

Anxiety r/t impaired verbal communication, ineffective airway clearance
Body image disturbance r/t abnormal opening in neck
Impaired verbal communication r/t presence of mechanical airway
Knowledge deficit r/t self-care, home maintenance management
Pain r/t edema, surgical procedure
Risk for aspiration r/t presence of tracheostomy
Risk for ineffective airway clearance r/t increased secretions, mucus plugs
Risk for infection r/t invasive procedure, pooling of secretions

Traction and Casts

Constipation r/t immobility
Diversional activity deficit r/t immobility
Impaired physical mobility r/t imposed restrictions on activity secondary to bone or joint disease injury
Pain r/t immobility, injury, or disease
Risk for disuse syndrome r/t mechanical immobilization
Risk for impaired skin integrity r/t contact of traction or cast with skin
Risk for peripheral neurovascular dysfunction r/t mechanical compression
Self-care deficit: feeding, dressing/grooming, bathing/hygiene, toileting r/t degree of impaired physical mobility, body area affected by traction or cast

Transient Ischemic Attack

Refer to TIA

Transposition of the Great Vessels

Refer to Congenital Heart Disease/Cardiac Anomalies

Transurethral Resection of the Prostate

Refer to TURP

Trauma, Risk for

Risk for trauma r/t internal: weakness, poor vision, balancing difficulties, reduced temperature and/or tactile sensation, reduced large or small muscle coordination, reduced hand-eye coordination, lack of safety education, lack of safety precautions, insufficient finances to purchase safety equipment or effect repairs, cognitive or emotional difficulties, history of previous trauma; external: slippery floors or walkways, unanchored rugs, bathtub without hand grip or antislip equipment, use of unsteady ladders or chairs, entering unlighted rooms, unsturdy or absent stair rails, unanchored electrical wires, litter or liquid spills on floors or stairways, high beds, children playing at the top of ungated stairs, obstructed passageways, unsafe window protection in home with young children, inappropriate call-for-aid mechanisms for bed-resting client, pot handles facing toward front of stove, bathing in very hot water, unsupervised bathing of young children, potentially ignitable gas leaks, delayed lighting of gas burner or oven, experimenting with chemicals or gasoline, unscreened fires or heaters, wearing plastic apron or flowing clothes around open flame, children playing with dangerous objects (e.g., matches, candles, or cigarettes), inadequately stored combustible items or corrosives, highly flammable children's toys or clothing, overloaded fuse box, contact with rapidly moving objects (e.g., machinery, industrial belts, or pulleys), sliding on coarse bed linen or struggling within bed restraints, faulty electrical plugs, frayed wires, defective appliances, contact with acids or alkalis, playing with fireworks or gunpowder, contact with intense cold, overexposure to sun or radiotherapy, misuse of sun lamps, use of cracked dishware or glasses, knives stored uncovered, guns or ammunition stored unlocked, large icicles hanging from the roof, exposure to dangerous machinery, children playing with sharp-edged toys, high crime neighborhood and vulnerable clients, driving a mechanically unsafe vehicle, driving after partaking of alcoholic beverages or drugs, driving at excessive speeds, driving without necessary visual aids, children riding in the front seat of car, smoking in bed or near oxygen, overloaded electrical outlets, grease waste collected on stoves, use of thin or worn potholders, misuse of necessary headgear for motorized cyclists, young children carried on adult bicycles, unsafe road or road-crossing conditions, playing or working near vehicle pathways, nonuse or misuse of seat restraints

Trauma in Pregnancy

Anxiety r/t threat to self or fetus, unknown outcome
Impaired skin integrity r/t trauma
Knowledge deficit r/t lack of exposure to situation
Pain r/t trauma
Risk for fetal injury r/t premature separation of the placenta
Risk for fluid volume deficit r/t blood loss
Risk for infection r/t traumatized tissue

Traumatic Brain Injury (TBI)

Refer to TBI; Intracranial Pressure, Increased

Traumatic Event

Post-trauma response r/t previously experienced trauma

Trembling of Hands

Anxiety/fear r/t threat to or change in health status, threat of death, situational crisis

Tricuspid Atresia

Refer to Congenital Heart Disease/Cardiac Anomalies

Truncus Arteriosus

Refer to Congenital Heart Disease/Cardiac Anomalies

TSE (Testicular Self-Examination)

Health-seeking behavior r/t procedure for doing self-testicular examinations

Tube Feeding

Risk for altered nutrition: less than body requirements r/t intolerance to tube feeding, inadequate calorie replacement to meet metabolic needs
Risk for aspiration r/t improperly administered feeding, improper placement of tube, improper positioning of client during and after feeding, excessive residual feeding or lack of digestion, altered gag reflex
Risk for fluid volume deficit r/t inadequate water administration with concentrated feeding

TURP (Transurethral Resection of the Prostate)

Knowledge deficit r/t postoperative self-care, home maintenance management
Pain r/t incision, irritation from catheter, bladder spasms, kidney infection
Risk for fluid volume deficit r/t fluid loss and possible bleeding
Risk for infection r/t invasive procedure; route for bacteria entry
Risk for urinary retention r/t obstruction of urethra or catheter with clots

Ulcer, Peptic or Duodenal

Altered health maintenance r/t lack of knowledge regarding health practices to prevent ulcer formation
Fatigue r/t loss of blood, chronic illness
Pain r/t irritated mucosa from acid secretion
Refer to GI Bleed

Ulcerative Colitis

Refer to Inflammatory Bowel Disease

Ulcers, Stasis

Refer to Stasis Ulcers

Unilateral Neglect of One Side of Body

Unilateral neglect r/t effects of disturbed perceptual abilities (e.g., hemianopsia), one-sided blindness, neurological illness or trauma

Unsanitary Living Conditions

Impaired home maintenance r/t impaired cognitive or emotional functioning, lack of knowledge, insufficient finances

Urgency to Urinate

Urge incontinence r/t decreased bladder capacity, irritation of bladder stretch receptors causing spasm, alcohol, caffeine, increased fluids, increased urine concentration, overdistention of bladder

Urinary Diversion

Refer to Ileal Conduit

Urinary Elimination, Altered

Altered urinary elimination r/t anatomical obstruction, sensory motor impairment, urinary tract infection

Urinary Incontinence

Refer to Incontinence of Urine

Urinary Retention

Urinary retention r/t high urethral pressure caused by weak detrusor, inhibition of reflex arc, strong sphincter, blockage

Urinary Tract Infection

Refer to UTI

Urolithiasis

Refer to Kidney Stone

Uterine Atony in Labor

Refer to Dystocia

Uterine Atony in Postpartum

Refer to Postpartum Hemorrhage

Uterine Bleeding

Refer to Hemorrhage; Shock; Postpartum Hemorrhage

UTI (Urinary Tract Infection)

Altered health maintenance r/t knowledge deficit regarding methods to treat and prevent UTIs
Altered pattern of urinary elimination: frequency r/t urinary tract infection
Pain: dysuria r/t inflammatory process in bladder

V

Vaginal Hysterectomy

Risk for altered urinary elimination r/t edema in area
Risk for infection r/t surgical site
Risk for perioperative positioning injury r/t lithotomy position
Urinary retention r/t edema at surgical site
Refer to Hysterectomy

Vaginitis

Altered health maintenance r/t knowledge deficit regarding self-care with vaginitis
Altered pattern of sexuality r/t abstinence during acute stage, pain
Pain: pruritis r/t inflamed tissues, edema
Risk for infection r/t spread of infection, risk of reinfection

Vagotomy

Refer to Abdominal Surgery

Value System Conflict

Potential for enhanced spiritual well-being r/t desire for harmony with self, others, and higher power/God
Spiritual distress r/t challenged value system

Varicose Veins

Altered health maintenance r/t knowledge deficit regarding health care practices, prevention, and treatment regimen
Altered tissue perfusion: peripheral r/t venous stasis
Chronic pain r/t impaired circulation
Risk for impaired skin integrity r/t altered peripheral tissue perfusion

Vascular Dementia (formerly Multi-infarct Dementia)

Refer to Dementia

Vascular Obstruction—Peripheral

Altered tissue perfusion: peripheral r/t interruption of circulatory flow
Anxiety r/t lack of circulation to body part
Pain r/t vascular obstruction
Risk for peripheral neurovascular dysfunction r/t vascular obstruction

Venereal Disease

Refer to STD

Ventilation, Inability to Sustain Spontaneous

Inability to sustain spontaneous ventilation r/t metabolic factors, respiratory muscle fatigue

Ventilator Client

Dysfunctional ventilatory weaning response r/t inability to sustain respirations without mechanical support
Fear r/t inability to breathe on own, difficulty communicating
Impaired gas exchange r/t ventilation perfusion imbalance
Impaired verbal communication r/t presence of endotracheal tube, decreased mentation
Inability to sustain spontaneous ventilation r/t metabolic factors, respiratory muscle fatigue
Ineffective airway clearance r/t increased secretions, decreased cough and gag reflex
Ineffective breathing pattern r/t decreased energy and fatigue secondary to possible alteration in nutrition (less than body requirements)
Powerlessness r/t health treatment regimen
Risk for infection r/t presence of endotracheal tube, pooled secretions
Social isolation r/t impaired mobility, ventilator dependence
Refer to Child with Chronic Condition; Hospitalized Child; Respiratory Conditions of the Neonate

Ventilatory, Dysfunctional Weaning Response (DVWR)

Dysfunctional ventilatory weaning response r/t inability to sustain respirations without mechanical support

Vertigo

Altered tissue perfusion: cerebral r/t decreased blood supply to brain
Risk for injury r/t altered sensory-perception
Sensory/perceptual alteration: kinesthetic r/t altered sensory reception, transmission, and/or integration; medications

Violent Behavior

Risk for violence: self-directed or directed at others r/t antisocial character, battered women, catatonic excitement, child abuse, manic excitement, organic brain syndrome, panic states, rage reactions, suicidal behavior, temporal lobe epilepsy, toxic reactions to medication

Vision Impairment

Fear r/t loss of sight
Risk for injury r/t sensory-perceptual alteration
Self-care deficit: specify r/t perceptual impairment
Sensory/perceptual alteration: visual r/t altered sensory reception related to impaired vision
Social isolation r/t altered state of wellness, inability to see

Vomiting

Altered comfort: nausea, retching r/t tension on abdominal muscles
Risk for altered nutrition: less than body requirements r/t inability to ingest food
Risk for fluid volume deficit r/t decreased intake, loss of fluids with vomiting

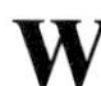

W

Weakness

Fatigue r/t decreased or increased metabolic energy production

Weight Gain

Altered nutrition: more than body requirements r/t excessive intake in relation to metabolic need

Weight Loss

Altered nutrition: less than body requirements r/t inability to ingest food due to biological, psychological, or economic factors

Wellness-Seeking Behavior

Health-seeking behavior r/t expressed desire for increased control of health practice

Wheezing

Ineffective airway clearance r/t tracheobronchial obstructions or secretions

Withdrawal from Alcohol

Refer to Alcohol Withdrawal

Withdrawal from Drugs

Refer to Drug Withdrawal

Wound Debridement

Impaired tissue integrity r/t debridement, open wound
Pain r/t debridement of wound
Risk for infection r/t open wound, presence of bacteria

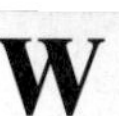

Wound Dehiscence, Evisceration

Altered nutrition: less than body requirements r/t inability to digest nutrients, need for increased protein for healing

Fear r/t client fear of body parts falling out, surgical procedure not going as planned

Risk for fluid volume deficit r/t inability to ingest nutrients, obstruction, fluid loss

Risk for injury r/t exposed abdominal contents

Wound Infection

Altered nutrition: less than body requirements r/t biological factors, infection, hyperthermia

Body image disturbance r/t dysfunctional open wound

Hyperthermia r/t increased metabolic rate, illness, infection

Impaired tissue integrity r/t wound, presence of infection

Risk for fluid volume deficit r/t increased metabolic rate

Risk for infection (spread of) r/t altered nutrition: less than body requirements

Section III

Guide to Planning Care

Activity intolerance

Linda Straight and Gwethalyn Edwards

Definition The state in which an individual has insufficient physiological or psychological energy to endure or complete required or desired daily activities.

Defining Characteristics

*Verbal report of fatigue or weakness; abnormal heart rate or blood pressure in response to activity; exertional discomfort or dyspnea; electrocardiographic changes reflecting dysrhythmias or ischemia; changes in skin color or moisture. (*Critical)

Related Factors (r/t)

Bedrest or immobility; generalized weakness; sedentary life-style; imbalance between oxygen supply and demand.

Client Outcomes/Goals

- Participates in prescribed physical activity with appropriate increases in heart rate, blood pressure, and breathing rate; monitor patterns (rhythm and ST segment) remain within normal limits.
- States symptoms of adverse effects of exercise and reports onset of symptoms immediately.
- Skin color remains normal and is warm and dry with activity.
- Verbalizes an understanding of the need to gradually increase activity based on testing, tolerance, and symptoms.
- Expresses an understanding of the need to balance rest and activity.
- Demonstrates increased activity tolerance.

Nursing Interventions and Rationales

- Determine cause of activity intolerance (refer to related factors) and determine if its cause is physical, psychological, or motivational.
  Determining the cause of a disease can help direct appropriate interventions.
- Monitor and record client's ability to tolerate activity; note pulse rate, blood pressure, monitor pattern, dyspnea, use of accessory muscles, and skin color before and after activity.
  If the following signs and symptoms of cardiac decompensation develop, activity should be stopped immediately:
  - *Excessive fatigue*
  - *Lightheadedness, confusion, ataxia, pallor, cyanosis, dyspnea, nausea, or any peripheral circulatory insufficiency*
  - *Onset of angina with exercise*
  - *Palpitations*
  - *Dysrhythmias (symptomatic supraventricular tachycardia, ventricular tachycardia, exercise-induced left bundle branch block, second or third degree atrioventricular block, frequent premature ventricular contractions*
  - *Exercise hypotension (>20 mm Hg drop in systolic blood pressure during exercise)*
  - *Excessive rise in blood pressure (systolic >220 mm Hg or diastolic >110 mm Hg) Note: these are upper limits; activity may be stopped before reaching these values*
  - *Inappropriate bradycardia (drop in heart rate greater than 10 beats/min) with no change or an increase in workload*
  - *Increased heart rate above the prescribed limit (Pate et al, 1991)*
- Instruct client to stop activity immediately and report to physician if he or she experiences the following symptoms: new or worsened intensity or increased frequency

of discomfort, tightness, or pressure in chest, back, neck, jaw, shoulders, and/or arms; palpitations; dizziness; weakness; unusual and extreme fatigue; excessive air hunger. *These are common symptoms of angina and are caused by a temporary insufficiency of coronary blood supply. Symptoms typically last for minutes as opposed to momentary twinges. If symptoms last longer than 5 to 10 minutes, the client should be evaluated by a physician (McGoon, 1993). The client should be evaluated before resuming activity (Thompson, 1988).*

- Teach client the need to pace activity and rest after meals. *Rest periods decrease oxygen consumption (Prizant-Weston, Castiglia, 1992).*
- Refer the cardiac client to cardiac rehabilitation for assistance in developing safe exercise guidelines based on testing and medications. *Cardiac rehabilitation personnel have expertise in helping clients safely maximize their exercise potential.*
- Ensure that the chronic pulmonary client has had O_2 saturation testing with exercise; use supplemental oxygen as prescribed when ambulating client. *Some clients need supplemental oxygen to safely ambulate; follow physician's guidelines.*
- Refer the chronic pulmonary client to a pulmonary rehabilitation program. *Pulmonary rehabilitation has been shown to improve exercise capacity, walking ability, and a sense of well-being (Fishman, 1994).*
- Observe for pain before activity and, if possible, treat pain before activity. *Pain restricts the client from achieving a maximum activity level and is often exacerbated by movement.*
- Obtain any necessary assistive devices or equipment needed before ambulating client (e.g., walkers, canes, crutches, portable oxygen). *Assistive devices can increase mobility by helping the client overcome limitations.*
- Use a walking belt when ambulating the client. *With a walking belt, the client can walk independently, yet the nurse can ensure safety if the client's knees buckle.*
- Refer to physical therapy for help in increasing activity levels.
- Work with client to set mutual goals that increase activity levels.
- Perform passive range-of-motion exercises if client is unable to tolerate activity. *Inactivity rapidly contributes to muscle shortening and changes in periarticular and cartilagenous joint structure. These factors contribute to contracture and limitation of motion (Creditor, 1993).*
- Encourage client to change position from supine to sitting several times daily and to avoid prolonged bedrest. *Immobilization and enforced bedrest in the supine position have considerable adverse effects on nearly every system in the body (Hoenig, Rubenstein, 1991).*

Geriatric

- Slow the pace of care; allow client extra time to carry out activities.
- When mobilizing the elderly client, watch for orthostatic hypotension accompanied by dizziness and fainting. *Orthostatic hypotension is common in the elderly as a result of cardiovascular changes, chronic diseases, and medication effects (Mobily, Kelley, 1991).*

Client/Family Teaching

- Instruct client in the use of relaxation techniques during activity.
- Teach client how to use assistive devices or medications before or during activity.
- Help client set up an activity log to record exercise and exercise tolerance.

REFERENCES

Casaburi R, Petty T: *Principles and practice of pulmonary rehabilitation*, Philadelphia, 1993, WB Saunders.

Convertino VA: Effect of orthostatic stress on exercise performance after bedrest: relation to in-hospital rehabilitation, *J Cardiac Rehabil* 3:660-663, 1983.

Creditor M: Hazards of hospitalization of the elderly, *Ann Intern Med* 149:825-833, 1994.

Fishman AP: Pulmonary rehabilitation research, *Resp Crit Care Med* 149:825-833, 1994.

Hoenig H, Rubenstein L: Hospital-associated deconditioning and dysfunction, *J Am Geriatr Soc* 39:220-222, 1991.

McGoon M: *Mayo Clinic heart book,* New York, 1993, William Morrow.

Mobily PR, Kelley LS: Iatrogenesis in the elderly: factors of immobility, *J Gerontol Nurs* 17(9):5-12, 1991.

Pate RR et al: *Guidelines for exercise testing and prescription,* ed 4, Philadelphia, 1991, Lea & Febiger.

Prizant-Weston M, Castiglia K: Hemodynamic regulation. In Bulecheck GM, McCloskey JC, editors: *Nursing interventions: essential nursing treatments,* Philadelphia, 1992, WB Saunders.

BIBLIOGRAPHY

Bolander VB: Meeting mobility needs. In *Sorensen and Luckmann's basic nursing: a psychophysiologic approach,* Philadelphia, 1994, WB Saunders.

MacVicar MG, Winningham ML, Nickel JL: Effects of aerobic interval training on cancer patients' functional capacity, *Nurs Res* 38:348-351, 1989.

Thompson P: The safety of exercise testing and participation. In Blair SN et al, editors: *Resource manual for guidelines for exercise testing and prescriptions,* Philadelphia, 1988, Lea & Febiger.

Risk for activity intolerance

Definition The state in which an individual is at risk of experiencing insufficient physiological or psychological energy to endure or complete required or desired daily activities.

Defining Characteristics

Presence of risk factors such as history of intolerance to activity; deconditioned status; presence of circulatory or respiratory problems; inexperience with activity.

Related Factors (r/t)

Refer to risk factors.

Client Outcomes/Goals, Nursing Interventions and Rationales, Client/Family Teaching

Refer to care plan for **Activity intolerance**.

Impaired adjustment

Gail Ladwig

Definition The state in which an individual is unable to modify his or her life-style or behavior in a manner consistent with a change in health status.

Defining Characteristics

Major Verbalized nonacceptance of health status change; nonexistent or unsuccessful involvement in problem solving or goal setting.

Minor Lack of movement toward independence; extended period of shock, disbelief, or anger regarding change in health status; lack of future-oriented thinking.

Related Factors (r/t)

Disability that requires change in life-style; inadequate support systems; impaired cognition; sensory overload; assault to self-esteem; altered locus of control; incomplete grieving.

Client Outcomes/Goals

- States acceptance of change in health status.
- Lists behaviors needed to adjust to change in health status.
- States personal goals for dealing with change in health status.
- Experiences a period of grief that is proportional to the actual or perceived effect of the loss.

Nursing Interventions and Rationales

- Monitor the physical and psychological degree of the change in health status.
  Knowing the degree of change helps determine appropriate interventions.
- Allow client time to express feelings about the change in health status.
  Verbalization of feelings leads to acceptance and understanding of changes. The client cannot be pushed into coping with the change in health status (Johnson, 1994).
- Help client work through the stages of grief. Denial is usually the initial response; acknowledge that grief takes time and give client permission to grieve; accept crying.
  Acceptance of feelings conveys empathy and promotes movement toward adjustment.
- Discuss with client resources that have worked previously in dealing with changes in life-style or health.
  Past successes can often be repeated, and the client needs to build on existing skills.
- Use open-ended questions to allow the client free expression (e.g., say to the client, "Tell me about your last hospitalization" or "How does this time compare?").
  Open-ended questions allow the client to be more actively involved in the interaction.
- Discuss client's current goals; if appropriate, have client list goals so he or she can refer to them and take steps to accomplish them.
  Self-monitoring serves an important role in the maintenance of internal standards of behavior (Fleury, 1991).
- List client activities that may require assistance and activities that can be performed independently.
  This list gives the client permission to ask for help and informs the client that outside resources are available.
- Allow client choices in daily care, particularly choices that result from the change in health status.
  To perceive ownership of change, the client needs to value the proposed change, feel able to carry it out, and accept responsibility for it (Fleury, 1991).
- Allow client time to adjust to new situation; introduce new material gradually to prevent overload; ask for frequent feedback.

The stress of changes in health care can be overwhelming. New material takes longer to learn and absorb; thus clarification of information and frequent repetition may be necessary.

- Give client positive feedback for accomplishments, no matter how small.
  Positive reinforcement encourages repetition.
- Manipulate environment to decrease stress.
  The change in health status is producing enough stress; thus the environment should be as trouble-free as possible.
- Maintain consistency and continuity in daily schedule.
  Such measures provide some constancy in the client's life.

Geriatric

- Assess for signs of depression resulting from illness-associated changes.
  The elderly are at risk of depression when living with a chronic illness (Badger, 1993).
- Monitor client for agitation.
  The elderly often use agitation to express an inability to accept change.

Client/Family Teaching

- Help client to list current strengths.
  Focusing on positives discourages negative thoughts.
- Allow client to proceed at own pace in learning; provide time for return demonstrations (e.g., self-injection of insulin). Use clear and distinct language free of medical jargon and meaningless values.
  Everyone learns at his or her own pace, and some clients need frequent repetition. A comfortable teaching atmosphere allows for openness and comfort when delivering disturbing information and facilitates trust (Hopkins, 1994).
- Initiate community referrals as needed (e.g., grief counseling, self-help groups).
  Groups help the client to know that he or she is "not alone."
- Involve significant others in planning and teaching.
  The support of significant others facilitates desired changes through their role in acknowledging and encouraging change. Through positive reinforcement and an expression of congruency in behavioral change, supportive others often serve as powerful external motivators (Fleury, 1991).

REFERENCES

Badger T: Physical health impairment and depression among older adults, *Image J Nurs Sch* 25:325-330, 1993.

Fleury D: Empowering potential: a theory of wellness motivation, *Nurs Res* 40:286-291, 1991.

Hopkins A: The trauma nurse's role with families in crisis, *Crit Care Nurse* 14(2):35-42, 1994.

Johnson J: Caring for the woman who's had a mastectomy, *Am J Nurs* 94(5):25-31, 1994.

Ineffective airway clearance

Gwethalyn Edwards and Betty Ackley

Definition The state in which an individual is unable to clear secretions or obstructions from the respiratory tract.

Defining Characteristics

Abnormal breath sounds (e.g., rales [crackles], rhonchi [wheezes]); changes in rate or depth of respiration; tachypnea; cough (effective or ineffective and with or without sputum); cyanosis; dyspnea.

Related Factors (r/t)

Decreased energy; fatigue; tracheobronchial infection; obstruction; secretions; perceptual or cognitive impairment; trauma.

Client Outcomes/Goals

- Demonstrates effective coughing and clear breath sounds; free of cyanosis and dyspnea.
- Maintains a patent airway at all times.
- Relates methods to enhance secretion removal.
- Relates the significance of changes in sputum to include color, character, amount, and odor.
- Free of signs of aspiration.

Nursing Interventions and Rationales

- Auscultate breath sounds q________h.
  Breathing sounds are normally clear or scattered fine crackles at bases that clear with deep breathing. The presence of course crackles during late inspiration indicates fluid in the airways; wheezing indicates an airway obstruction.
- Monitor respiratory patterns to include rate, depth, and effort.
  A normal respiratory rate for the adult without dyspnea is 12-16.
- Monitor blood gas values.
  Normal blood gas values are Po_2 *80 to 100 and* Pco_2 *35 to 45. Hypoxemia can result from diffusion defects or ventilation perfusion mismatches secondary to secretions.*
- Position client to optimize respiration (e.g., elevate head of bed 30 to 45 degrees and reposition at least every 2 hours).
  An upright position allows for maximal air exchange and lung expansion; lying flat causes abdominal organs to shift toward the chest, which crowds the lungs and makes it more difficult to breathe.
- If the client has unilateral lung disease, alternate a semi-Fowler's position with a lateral position (with a 10 to 15 degree elevation and "good lung down") for 60 to 90 min; this method is contraindicated for the client with a pulmonary abscess or hemorrhage or interstitial emphysema.
  Gravity and hydrostatic pressure allow the dependent lung to become better ventilated and perfused, which increases oxygenation (Yeaw, 1992).
- Help client to deep breathe and cough.
  Controlled coughing uses the diaphragmatic muscles, which makes the cough more forceful and effective.
- Suction as needed on the basis of changes in lung sounds. Hyperoxygenate before, between, and after endotracheal suction sessions, even if using a closed tracheal suction system. Avoid using saline instillation during suctioning.
  Nursing research has demonstrated that the client should be hyperventilated when suctioning if using either the open- or closed-suction system (Winslow, 1993). Saline

instillation before suctioning has an adverse effect on oxygen saturation (Ackerman, 1993).

- Document results of coughing and suctioning, particularly client tolerance and secretion characteristics.
- Encourage activity and ambulation as tolerated; if unable to ambulate client, turn client from side to side at frequent intervals.
  Body movement helps mobilize secretions.
- Encourage fluids if not contraindicated.
  Fluids help minimize mucosal drying and maximize ciliary action to move secretions (Carroll, 1994).
- Administer oxygen as ordered.
  Oxygen has been shown to correct hypoxemia.
- Administer medications such as bronchodilators if ordered; watch for side effects such as tachycardia or anxiety.
  Bronchodilators decrease airway resistance secondary to bronchoconstriction.

Geriatric

- Encourage ambulation as tolerated without causing exhaustion.
  Immobility is often harmful to the elderly because it decreases ventilation and increases stasis of secretions, which leads to atelectasis or pneumonia (Hoyt, 1992).
- Actively encourage the elderly to deep breathe and cough.
  Cough reflexes are blunted, and coughing is decreased in the elderly (Sparrow, Weiss, 1988).
- Ensure adequate hydration within cardiac and renal reserves.
  The elderly are prone to dehydration, and therefore more viscous secretions, because they frequently use diuretics or laxatives and forget to drink adequate amounts of water (Hoyt, 1992).

Client/Family Teaching

- Teach client how to deep breathe and cough effectively.
  Controlled coughing uses the diaphragmatic muscles, which makes the cough more forceful and effective.
- Teach client the significance of rest periods between short periods of exertion.
- Educate client and family about the significance of changes in sputum production, including color, character, amount, and odor.
  With this knowledge the client and family can identify signs of infection early and seek treatment before acute illness occurs.

REFERENCES

Ackerman MI: Ask the experts, *Crit Care Nurse*, 13(3):103-104, 1993.
Carroll P: Safe suctioning prn, *RN* 57(5):32-37, 1994.
Hoyt MM: Impaired gas exchange in the elderly, *Geriatr Nurs* 13(5):262-268, 1992.
Sparrow D, Weiss S: Pulmonary system. In Rose JW, Besdine RS, editors: *Geriatric medicine*, Boston, 1988, Little, Brown.
Winslow EH: Open-and-closed debate on hyperoxygenation: working smart, *Am J Nurs* 13:16, 1993.
Yeaw P: Good lung down, *Am J Nurs* 92(3):27-32, 1992.

BIBLIOGRAPHY

Dam V, Wild MC, Baun MM: Effect of oxygen insufflation during endotracheal suctioning on arterial pressure and oxygenation in coronary artery bypass graft patients, *Am J Crit Care* 3:191-197, 1994.
Redick EL: Closed-system, in-line endotracheal suctioning, *Crit Care Nurse* 13:47-51, 1993.

Altered family process: alcoholism

Jane Curtis

Definition The state in which the psychosocial, spiritual, and physiological functions of the family unit are chronically disorganized, which leads to conflict, denial of problems, resistance to change, ineffective problem solving, and a series of self-perpetuating crises.

Defining Characteristics

Major *Feelings*: Decreased self-esteem; worthlessness; anger; suppressed rage; frustration; powerlessness; anxiety; tension; distress; insecurity; repressed emotions; responsibility for alcoholic's behavior; lingering resentment; shame; embarrassment; hurt; unhappiness; guilt; emotional isolation; loneliness; vulnerability; mistrust; hopelessness; rejection.

Roles and Relationships: Deterioration in family relationships; disturbed family dynamics; ineffective spouse communication; marital problems; altered role function; disruption of family roles; inconsistent parenting; low perception of parental support; family denial; intimacy dysfunction; chronic family problems; closed communication systems.

Behaviors: Inappropriate expression of anger; difficulty with intimate relationships; loss of control of drinking; impaired communication; ineffective problem-solving skills; enabling to maintain drinking; inability to meet emotional needs of family members; manipulation; dependence; criticizing; alcohol abuse; broken promises; rationalization; denial of problems; refusal to get help; inability to appropriately accept and receive help; blaming; inadequate understanding or knowledge of alcoholism.

Minor *Feelings*: Feeling different from other people; depression; hostility; fear; emotional control by others; confusion; dissatisfaction; loss; misunderstood; abandonment; confused love and pity; moodiness; failure; being unloved; lack of identity.

Roles and Relationships: Triangulating family relationships/reduced ability of family members to relate to each other for mutual growth and maturation; lack of skills necessary for relationships; lack of cohesiveness; disrupted family rituals; inability of family to meet security needs of its members; lack of respect for individuality and autonomy of family members; patterns of rejection; economic problems; neglected obligations.

Behaviors: Inability to meet spiritual needs of its members; inability to express or accept a wide range of feelings; orientation to tension relief rather than achievement of goals; alcohol-centered family special occasions; escalating conflict; lying; contradictory or paradoxical communication; lack of dealing with conflict; harsh self-judgment; isolation; nicotine addiction; difficulty having fun; self-blaming; unresolved grief; controlled communication; power struggles; inability to adapt to change; immaturity; stress-related physical illnesses; inability to constructively deal with traumatic experiences; seeking of approval and affirmation; lack of reliability; disturbances in academic performance in children; disturbances in concentration; chaos; abuse of substances other than alcohol; failure to accomplish current or past developmental tasks; difficulty with life cycle transitions; verbal abuse of spouse or parent; agitation; diminished physical contact.

Related Factors (r/t)

Abuse of alcohol; family history of alcoholism; resistance to treatment; inadequate coping skills; genetic predisposition; addictive personality; lack of problem-solving skills; biochemical influences.

Client Outcomes/Goals

- Family members develop a relationship with the nurse that demonstrates at least a minimal level of trust.

- Family members demonstrate an understanding of alcoholism as a family illness and the severity of the threat to emotional and physical health of family members.
- Family members develop a belief in the feasibility and effectiveness of efforts to address the alcoholism.
- Family begins to change dysfunctional patterns by moving from inappropriate to appropriate role relationships, improving cohesion among family members, decreasing conflict and social isolation, and improving coping behaviors.
- Family maintains improvements.

Nursing Interventions and Rationales

- Demonstrate high levels of empathy and expectancy of positive outcomes in interactions with family members.
  Empathy as evidenced by respect, warmth, sympathetic understanding, supportiveness, caring, concern, commitment, and interest has been found to be the most important caregiver trait that affects motivation for treatment among alcoholic clients. The client's perception that the caregiver wants to help and that a positive outcome can be achieved increases commitment and willingness to be influenced (Miller, 1985). Presenting families with realistic facts in a nonjudgmental manner facilitates participation in treatment (Task Force, ANA, 1987).
- Educate family members about alcoholism and the available educational and support programs (e.g., Al-Anon, Al-A-Teen, community education, individual or group therapy) and encourage participation. Stress individual self-focus as a first step in problem resolution.
  Health Beliefs Model Research confirms that client understanding of the severity of the threat to personal and family health and a belief in the feasibility and effectiveness of treatment are important motivating factors in changing health-related behavior (Damrosch, 1991; Giuffra, 1993). Family members can benefit themselves, the family, and the client through self-focus and participation in education and support activities (Williams, 1989; Captain, 1989). The perception of choice enhances motivation and improves compliance and outcome (Miller, 1985).
- When completing a family assessment, include demographic data, physical and emotional health of individuals, current family structure and roles, communication patterns, relationships among members, current stressors and conflicts, family cohesion, coping behaviors, shared interests and activities, resources and supports, knowledge of the problem, and expectations for recovery.
  NOTE: Assessment factors are included under interventions because it has been noted that assessment questions initiate a family process of self-examination and family problem solving and also provide assessment data (Craft, Willadsen, 1992).
  Most families are not aware of their adjustment to the addictive behavior, and family structure and function may be altered (e.g., a child assuming a parent's role in absence of parent appropriateness). In addition, individual family members or the family unit itself may be experiencing biological, cognitive, or spiritual responses that require separate interventions (Task Force, ANA, 1987; Captain, 1989). The range of possible nursing interventions required for the family members is extremely broad, and the nurse is advised to consult Standards of Addictions Nursing for assistance (Task Force, ANA, 1987).
- Help family to restructure family patterns of interaction and function that support the development of consistency, a predictable environment, emotional nurturance, and positive modeling.

Studies indicate that consistency, a predictable environment, emotional nurturance, and positive social modeling may act as ameliorating factors in the dysfunctional environment (Roberts, 1992; Sielhamer, Jacob, Dunn, 1993). Clinical reports and research also indicate that recovery is partially contingent on the restructuring of family interaction patterns. In assisting the family, the generalist nurse becomes a role model, counselor, educator, and promoter of effective interactions, self-care, and referral sources by using principles of nursing care derived from medical, surgical, psychiatric, and community health nursing. The nurse specialist, who has had specialty training and advanced education, may serve as family therapist (Task Force, ANA, 1987).

- Assist with stabilization and maintenance of positive change in the family. Focus on the continued use of resources, including the need for more extensive resources such as marital counseling, which may become apparent as family dynamics change. To form a basis for realistic and objective evaluation of family changes, continue to provide education pertinent to the appropriate stage of family improvement. Support increasing social contacts and family recreational activities, and use contracting or homework assignment techniques to encourage positive behaviors. Monitor family closely for return to old patterns of behavior.
  The improvement of family interaction is an important condition for maintaining change. Family cohesion is fostered through the sharing of positive and fun experiences and is a critical factor in lasting recovery (Captain, 1989). A return to previous behavior patterns, termed relapse, occurs most frequently within the first 3 months. Factors that have been useful in relapse prevention are education, social support, skills training, reinforcement, recreational activities, and the practice of new behaviors (Jones, 1990). Continuation and compliance are behaviors that are influenced by maintaining contact with an empathetic caregiver (Miller, 1985). There is evidence that success is achieved only after several relapses, and the effort to succeed is enhanced by knowledge, skills training, support and self-help groups, and other techniques (Damrosch, 1991).

REFERENCES

Captain C: Family recovery from alcoholism, mediating family factors, *Nurs Clin North Am* 24:55-67, 1989.

Craft MJ, Willadsen JA: Interventions related to family, *Nurs Clin North Am* 27:517-527, 1992.

Damrosch S: General strategies for motivating people to change their behavior, *Nurs Clin North Am* 26:833-843, 1991.

Giuffra MJ: Nursing strategies with alcohol and drug problems in the family. In Naegle MA, editor: *Substance Abuse in Education in Nursing Vol. III,* National League for Nursing Press, New York, Publication No. 15-2464.

Jones, J: A proposed model of relapse prevention for adolescents who abuse alcohol, *J Child Adol Psychiatr Ment Health Nurs* 3:139-143, 1990.

Miller WR: Motivation for treatment: a review with special emphasis on alcoholism, *Psychol Bull* 98:84-107, 1985.

Roberts BJ: Adult children of alcoholics, *J Am Acad Nurse Pract* 4:22-26, 1992.

Sielhamer RA, Jacob T, Dunn NJ: The impact of alcohol consumption on parent-child relationships in families of alcoholics, *J Stud Alcohol* 54:189-198, 1993.

Task Force on Substance Abuse Nursing Practice: *The care of clients with addictions, dimensions of nursing practice,* American Nurses Association, 2420 Pershing Road, Kansas City, Mo, 1987.

Williams, E: Strategies for intervention, *Nurs Clin North Am* 24:95-107, 1989.

BIBLIOGRAPHY

Task Force on Substance Abuse Nursing Practice: *Standards of addictions nursing practice with selected diagnosis and criteria,* American Nurses Association, 2420 Pershing Road, Kansas City, Mo, 1988.

Anxiety

Pam Bifano Schweitzer

Definition A vague, uneasy feeling whose source is often nonspecific or unknown to the individual.

Defining Characteristics

Subjective Increased tension; apprehension; painful and persistent feelings; increased helplessness; uncertainty; fear; regret; overexcitement; rattled, distressed, or jittery feelings; feelings of inadequacy; shakiness; fear of unspecific consequences; expressed concerns regarding changes in life events; worry; anxiety.

Objective Sympathetic stimulation evidenced by cardiovascular excitation, superficial vasoconstriction, or pupil dilation; restlessness; insomnia; darting glances; poor eye contact; trembling or hand tremors; extraneous movement (e.g., foot shuffling, hand or arm movements); facial tension; quivering voice; self-focusing; increased wariness; increased perspiration.

Related Factors (r/t)

Unconscious conflict regarding essential values or goals of life; threat to self-concept; threat of death; threat to or change in health status; threat to or change in environment; threat to or change in interaction patterns; situational or maturational crises; interpersonal transmission of contagion; unmet needs.

Client Outcomes/Goals

- Identifies and verbalizes symptoms of anxiety.
- Identifies, verbalizes, and demonstrates techniques to control anxiety.
- Verbalizes absence of or decrease in subjective distress.
- Vital signs reflect baseline or decreased sympathetic stimulation.
- Posture, facial expressions, gestures, and activity levels reflect decreased distress.
- Demonstrates improved concentration and accuracy of thoughts.
- Identifies and verbalizes anxiety precipitants, conflicts, and threats.
- Demonstrates return of basic problem-solving skills.
- Demonstrates increased external focus.
- Demonstrates some ability to reassure self.

Nursing Interventions and Rationales

- Assess client's level of anxiety and physical reactions to anxiety (e.g., tachycardia, tachypnea, nonverbal expressions of anxiety); validate observations by saying to client, "Are you feeling anxious now?"
  Anxiety is a highly individualized, normal, physical, and psychological response to internal or external life events (Badger, 1994).
- Use presence, touch (with permission), verbalization, or demeanor to remind client that he or she is not alone and to encourage expression or clarification of needs, concerns, unknowns, and questions.
  Being supportive and approachable encourages communication.
- Accept client's defenses; do not confront, argue, or debate.
  If defenses are not threatened, the client may feel safe enough to look at behavior (Clunn, Payne, 1982).
- Allow and reinforce client's personal reaction to or expression of pain, discomfort, or threats to well-being (e.g., talking, crying, walking, other physical or nonverbal expressions).
  Talking or otherwise expressing feelings sometimes reduces anxiety.

- Help client identify precipitants of anxiety, which may indicate interventions.
  Gaining insight enables the client to reevaluate the threat or identify new ways to deal with the threat (Beck, Emery, 1985).
- If the situational response is rational, use empathy to encourage client to interpret the anxiety symptoms as normal.
  Anxiety is a normal response to actual or perceived danger (Peplau, 1963).
- If irrational thoughts or fears are present, offer client accurate information.
  Correcting mistaken beliefs reduces anxiety.
- Avoid excessive reassurance, which may reinforce undue worry.
  "Reassurance is not helpful for the anxious individual" (Clunn, Payne, 1982, p. 105).
- Intervene when possible to remove sources of anxiety.
  Anxiety is a normal response to actual or perceived danger; if the threat is removed, the response will stop.
- Explain all activities, procedures, and issues that involve the client; use nonmedical terms and calm, slow speech. Do this in advance of procedures when possible, and validate client's understanding.
  Uncertainty and lack of predictability contribute to anxiety.
- Explore coping skills previously used by client to relieve anxiety; reinforce these skills and explore other outlets.
  Methods of coping with anxiety that have been successful in the past are likely to be helpful again.
- Rule out withdrawal from alcohol, sedatives, or smoking as the cause of anxiety.
  Withdrawal from these substances is characterized by anxiety (Badger, 1994).
- Identify and limit, discontinue, or be aware of the use of any stimulants such as caffeine, nicotine, theophylline, terbutaline sulfate, amphetamines, and cocaine.
  Many substances cause or potentiate anxiety symptoms.

Geriatric

- Monitor client for depression; use appropriate interventions.
  Anxiety often accompanies or masks depression in elderly adults.
- Provide a protective and safe environment; use consistent caregivers and maintain the accustomed environmental structure.
  Elderly clients tend to have more perceptual impairments and adapt to changes with more difficulty, especially during an illness.
- Observe for adverse changes if antianxiety drugs are taken.
  Age renders clients more sensitive to both the clinical and toxic effects of many agents.
- Provide a quiet environment with diversion.
  Excessive noise increases anxiety; involvement in a quiet activity can be soothing to the elderly.

Client/Family Teaching

- Teach client and family symptoms of anxiety.
  If client and family can identify anxious responses, they can intervene earlier.
- Help client to define anxiety levels (from "easily tolerated" to "intolerable") and select appropriate interventions.
  Mild anxiety enhances learning and adaptation, but moderate to severe anxiety may impede or immobilize progress (Peplau, 1963).
- If antianxiety medications have been prescribed, teach client how to use them appropriately.
- Teach client to identify and use distraction or diversion tactics when possible.
  Early interruption of the anxious response prevents escalation.

- Teach client to allow anxious thoughts and feelings to be present until they dissipate.
  Allowing and even devoting time and energy to a thought, purposefully and repetitively, reduces associated anxiety (Beck, Emery, 1985).
- Teach progressive muscle relaxation techniques.
- Teach relaxation breathing for occasional use; teach client to breathe in through nose, fill slowly from abdomen upward, and think "re," and then breathe out through mouth, from chest downward, and think "lax."
- Teach to visualize or fantasize absence of anxiety or pain, successful experience of the situation, resolution of conflict, or outcome of procedure.
- Teach relationship between a healthy physical and emotional life-style and a realistic mental attitude.
  Health and well-being are influenced by how well defined and met needs are in areas of safety, diet, exercise, sleep, work, pleasure, and social belonging.
- Teach use of appropriate community resources in emergency situations such as hotline, emergency rooms, law enforcement, and judicial systems.
- Encourage use of appropriate community resources in emergency situations such as family, friends, neighbors, self-help and support groups, volunteer agencies, churches, clubs and centers for recreation, and others with similar interests.

REFERENCES

Badger JM: Calming the anxious patient, *Am J Nurs* 94(5):46-50, 1994.

Beck AT, Emery G: *Anxiety disorders and phobias: a cognitive perspective*, New York, 1985, Basic Books.

Clunn PA, Payne DB: *Psychiatric mental health nursing*, Garden City, NJ, 1982, Medical Examination Publishing.

Peplau H: A working definition of anxiety. In Burd S, Marshall M, editors: *Some clinical approaches to psychiatric nursing*, New York, 1963, MacMillan.

BIBLIOGRAPHY

Bandura A: Self-efficacy: toward a unified theory of behavior change, *Psychol Serv* 84:191, 1977.

Beck AT: Theoretical perspectives on clinical anxiety. In Tuma SH, Maser J, editors: *Anxiety and the anxiety disorders*, Hillsdale, 1985, Lawrence Erlbaum Associates.

Griest JH, Jefferson JW, Marks IM: *Anxiety and its treatment: help is available*, District of Columbia, 1986, American Psychiatric Press.

Wolpe J: *The practice of behavior therapy*, New York, 1970, Pergamon.

Risk for aspiration

Betty Ackley

Definition The state in which an individual is at risk for entry of gastrointestinal secretions, oropharyngeal secretions, or solids or fluids into the tracheobronchial passages.

Defining Characteristics

Presence of risk factors such as reduced level of consciousness; depressed cough and gag reflexes; presence of tracheostomy or endotracheal tube; incomplete lower esophageal sphincter; gastrointestinal tubes; tube feeding; medication administration; situations hindering elevation of upper body; increased gastrointestinal motility; delayed gastric emptying; impaired swallowing; facial, oral, or neck surgery or trauma; wired jaws.

Related Factors (r/t)

Refer to risk factors.

Client Outcomes/Goals

- Swallows and digests oral, nasogastric, or gastric feeding without aspiration.
- Maintains patent airway and clear lung sounds.

Nursing Interventions and Rationales

- Monitor respiratory rate, depth, and effort; note any signs of aspiration such as dyspnea, cough, cyanosis, wheezing, or fever.
  Signs of aspiration should be detected as soon as possible to prevent further aspiration and to initiate treatment that can be lifesaving. Because of laryngeal pooling and residue in the client with dysphagia, silent aspiration that is not manifested by choking or coughing may occur.
- Auscultate lung sounds q_______h and before and after feedings; note any new onset of crackles or wheezing.
- Take vital signs q_______h.
- Before initiating oral feeding, check client's gag reflex and ability to swallow by feeling above and below the thyroid cartilage as the client attempts to swallow.
  It is important to check the client's ability to swallow before feeding. A client can aspirate even with an intact gag reflex (Baker, 1993).
- When feeding client, watch for signs of impaired swallowing or aspiration, including coughing, choking, spitting food, or excessive drooling. If client is having problems swallowing, refer to nursing interventions for **Impaired swallowing**.
- Have suction machine available for high-risk clients.
- Keep head of bed elevated when feeding and for at least a half hour afterwards.
  This position helps keep food in the stomach and decreases aspiration.
- Note presence of any nausea, vomiting, or diarrhea.
- Listen to bowel sounds q_______h, listening for decreased, absent, or hyperactive bowel sounds.
  Decreased or absent bowel sounds can indicate an ileus with possible vomiting and aspiration; increased high-pitched bowel sounds can indicate mechanical bowel obstruction with possible vomiting and aspiration.
- Note new onset of abdominal distention or increased rigidity of abdomen.
  Abdominal distention or rigidity can be associated with paralytic or mechanical obstruction and an increased likelihood of vomiting and aspiration.
- If client has a tracheostomy, check for inflation of the tracheostomy cuff before initiating feeding per physician's order; avoid overinflating the cuff.

The presence of a tracheostomy tube increases the incidence of aspiration; inflating the cuff may help decrease aspiration, but overinflating the cuff predisposes the client to aspiration by compression of the esophagus (Elpern, Jacobs, Bone, 1987).

- Feed or hydrate client only during formal rest periods from restraints.
- If client shows symptoms of nausea and vomiting, position on side.
- If client needs to be fed, feed slowly and allow adequate time for chewing and swallowing.

Enteral Feedings

- Check to make sure initial feeding tube placement was confirmed by x-ray, especially if a small-bore feeding tube is used; keep feeding tube securely taped.
  X-ray verification of placement is the only consistently reliable method to detect inadvertent respiratory placement (Metheny et al, 1990).
- Determine placement of feeding tube before each feeding or every 4 hours if continuous feeding. Check pH of aspirate; do not rely on air insufflation method.
  The auscultatory air insufflation method is often not reliable in differentiating between gastric or respiratory placement. pH testing can generally predict feeding tube position in the gastrointestinal tract (Metheny et al, 1990; Metheny et al, 1993).
- Check for gastric residual at least every 8 hours and before feedings; if greater than 100 ml, follow institutional protocol on holding feeding.
  Increased intragastric pressure can result in regurgitation and aspiration.
- If ordered by physician, put several drops of blue or green food coloring in tube feeding to help indicate aspiration.
  Colored secretions suctioned or coughed from the respiratory tract indicate aspiration (Ackerman, 1993).
- During feeding, position client with head of bed elevated at least 30 degrees, preferably higher; maintain for 30 to 45 minutes after feeding.
  Keeping the client's head elevated helps keep food in stomach and decreases incidence of aspiration.
- Stop continual feeding temporarily when turning or moving client.
  It is difficult to keep the head elevated when turning or moving a client.

Geriatric

- Carefully check elderly client's gag reflex and ability to swallow before feeding.
  Laryngeal nerve endings are reduced in the elderly, which diminishes the gag reflex (Close, Woodson, 1989).
- Use central nervous system depressants cautiously; the elderly client may have an increased incidence of aspiration with altered levels of consciousness.
  Elderly clients have altered metabolism, distribution, and excretion of drugs; some medications can interfere with the swallowing reflex.

Client/Family Teaching

- Teach client and family signs of aspiration and the precautions needed to prevent aspiration.
- Teach client and family how to safely administer tube feeding.

REFERENCES

Ackerman MI: Ask the experts, *Crit Care Nurse*, 13(3):103-104, 1993.

Baker DM: Assessment and management of impairments in swallowing, *Nurs Clin North Am* 28:793-805, 1993.

Close LG, Woodson GE: Common upper airway disorders in the elderly and their management, *Geriatrics* 44(1):67-72, 1989.

Elpern EH, Jacobs ER, Bone RC: Incidence of aspiration in tracheally intubated adults, *Heart Lung* 16:527-531, 1987.

Metheny N et al: Detection of inadvertent respiratory placement of small-bore feeding tubes: a report of 10 cases, *Heart Lung* 19:631-638, 1990.

Metheny N et al: Effectiveness of pH measurements in predicting feeding tube placement: an update, *Nurs Res* 42:324-331, 1993.

Metheny N et al: Effectiveness of the auscultatory method in predicting feeding tube location, *Nurs Res* 39:262-267, 1990.

BIBLIOGRAPHY

DePippo KL, Holas MA, Reding MJ: Validation of the 3-oz water swallow test for aspiration following stroke, *Arch Neurol* 49:1259-1261, 1992.

Johnson ER, McKenzie SW, Sievers A: Aspiration pneumonia in stroke, *Arch Phys Med Rehabil* 74:973-976, 1993.

Moore K: Stroke: the long road back, *RN* 57:50-55, 1994.

Odom JL: Airway emergencies in the post anesthesia care unit, *Post Anesth Care Nurs* 28:483-490, 1993.

Rakel BA, Titler M, Goode C: Nasogastric and nasointestinal feeding tube placement: an integrative review of research, *AACN Clin Issues* 5:194-206, 1994.

Body image disturbance

Gail Ladwig

Definition Disruption in the way one perceives one's body image.

Defining Characteristics

Objective Missing body part; actual change in structure or function; avoidance of looking at or touching body part; intentional or unintentional hiding or overexposure of body part; trauma to nonfunctioning part; change in social involvement; change in ability to estimate spatial relationship of body to environment.

Subjective Change in life-style; fear of rejection or reaction by others; focus on past strength, function, or appearance; negative feelings about body; feelings of helplessness, hopelessness, or powerlessness; preoccupation with change or loss; emphasis on remaining strengths and heightened achievement; extension of body boundary to incorporate environmental objects; personalization of part or loss by name; depersonalization of part or loss by impersonal pronouns; refusal to verify actual change.

Related Factors (r/t)

Biophysical, cognitive, perceptual, psychosocial, cultural, or spiritual factors.

Client Outcomes/Goals

- States or demonstrates acceptance of change or loss and an ability to adjust to life-style change.
- Calls body part or loss by appropriate name.
- Looks at and touches changed or missing body part.
- Cares for changed or nonfunctioning part without inflicting trauma.
- Returns to previous social involvement.
- Correctly estimates relationship of body to environment.

Nursing Interventions and Rationales

- Observe client's usual coping mechanisms under extreme times of stress and reinforce their use in this crisis.
  Clients are in shock during acute phase, and their own value system must be considered; clients deal better with change over time (Price, 1992).
- Acknowledge denial, anger, or depression as normal feelings in adjusting to changes in body and life-style. Do not ask client to explore feelings unless he or she has indicated a need to do so.
  There is a period of grief associated with a change in body image, and these are normal grief responses. Complicated and emotionally powerful issues involving an altered body image take time to work through and express (Johnson, 1994).
- Encourage client and family to discuss and share feelings regarding the health problem and its treatment, progress, and prognosis.
  The expression of feelings is therapeutic, and the acknowledgment of feelings conveys acceptance and helps establish trust.
- Explore strengths and resources with client; discuss possible changes and weight and hair loss; select a wig before hair loss occurs.
  Emphasizing strengths promotes a positive self-image; planning for an event such as hair loss helps to decrease the sudden change in appearance.
- Encourage client to discuss interpersonal and social conflicts that may arise.
  Open communication is important for adaptation.
- Encourage client to make own decisions, participate in plan of care, and accept both inadequacies and strengths.

Active participation in self-care enables the client to adapt to actual or perceived changes in structure or function.

- Help client accept help from others; provide a list of appropriate community resources (e.g., Reach to Recovery, Ostomy Association).
  Support groups help the client realize that he or she is "not alone."
- Help client describe self-ideal, identify self-criticisms, and be accepting of self.
  These exercises help the client to accept reality, and they discourage negative self-image.
- Allow client sufficient time to accept change; reinforce client's strengths.
  The grief process varies for each individual, and all clients need sufficient time to grieve.
- Avoid a look of distaste when caring for the client with a disfiguring surgery or injury; provide privacy.
  A client with a change in body image is very aware of nonverbal responses; to preserve the client's dignity, care of the changed body should be completed without unnecessary exposure.
- Encourage client to continue the same personal care routine that he or she followed before the change in body image; this care should be completed preferably in the bathroom and not in bed.
  This routine gives the client privacy and also prevents the client from settling into an "invalid" role. Research has shown that women who resume familiar routines and habits heal better and suffer less depression than those who settle into the role of patient (Johnson, 1994).
- Assist with the resolution of an alteration in body image by encouraging client to look at the change and touch it if appropriate.
  This exercise promotes acceptance of change in a safe and supportive environment.

Geriatric

- Focus on abilities that remain after the change.
  Motivation and self-worth are increased in the elderly by highlighting their capabilities. Even a severely disabled client is usually capable of doing something.

Client/Family Teaching

- Teach appropriate care of altered body part (e.g., mastectomy, amputation, ostomy).
- Inform client of available community support groups; offer to make initial phone call.
- Encourage significant others to offer support.
  Social support from significant others enhances both emotional and physical health (Badger, 1990).

REFERENCES

Badger V: Men with cardiovascular disease and their spouses, coping, health and marital adjustment, *Arch Psychiatr Nurs* 4:319-324, 1990.

Johnson J: Caring for the woman who's had a mastectomy, *Am J Nurs* 94(5):25-31, 1994.

Price B: Living with altered body image: the classic patient experience, *Br J Nurs* 25:641-645, 1992.

BIBLIOGRAPHY

McFarland K, McFarlane E: *Nursing diagnosis and intervention: planning for patient care*, ed 2, St Louis, 1993, Mosby.

Effective breast-feeding

Vicki McClurg and Virginia Wall

Definition The state in which a mother-infant dyad exhibits adequate proficiency and satisfaction with the breast-feeding process.

Defining Characteristics

Major: Mother's ability to position infant at breast to promote a successful latch-on response; infant contentment after feeding; regular and sustained suckling and swallowing at the breast; age-appropriate infant weight patterns; effective mother-infant communication patterns (e.g., infant cues, maternal interpretation and response).

Minor: Signs or symptoms of oxytocin release (let-down or milk ejection reflex); age-appropriate infant elimination patterns; eagerness of infant to nurse; maternal verbalization of satisfaction with the breast-feeding process.

Related Factors (r/t)

Basic breast-feeding knowledge; normal maternal breast structure; normal infant oral structure; infant gestational age greater than 34 weeks; support sources (e.g., encouraging partner, history of positive breast-feeding experiences among relatives and friends, access to support groups such as La Leche League); maternal confidence; breast-feeding within first hour after birth; exclusive and frequent breast-feeding until milk supply established; maternal determination to breast-feed.

Client Outcomes/Goals

- Maintains effective breast-feeding.
- Infant maintains normal growth patterns.
- Mother verbalizes satisfaction with the breast-feeding process.

Nursing Interventions and Rationales

- Assess knowledge base regarding basic breast-feeding.
  Support and teaching must be individualized to the client's level of understanding. "Much of the process of preparing to breastfeed consists of acquiring information and becoming cognitively and emotionally ready" (Chute, 1992, p. 570).
- Assess breast and nipple structure.
  Normal nipple and breast structure or early detection and treatment of abnormalities is important for successful breast-feeding (Jensen, Wallace, Kelsay, 1994).
- Assist client with the first attachment at the breast within the first hour after birth.
  During the quiet-alert state in the first hour following birth, the infant is most likely to latch on successfully. Early breast-feeding has a positive effect on lactation performance. A successful first feeding boosts maternal confidence (Chute, 1992).
- Assess client's knowledge of prevention and treatment of common breast-feeding problems.
  Most common problems that can lead to early termination of breast-feeding are preventable (Chute, 1992).
- Monitor the breast-feeding process.
  The nurse's presence and involvement allows for early detection of difficulties and fosters success (Shrago, 1992).
- Encourage rooming-in and breast-feeding on demand.
  Rooming-in and breast-feeding on demand are positively associated with breast-feeding success (Perez-Escamilla et al, 1994).
- Evaluate adequacy of infant intake.

Infant intake can be measured by objective criteria such as number and quality of feedings, infant elimination patterns (should have six voidings of light yellow urine per day), and infant weight gain (Hill, 1992).

- Avoid supplemental bottle feedings.
  Supplemental feedings can interfere with the infant's desire to breast-feed, increase the risk of allergies, and convey the subtle message that the mother's breastmilk is not adequate (Chute, 1992; Hill, 1992).
- Avoid nipple shields.
  The amount of milk an infant can get through a nipple shield is diminished (Riordan, Auerbach, 1993).
- Assess support person network.
  Social support is important in ensuring the success of breast-feeding (Chute, 1992; Gamble, Morse, 1993; Sears, 1992).
- Give praise for positive mother-infant interactions related to breast-feeding.
  "Strategies that promote not only the initiation, but also the successful continuation of breastfeeding, are particularly important in helping the mother achieve competence and mastery in this important aspect of mothering" (Chute, 1992, p. 570).
- Do not provide samples of formula at discharge.
  Commercial discharge packs are associated with poor lactation success, especially in vulnerable subgroups such as first time mothers and low income women (Perez-Escamilla et al, 1994).
- Provide a nurse-initiated phone call within 2 days of discharge from hospital.
  Outreach of this type is associated with breast-feeding success (Bernard-Bonnin et al, 1989).

Client/Family Teaching

- Teach client to observe for infant's subtle hunger cues (e.g., quiet-alert state, rooting, sucking, hand-to-mouth activity) and to nurse whenever signs are apparent.
  Feedings are initiated more easily when the infant is hungry and in the quiet-alert state (Shrago, 1992).
- Review guidelines for frequency of feedings (every 2 to 3 hours or at least eight feedings per 24 hours).
  In the first few days frequent and regular stimulation of the breasts is important to establish an adequate milk supply.
- Review guidelines for duration of feeding (e.g., until suckling and swallowing slow down).
  The mother should be taught to use infant cues of satiety rather than arbitrary time limits.
- Provide anticipatory guidance about common breast-feeding problems.
  Lack of knowledge about detection, prevention, and treatment of problems can lead to premature termination of breast-feeding.
- Provide anticipatory guidance about common infant behaviors.
  Lack of knowledge regarding infant growth spurts, temperament, sleep-wake cycles, and introduction of other foods can create parental anxiety and lead to premature termination of breast-feeding (Hill, 1992; Shrago, 1992).
- Provide information about additional breast-feeding resources.
  Breast-feeding classes, books, materials, and support groups can provide current and accurate information and enhance maternal success and satisfaction with the breast-feeding process.

REFERENCES

Bernard-Bonnin A et al: Hospital practices and breastfeeding duration: a meta-analysis of controlled clinical trials, *Birth* 16:64-66, 1989.

Chute GE: Promoting breastfeeding success: an overview of basic management, *NAACOG's Clin Issues Perinatal Women Health Nurs* 3:570, 1992.

Gamble D, Morse JB: Fathers of breastfed infants: postponing and types of involvement, *JOGNN* 22:358-365, 1993.

Hill PD: Insufficient milk supply syndrome, *NAACOG's Clin Issues Perinatal Women Health Nurs* 3:605-612, 1992.

Jensen D, Wallace S, Kelsay P: LATCH: a breastfeeding charting system and documentation tool, *JOGNN*, 23:27-32, 1994.

Perez-Escamilla R et al: Infant feeding policies in maternity wards and their effect on breastfeeding success: an analytical overview, *Am J Public Health* 84:89-97, 1994.

Riordan J, Auerbach KG: *Breastfeeding and human lactation*, Boston, 1993, Jones and Bartlett.

Sears W: The father's role in breastfeeding, *NAACOG's Clin Issues Perinatal Women Health Nurs* 3:713-716, 1992.

Shrago LC: The breastfeeding dyad: early assessment, documentation, and intervention, *NAACOG's Clin Issues Perinatal Women Health Nurs* 3:583-597, 1992.

BIBLIOGRAPHY

North American Nursing Diagnosis Association. (Revised 1990). Taxonomy 1. St Louis, MO, NANDA.

Ineffective breast-feeding

Vicki McClurg and Virginia Wall

Definition The state in which a mother, infant, or child experiences dissatisfaction or difficulty with the breast-feeding process.

Defining Characteristics

Major Unsatisfactory breast-feeding process.

Minor Actual or perceived inadequate milk supply; infant's inability to attach on to maternal breast correctly; no observable signs of oxytocin release (let-down or milk ejection reflex) either during feeding (uterine cramping, increased lochia flow, dripping from contralateral breast, tingling sensation in breasts, sound of infant swallowing) or after feeding (noticeable softening of breasts); observable signs of inadequate infant intake (e.g., inadequate weight gain, inadequate elimination patterns, dehydration); nonsustained suckling or swallowing at the breast; insufficient emptying of each breast at each feeding; persistence of sore nipples beyond the first week of breast-feeding or for the duration of a feed in the first week after birth; insufficient opportunity for suckling at the breast; infant fussiness and crying within the first hour after breast-feeding; infant unresponsiveness to other comfort measures; infant arching and crying at the breast; maternal reluctance to put infant to breast; infant resistance to latch on; sleepiness at the breast.

Related Factors (r/t)

Maternal Breast anomaly (e.g., inverted nipple); drugs; engorgement; fatigue; history of breast-feeding failure; previous breast surgery; sore nipples; anxiety or ambivalence; depression; knowledge deficit; nonsupportive partner, family, or health care provider.

Infant Anomaly (e.g., abnormal oral structure); delayed initiation of breast-feeding; illness; inability to modulate states (sleep-wake cycles); poor sucking reflex; prematurity; supplemental feedings with artificial nipple.

Client Outcomes/Goals

- Achieves effective breast-feeding.
- Verbalizes or demonstrates techniques to manage breast-feeding problems.
- Infant manifests signs of adequate intake at the breast.
- Manifests positive self-esteem in relation to the infant feeding process.
- Explains a safe alternative method of infant feeding if unable to continue exclusive breast-feeding.

Nursing Interventions and Rationales

- Assess for presence or absence of related factors or conditions that would preclude breast-feeding.
  Some conditions (e.g., maternal drug use, maternal HIV-positive status, infant cleft palate) may preclude breast-feeding and necessitate a safe alternative method of feeding (Riordan, 1993).
- Evaluate and record the mother's ability to position; give cues and help the infant latch on.
  "Correct positioning is perhaps the most critical single measure for getting breastfeeding off to a good start" (Chute, 1992, p. 572).
- Evaluate and record the infant's ability to properly grasp and compress the areola with its lips, tongue, and jaw.
  "For the infant to obtain milk from the breast, the jaws must compress the milk sinuses beneath the areola," and the jaws must be well back on the areola, the tongue over the lower gum, forming a trough around the breast, the lips flanged and sealed around the breast (Chute, 1992, p. 575).

- Evaluate and record the infant's suckling and swallowing pattern at the breast.
When the infant sucks adequately, there is visible muscular movement above the ears. When breastmilk is actively flowing, infants suck at a rate of once per second, and swallowing increases as milk supply increases (Shrago, 1992).
- Evaluate and record signs of oxytocin release.
The letdown reflex (tingling sensation in the breasts, milk dripping from the breasts, and uterine cramping) is an indication of oxytocin release and is necessary for transfer of milk to the infant (Bobak, Jensen, 1993; Hill, 1992).
- Evaluate and record infant's state at the time of feeding.
Infants breast-feed best when in the quiet-alert state. Difficulties arise when trying to breast-feed a sleepy, ravenously hungry, or crying infant (Shrago, 1992).
- Assess knowledge regarding psychophysiology of lactation and specific treatment measures for underlying problems.
Support and teaching must be individualized to the client's level of understanding. The mother must acquire knowledge and become cognitively and emotionally ready (Chute, 1992; Ziemer, Pigeon, 1993).
- Assess psychosocial factors that may contribute to ineffective breast-feeding (e.g., anxiety, goals, values, and life-style that contribute to ambivalence about breast-feeding).
"The attitude of the mother toward breastfeeding (positive, doubtful, or negative) is a powerful factor in achieving successful lactation, influencing milk production, and facilitating the art of breastfeeding" (Bobak, Jensen, 1993, p. 625).
- Promote comfort and relaxation to reduce pain and anxiety.
Discomfort associated with breast-feeding can cause some women to discontinue breast-feeding prematurely. Promoting comfort and relaxation can lead to more successful breast-feeding (Buchko et al, 1994; Chute, 1992; Ziemer, Pigeon, 1993).
- Bring the infant to a quiet-alert state through alerting techniques (e.g., provide variety in auditory, visual, and kinesthetic stimuli by unwrapping the infant, placing the infant upright, or talking to the infant) or consoling techniques as needed.
A variety of stimuli can bring the infant to a quiet-alert state. Repetition can soothe a crying baby, thus making it easier to initiate breast-feeding (Shrago, 1992).
- Enhance the flow of milk; teach mother to massage breast or burp infant and switch to other breast when infant's swallowing slows down.
The perception of inadequate milk supply can lead to early weaning. Infants should breast-feed from both breasts at each feeding. Breast massage can enhance the flow of milk and stimulate production (Hill, 1992; Riordan, Auerbach, 1993).
- Evaluate adequacy of infant intake.
Infant intake can be measured by objective criteria such as number and quality of feedings, infant elimination patterns (should have six voidings per day of light yellow urine), and infant weight gain (Hill, 1992).
- Discourage supplemental bottle feedings and encourage exclusive and effective breast-feeding.
Supplemental feedings can interfere with the infant's desire to breast-feed, increase the risk of allergies, and convey the subtle message that the mother's breastmilk is not adequate (Chute, 1992; Hill, 1992).
- Acknowledge mother's feelings and support her decision to continue breast-feeding or to choose an alternate plan.

Mastering infant feeding is an important first step in mothering; the mother needs to be empowered so that she feels competent and capable of making intelligent decisions (Chute, 1992).

- Make appropriate referrals.
  Collaborative practice with neonatal nutritionists, physical or occupational therapists, or lactation specialists helps ensure feeding and parenting success (Meier et al, 1993).
- If client is unsuccessful in achieving effective breast-feeding, help her to accept and learn an alternate method of infant feeding.
  Once the decision has been made to provide an alternate method of infant feeding, the mother needs support and education.

Client/Family Teaching

- Provide instruction in correct positioning.
  "Correct positioning is perhaps the most critical single measure for getting breastfeeding off to a good start. Many problems can be attributed to carelessness or inattention to this simple aspect of breastfeeding" (Chute, 1992, p. 572).
- Reinforce and add to knowledge base regarding underlying problems and specific treatment measures.
  If the mother understands the rationale for recommended treatment, she may be more likely to comply with recommendations and less likely to perceive the problem as insurmountable.
- Provide education to support persons as needed.
  Informational support providers help the mother achieve a more positive outcome (McNatt, Freston, 1992).

REFERENCE

Bobak IM, Jensen MD: *Maternity and gynecologic care: the nurse and the family*, ed 5, St Louis, 1993, Mosby.

Buchko BL et al: Comfort measures in breastfeeding: primiparous women, *JOGNN* 23:46-52, 1994.

Chute GE: Promoting breastfeeding success: an overview of basic management, *NAACOG's Clin Issues Perinatal Women Health Nurs* 3:570-582, 1992.

Hill PD: Insufficient milk supply syndrome, *NAACOG's Clin Issues Perinatal Women Health Nurs* 3:605-612, 1992.

McNatt MH, Freston MG: Social support and lactation outcomes in postpartum women, *J Human Lact* 8:73-77, 1992.

Meier PP et al: Breastfeeding support services in the neonatal intensive-care unit, *JOGNN* 22:338-347, 1993.

Riordan J: AIDS and breastfeeding: the ultimate paradox, *J Human Lact* 9:3-4, 1993.

Riordan J, Auebach KG: *Breastfeeding and human lactation*, Boston, 1993, Jones and Bartlett.

Shrago LC: The breastfeeding dyad: early assessment, documentation, and intervention, *NAACOG's Clin Issues Perinatal Women Health Nurs* 3:583-597, 1992.

Ziemer MM, Pigeon JG: Skin changes and pain in the nipple during the first week of lactation, *JOGNN* 22:247-256, 1993.

BIBLIOGRAPHY

North American Nursing Diagnosis Association. (Revised 1990.) Taxonomy 1. St Louis, MO, NANDA.

Stutte PC, Bowles, BC, Morman GY: The effects of breast massage on volume and fat content of human milk. *Genesis* 10:22-24, 1988.

Interrupted breast-feeding

Vicki McClurg and Virginia Wall

Definition A break in the continuity of the breast-feeding process as a result of inability or inadvisability to put baby to breast for feeding.

Defining Characteristics

Major Infant does not receive nourishment at the breast for some or all feedings.

Minor Maternal desire to maintain lactation and provide (or eventually provide) her breastmilk for her infant's nutritional needs; separation of mother and infant; lack of knowledge regarding expression and storage of breastmilk.

Related Factors (r/t)

Maternal or infant illness; prematurity; maternal employment; contraindications to breast-feeding (e.g., drugs, true breastmilk jaundice); need to abruptly wean infant (with intent to resume at later date).

Client Outcomes/Goals

Infant
- Receives mother's breastmilk if not contraindicated by maternal conditions (e.g., certain drugs, infections) or infant conditions (e.g., true breastmilk jaundice).

Maternal
- Initiates or maintains lactation.
- Achieves effective breast-feeding or satisfaction with the breast-feeding experience.
- Demonstrates effective methods of breastmilk collection and storage.

Nursing Interventions and Rationales

- Evaluate and record mother's desire to begin or continue breast-feeding.
  Maternal commitment to breast-feed is associated with breast-feeding success (Bottorf, 1990; Coates, Riordan, 1992; Coreil, Murphy, 1988).
- Evaluate advisability of initiating or reinstituting breast-feeding.
  Some conditions (e.g., maternal drug use, HIV-positive status) may be contraindications to breast-feeding. Some conditions (e.g., infant cleft palate, maternal breast surgery) may make it impossible to breast-feed (Riordan, 1993).
- Evaluate infant's ability to breast-feed and interest in breast-feeding.
  The infant must be able to demonstrate ability and interest in breast-feeding for the mother to resume breast-feeding (Danner, 1992).
- Evaluate mother's social support for continuing to breast-feed.
  Relactating after an interruption is often stressful; the mother will benefit from social support of her efforts (McNatt, Freston, 1992).
- Assess mother's emotional response to the events that caused the interruption.
  Feelings of grief, guilt, anxiety, and failure are common and may need to be addressed before breast-feeding can be successful (Driscoll, 1992).
- Develop with mother a satisfactory feeding plan to allow for continued breast-feeding.
  Involvement of the mother in planning helps her feel able to participate in caretaking.
- Assess and record mother's knowledge of breastmilk expression techniques.
  During interruption, the mother needs to maintain lactation by expressing milk via either hand expression or manual or electric breast pumping.
- Assess and record mother's knowledge regarding how to handle, store, and transport breastmilk safely.
  If expressed breastmilk is to be fed to an infant, the mother must demonstrate proper storage and handling techniques to ensure that milk remains fresh and uncontaminated (Human Milk Banking Association of North America, 1993; Mohandes et al, 1993).

- Assess equipment needs.
  "The health care professional needs to base pumping recommendations on many factors and take into account each mother's situation" (Riordan, Auerbach, 1993, p. 305).
- Provide resource information (e.g., support groups, equipment and supply rental or sales).
  The mother needs this information to enable her to follow through with care plan and receive support as needed.
- Promote emotional resolution by encouraging mother to verbalize frustrations and disappointments.
  Resolution of frustrations and disappointments are important for a satisfactory breast-feeding experience (Driscoll, 1992).

Client/Family Teaching

- Teach mother effective methods for expressing breastmilk.
  The mother needs to be taught how to continue lactation during the interruption of breast-feeding.
- Teach mother safe breastmilk handling techniques.
  The mother needs to be taught how to handle breastmilk to provide a safe product for her infant (Mohandes et al, 1993).
- Provide anticipatory guidance for common problems associated with interrupted breast-feeding (e.g., diminishing milk supply, infant difficulty with resuming breast-feeding).
  Knowing what to expect helps the mother cope with any difficulties that may arise.
- Provide education to support persons as needed.
  Informational support providers help the mother achieve a more positive outcome (McNatt, Freston, 1992).

REFERENCES

Bottorff JL: Persistence in breastfeeding: a phenomenological investigation, *J Adv Nurs* 15:201-209, 1990.

Coates M, Riordan J: Breastfeeding during maternal or infant illness, *NAACOG's Clin Issues Perinatal Women Health Nurs* 3:683-693, 1992.

Coreil J, Murphy JE: Maternal commitment, lactation practices, and breastfeeding duration, *JOGNN* 17:273-278, 1988.

Danner SC: Breastfeeding the neurologically impaired infant, *NAACOG's Clin Issues Perinatal Women Health Nurs* 3:640-646, 1992.

Driscoll JW: Breastfeeding success and failures: implications for nurses, *NAACOG's Clin Issues Perinatal Women Health Nurs* 3:565-569, 1992.

Human Milk Banking Association of North America (HMBANA): *Recommendations for collection, storage, and handling of a mother's milk for her own infant in the hospital setting*, West Hartford, Conn, 1993, Human Milk Banking Association of North America.

McNatt MH, Freston MG: Social support and lactation outcomes in postpartum women, *J Human Lact* 8:73-77, 1992.

Mohandes AE et al: Bacterial contaminants of collected and frozen human milk used in an intensive care nursery, *Am J Infect Control* 21:226-230, 1993.

Riordan J: AIDS and breastfeeding: the ultimate paradox, *J Human Lact* 9:3-4, 1993.

Riordan J, Auerbach KG: *Breastfeeding and human lactation*, Boston, 1993, Jones and Bartlett.

Ineffective breathing pattern

Betty Ackley

Definition The state in which an individual's inhalation and/or exhalation pattern does not enable adequate pulmonary inflation or emptying.

Defining Characteristics

Dyspnea; shortness of breath; tachypnea; fremitus; abnormal arterial blood gas; cyanosis; cough; nasal flaring; respiratory depth changes; assumption of three-point position; pursed-lip breathing; prolonged expiratory phase; increased anteroposterior diameter; use of accessory muscles; altered chest excursion.

Related Factors (r/t)

Neuromuscular impairment; musculoskeletal impairment; perceptual or cognitive impairment; pain; anxiety; decreased energy; fatigue.

Client Outcomes/Goals

- Demonstrates a breathing pattern that supports blood gas results within the client's normal parameters.
- Reports ability to breathe comfortably.
- Demonstrates ability to perform pursed-lip breathing and relaxation techniques.

Nursing Interventions and Rationales

- Monitor respiratory rate, depth, and ease of respiration.
  Normal respiratory rate is 12 to 16 breaths/min in the adult.
- Note pattern of respiration.
  Normal respiratory pattern is regular in the healthy adult.
- Note use of accessory muscles, abdominal breathing, nasal flaring, retractions, irritability, confusion, or lethargy.
  These symptoms signal increasing respiratory difficulty and decreasing Po_2.
- Observe color of tongue, oral mucosa, and skin color.
  Cyanosis in the tongue and oral mucosa is central cyanosis and generally represents a medical emergency. Peripheral cyanosis of nailbeds or lips may or may not be serious (Carpenter, 1993).
- Observe sputum, noting color, odor, and volume.
  Normal sputum is clear or grey and minimal; abnormal sputum is green, yellow, or bloody and is also malodorous and often copious.
- Auscultate breath sounds noting decreased or absent sounds, crackles, or wheezes.
  These sounds can indicate a respiratory pathology associated with an altered breathing pattern.
- Monitor client's O_2 saturation and blood gases.
  O_2 saturation <90% (normal 95% to 100%) or Po_2 <80 (normal 80 to 100) indicates significant oxygenation problems.
- Monitor for presence of pain and provide pain medication for comfort as needed.
  Pain causes the client to hypoventilate and avoid taking deep breaths.
- Position client in an upright or semi-Fowler's position, or provide an over-bed table for client to lean on.
  An upright position facilitates lung expansion.
- If client has unilateral lung disease, alternate semi-Fowler's position with lateral position (with a 10 to 15 degree elevation and "good lung down") for 60 to 90 min (contraindicated for pulmonary abscess or hemorrhage or interstitial emphysema).
  Gravity and hydrostatic pressure allow the dependent lung to become better ventilated and perfused, which increases oxygenation (Yeaw, 1992).

- Increase client's activity up to walking 3 to 4 times daily as tolerated. Refer to nursing interventions for **Activity intolerance**.
  Body movement helps mobilize respiratory secretions.
- Schedule rest periods before and after activity.
  Respiratory clients are easily exhausted and need additional rest.
- Provide small, frequent feedings.
  Small feedings are given to avoid compromising ventilatory effort and to conserve energy.
- Encourage client to take deep breaths at prescribed intervals or use incentive spirometry; reinforce client's progress.
- In acute dyspneic state, ensure that client has received the medications or treatment needed and then stay to provide support.
  Anxiety can exacerbate dyspnea, causing the client to enter into a dyspneic panic state. The nurse's presence, reassurance, and help in controling the client's breathing with slower pursed-lip breathing is helpful.
- If chronic pulmonary disease is interfering with quality of life, refer for pulmonary rehabilitation.
  Pulmonary rehabilitation has been shown to improve exercise capacity, ability to walk, and sense of well-being (Fishman, 1994).

Geriatric

- Encourage ambulation as tolerated.
  Immobility is often harmful to the elderly because it decreases ventilation and increases stasis of secretions (Foyt, 1992).
- Encourage elders to sit upright or stand and to avoid lying down during the day.
  Thoracic aging results in decreased lung expansion; an erect position fosters maximal lung expansion.

Client/Family Teaching

- Teach pursed-lip breathing techniques, controlled breathing techniques, and incentive spirometry (McConnell, 1992).
  Pursed-lip breathing helps keep alveoli inflated longer to increase oxygenation.
- Using a prerecorded tape, teach client progressive muscle relaxation techniques.
  Relaxation therapy can help reduce dyspnea and anxiety (Gift et al, 1992).
- Teach about the dosage, actions, and side effects of medications.
  Bronchodilators can have undesirable side effects, especially when taken in inappropriate doses.
- Teach the need to monitor sputum for changes in color, amount, or consistency.
  Such knowledge helps the client identify infections earlier.

REFERENCES

Carpenter, KD: A comprehensive review of cyanosis, *Crit Care Nurse* 13:66-72, August 1993.

Fishman AP: Pulmonary rehabilitation research, *Respir Crit Care Med* 149:825-833, 1994.

Foyt MM: Impaired gas exchange in the elderly, *Geriatr Nurs* 13(5):262-268, 1992.

Gift A, Moore T, Soeken K: Relaxation to reduce dyspnea and anxiety in COPD patients, *Nurs Res* 41(4):242-250, 1992.

McConnell : Performing pursed-lip breathing, *Nursing* 22:18, 1992.

Yeaw P: Good lung down, *Am J Nurs* 92(3):27-32, 1992.

BIBLIOGRAPHY

Kim MJ et al: Inspiratory muscle training in patients with chronic obstructive pulmonary disease, *Nurs Res* 42:356-362.

McCord M, Cronin-Stubbs D: Operationalizing dyspnea: focus on measurement, *Heart Lung* 21:167-179, 1992.

Decreased cardiac output

Betty Ackley

Definition The state in which the blood pumped by an individual's heart is sufficiently reduced so that it is inadequate to meet the needs of the body's tissues.

Defining Characteristics

Variations in blood pressure; dysrhythmias; fatigue; jugular vein distention; color changes of skin and mucous membranes; oliguria; decreased peripheral pulses; cold, clammy skin; crackles; dyspnea; orthopnea; change in mental status; shortness of breath; syncope; vertigo; edema; cough; frothy sputum; gallop rhythm; weakness.

Related Factors (r/t)

Myocardial infarction or ischemia; valvular disease; cardiomyopathy; serious dysrhythmias; ventricular damage; altered preload or afterload; pericarditis; sepsis; congenital heart defects; vagal stimulation; stress; anaphylaxis; cardiac tamponade.

Client Outcomes/Goals

- Demonstrates adequate cardiac output as evidenced by a blood pressure and pulse rate and rhythm within normal parameters; strong peripheral pulses; and an ability to tolerate activity without symptoms of dyspnea, syncope, or chest pain.
- Free of side effects from the medications used to accomplish adequate cardiac output.
- Explains actions and precautions to take to live with cardiac disease.

Nursing Interventions and Rationales

- Observe for chest pain; note location, radiation, severity, quality, duration, and precipitating and relieving factors.
  Chest pain is often indicative of an inadequate blood supply to the heart, which can compromise cardiac output.
- If chest pain is present, monitor cardiac rhythm, run a strip, medicate for pain, and notify the physician.
- Listen to heart sounds—rate, rhythm, S_3, S_4, rub, new onset of systolic murmur.
  The new onset of a gallop rhythm plus tachycardia and fine crackles in lung bases can indicate onset of congestive heart failure.
- Observe for diminished quality of peripheral pulses, cool skin and extremities, increased respiratory rate, increased heart rate, and decreased level of consciousness.
  These symptoms are additional signs of cardiac output decline (Murphy, Bennett, 1992).
- Monitor for dysrhythmias.
- Monitor hemodynamic parameters for increases in pulmonary wedge pressure, increases in systemic vascular resistance, or decreases in cardiac index.
  Hemodynamic parameters can give a good indication of cardiac function.
- Monitor intake and output; observe for decreased output.
  Decreased cardiac output results in decreased perfusion of the kidneys, with a resultant decrease in urine output.
- Note test results to correlate with severity of disease and the need for restrictions—creatine phosphokinase-MB, lactate dehydrogenase, white blood cell, arterial blood gases, electrocardiogram, echocardiogram.
  Diagnostic testing can give a good indication of the seriousness of the cardiac condition.
- Administer oxygen as needed per physician's order.

"Supplemental oxygen increases oxygen availability to the myocardium" (Prizant-Weston, Castiglia, 1992, p. 549).

- Titrate inotropic and vasoactive medications within defined parameters to maintain contractility, preload, and afterload per physician's order.
  By following parameters the nurse ensures maintenance of the delicate balance of medications to stimulate the heart and maintain adequate perfusion of the body.
- Serve smaller meals of low sodium and low cholesterol. May give small amounts of caffeine (one or two cups in 24 hours) if tolerated without dysrhythmias.
  Clients with cardiac disease tolerate smaller meals better because they require less cardiac output to digest. One cup of caffeinated coffee has generally not been found to have any significant effects (Powell, 1993; Schneider, 1987).
- Schedule periods of rest between activities.
  Rest periods decrease oxygen consumption (Prizant-Weston, Castiglia, 1992).

Geriatric

- Observe for atypical pain; the elderly often have jaw pain instead of chest pain or may have silent myocardial infarctions with symptoms of dyspnea or fatigue.
  The elderly have altered pain pathways and often do not experience the usual chest pain of cardiac patients (Carnevali, Patrick, 1993).
- Observe for syncope, dizziness, palpitations, or feelings of weakness with cardiac disease.
  Dysrhythmias are common in the elderly (Carnevali, Patrick, 1993).
- Observe for side effects from cardiac medications.
  The elderly have difficulty with metabolism and excretion of medications; therefore toxic effects are more common in the elderly.
- Refer client to cardiac rehabilitation program for education, evaluation, and guided support to increase activity and rebuild life.

Client/Family Teaching

- Teach symptoms of cardiovascular disease and the appropriate actions to take if client becomes symptomatic.
- Teach stress reduction (e.g., imagery, controlled breathing, muscle relaxation techniques).
- Explain necessary restrictions, including diet, fluids, and the avoidance of Valsalva's maneuver; teach exercise designed for client and the importance of pacing activities and resting between activities.
- Teach client the actions and side effects of cardiovascular medications.
- Instruct family regarding cardiopulmonary resuscitation.

REFERENCES

Carnevali DL, Patrick M: *Nursing management for the elderly*, ed 3, Philadelphia, 1993, JB Lippincott.

Murphy T, Bennett EJ: Low-tech, high touch perfusion assessment, *Am J Nurs* 92(5):36-40, 1992.

Powell AH: What's that brewing in the CCU?: working smart, *Am J Nurs* 93(12):16, 1993.

Prizant-Weston M, Castiglia K: *Hemodynamic regulation.* In Bulechek GM, McCloskey JC, editors: *Nursing interventions: essential nursing treatments*, Philadelphia, 1992, WB Saunders.

Schneider JR: Effects of caffeine ingestion on heart rate, blood pressure, myocardial oxygen consumption, and cardiac rhythm in acute myocardial infarction patients, *Heart Lung* 16:167-174, 1987.

BIBLIOGRAPHY

Folta A, Potempa KM: Reduced cardiac output and exercise capacity in patients after MI, *J Cardiovasc Nurs* 6:71-77, 1992.

Kern L, Omery A: Decreased cardiac output in the critical care setting, *Nurs Diag* 3:94-105, 1992.

Caregiver role strain

Betty Ackley

Definition

A caregiver's felt difficulty in performing the family caregiver role.

Defining Characteristics*

Not enough resources (e.g., time, emotional strength, physical energy, help from others) to provide the care needed; difficulty performing specific caregiving activities such as bathing, cleaning up after incontinence, and managing behavioral problems and pain; worry regarding such things as the care receiver's health and emotional state, putting the care receiver in an institution, and caring for the care receiver if something should happen to the caregiver; feelings that caregiving interferes with other important roles such as being a worker, parent, spouse, or friend; feelings of loss because the care receiver is like a different person compared to before caregiving began; in the case of a child, feelings that the care receiver was never the child the caregiver expected; family conflict regarding issues of providing care; other family members do not do their share in providing care to the receiver; feelings that not enough appreciation is shown for what the caregiver does; stress or nervousness in the relationship with the care receiver; depression.

Related Factors (r/t)

Pathophysiological

Illness severity of the care receiver; addiction or codependency; premature birth or congenital defect; discharge of family member with significant home-care needs; caregiver health impairment; unpredictable illness course or instability in care receiver's health; caregiver is female; psychological or cognitive problems of care receiver.

Developmental

Caregiver not developmentally ready for caregiver role (e.g., young adult providing care for a middle-aged parent); developmental delay or retardation of the care receiver or caregiver.

Psychosocial

Marginal family adaptation or dysfunction before the caregiving situation; marginal caregiver coping patterns; past history of poor relationship between caregiver and care receiver; caregiver is spouse; care receiver exhibits deviant or bizarre behavior.

Situational

Presence of abuse or violence; presence of situational stressors that normally affect families such as significant loss, disaster, crisis, poverty, economic vulnerability, or major life events (e.g., birth, hospitalization, leaving home, returning home, marriage, divorce, employment, retirement, death); duration of caregiving required; inadequate physical environment for providing care (e.g., housing, transportation, community services, equipment); family or caregiver isolation; lack of respite and recreation for caregiver; inexperience with caregiving; caregiver's competing role commitments; complexity or amount of caregiving tasks.

Client Outcomes/Goals

- Caregiver is physically and psychologically healthy.
- Caregiver is able to identify resources available to help in giving care.
- Care receiver is receiving appropriate care.

Nursing Interventions and Rationales

- Monitor quality of care for adequacy and need for improvement.
- Determine physical and psychological health of caregiver and watch for signs of depression; refer to resources as needed.

  Caregiving may weaken the immune system and predispose the caregiver to illness in some situations; the incidence of depression in family caregivers is estimated to be 40% to 50% (Stevens, Walsh, Baldwin, 1993).

*Eighty percent of caregivers report one or more of these defining characteristics.

- Observe for signs of addiction or codependency in caregiver or care receiver.
- Provide for home health services as needed to help with significant home care needs.
- Arrange for intervals of respite care for caregiver.
- Help caregiver to identify supports and decide how to best use them.
- Encourage caregiver to grieve over loss of care receiver's function. Refer to nursing interventions for **Grieving.**
  Caregivers grieve the loss of function of their loved one, especially when dementia is involved (Liken, Collins, 1993).
- Identify with caregiver those things he or she has control over.
- Help caregiver find personal time to meet own needs.
- Encourage caregiver to talk about feelings, concerns, and fears.
- Acknowledge frustration associated with caregiver responsibilities.
- Give caregiver permission to share angry feelings in a safe environment.
- Give caregiver permission to arrange custodial care in an extended care facility if necessary; support both caregiver and care receiver during this difficult transition.
  Placing a loved one in an extended care facility can relieve the burden of care but does not relieve the stress resulting from financial concerns, guilt, loss of control, or lack of support (Stevens, Walsh, Baldwin, 1993).

Geriatric

- Monitor for psychological distress and signs of depression in caregiver, especially if caring for a mentally impaired elder.
  Those caring for a mentally impaired elder for an extended time with minimal social support are at a high risk for psychological distress or depression (Baille et al, 1988).
- Observe for any evidence of caregiver or care receiver violence; if evidence is present, speak with caregiver and care receiver separately.
  Caregiver violence is possible, especially if the care receiver was violent to caregiver in the past (Clinical News, Am J Nurs 1993).
- Recognize that it is hard for the elderly to accept any change in caregivers or in the environment.
- Help caregiver identify ways to equitably distribute workload among family or significant others.
- Arrange for follow-up care following discharge, including a nursing-social work team, to provide medical and social services to the caregiver and client.
  A posthospital support program that supports the elderly and the caregiver has been shown to delay nursing home placements, possibly delay some deaths, and save money (Oktay, Volland, 1990).

Client/Family Teaching

- Teach caregiver methods for managing behavioral symptoms.
- Refer to counseling or support groups to assist in adjusting to caregiver role.

REFERENCES

Baille V, Norbeck JS, Barnes LE: Stress, social support, and psychological distress of family caregivers of the elderly, *Nurs Res* 37(4):217-222, 1988.

Liken MA, Collins CE: Grieving: facilitating the process for dementia caregivers, *J Psychosoc Nurs Ment Health Serv* 31(1):21-26, 1993.

Oktay JS, Volland PT: Post-hospital program for the frail elderly and their caregivers: a quasi-experimental evaluation, *Am J Public Health* 80:39-46, 1990.

What makes caregivers become violent. (Clinical News), *Am J Nurs* 93(2):12-13, 1993.

Stevens GL, Walsh RA, Baldwin BA: Family caregivers of institutionalized and noninstitutionalized elderly individuals, *Nurs Clin North Am* 28:349-362, 1993.

BIBLIOGRAPHY

Thomas VM et al: Caring for the person receiving ventilatory support at home: caregivers' needs and involvement, *Heart Lung* 21:180, 1992.

Risk for caregiver role strain

Definition A caregiver is vulnerable to experiencing difficulty in performing the family caregiver role.

Related Factors (r/t)

Refer to related factors for **Caregiver role strain**.

Client Outcomes/Goals, Nursing Interventions and Rationales, and Client/Family Teaching

Refer to **Caregiver role strain**.

Altered comfort

Betty Ackley

Definition The state in which an individual experiences an uncomfortable sensation in response to a noxious stimulus (Carpenito).

Defining Characteristics

Major Verbalization or demonstration of discomfort.

Minor Guarded position; cutaneous irritation; abdominal heaviness; itching; retching.

Related Factors (r/t)

Visceral disorders; inflammation; musculoskeletal disorders; treatments; personal situations (e.g., pregnancy, overactivity); chemical irritants (adapted from Carpenito).

Client Outcomes/Goals

- States is comfortable.
- Explains methods to decrease itching.
- States relief of discomfort of nausea.

Nursing Interventions and Rationales

Pruritis

- Determine cause of pruritis (e.g., dry skin, contact with irritating substance, medication side effect, insect bite, infection, symptom of systemic disease).
  Etiology of pruritis helps direct treatment.
- Apply soaks with washcloths wrung out in cool water or ice water as needed.
  The application of cool or cold washcloths can depress the itching sensation.
- Keep client's fingernails short; have client wear mitts if necessary.
  Scratching with fingernails can excoriate the area and increase skin damage.
- Leave pruritic area open to the air if possible.
  Covering the area with a nonventilated dressing can increase warmth in the area and the itching sensation.
- Use nonallergenic mild soap sparingly.
  Many soaps can be irritating to the skin and increase the itching sensation.
- Keep skin well lubricated; apply nonallergenic creams after bathing while the skin is still moist.
  These agents lubricate the skin surface and make the skin feel smoother and less dry (Hardy, 1992).
- If pruritis areas are open and weeping, apply a shake solution such as calamine to the area.
  When they evaporate, these solutions cool the skin and dry weeping lesions (DeWitt, 1990).
- Provide distraction techniques such as music or television.
  These activities help to temporarily distract the client from the itching sensation.
- Consult with physician for medication to relieve itching.
  Medications such as antihistamines can be helpful for pruritis (DeWitt, 1990).

Geriatric

- Limit number of complete baths to two or three per week and alternate with partial baths. Use a tepid water temperature at 90° to 105° F for bathing.
  Excessive bathing, especially in hot water, depletes aging skin of moisture and increases dryness.
- Use superfatted soap such as Dove, Tone, or Caress.
  Superfatted soaps help retain moisture in dry, elderly skin (Hardy, 1992).
- Increase fluid intake within cardiac or renal limits to a minimum of 1500 ml/day.
  Dry skin is caused by loss of fluid in the skin; increasing fluid intake hydrates the skin.

- Use a humidifier or a container of water on warm environment to increase humidity in the environment, especially during the winter.
  Increasing moisture in the air helps to keep moisture in the skin (Fenske, Grayson, Newcomer, 1989).

Nausea/Vomiting

- Determine cause of nausea and vomiting (e.g., medication effects, viral illness, food poisoning, extreme anxiety, pregnancy).
- Keep a clean emesis basin and tissues within client's reach.
- Provide oral care after client vomits.
  Oral care helps remove the taste and smell of vomitus, thus reducing the stimulus for further vomiting.
- Stay with client to give support; place hand on shoulder; hold the emesis basin.
  Human support can be helpful and comforting to the client at this frightening time.
- Provide distraction from sensation of nausea, using soft music, television, and videos per client preference.
  Distraction can help direct attention away from the sensation of nausea.
- Maintain a quiet, well-ventilated environment.
  Odors from a kitchen or bathroom can trigger nausea (Pervan, 1990).
- Avoid sudden movement for the client; allow client to lie still.
  Movement can trigger further nausea and vomiting.
- If client is pregnant, suggest she sit down when experiencing nausea.
  Sitting down reduced nausea up to 80% of the time in pregnant women (Dilorio, van Lier, 1989).
- Consult with physician regarding need for antiemetic medications.
- After vomiting is controlled and nausea abates, begin feeding client small amounts of clear fluids such as soda or broth, then crackers; progress to a soft diet.
- Remove cover of food tray before bringing it into client's room.
  The sudden, concentrated food odors that come when the cover is removed in front of the client can trigger nausea (Pervan, 1990).

Client/Family Teaching

- Teach techniques to use when uncomfortable, including relaxation techniques, guided imagery, hypnosis, and music therapy (Jablonski, 1993; Pervan, 1993).
- Teach the client with pruritis to substitute rubbing, pressure, or vibration for scratching when itching is severe and irrepressible.

REFERENCES

Carpenito JL: *Nursing diagnosis: application to clinical practice*, ed 5, Philadelphia, 1993, JB Lippincott.

DeWitt S: Nursing assessment of the skin and dermatologic lesions, *Nurs Clin North Am*, 25:235-242, 1990.

Dilorio CK, van Lier DJ: Nausea and vomiting in pregnancy. In Funk SG et al, editors: *Key aspects of comfort: management of pain, fatigue, and nausea*, New York, 1989, Springer.

Fenske NA, Grayson LD, Newcomer VD: Common problems of aging skin, *Patient Care* 23:225, 1989.

Hardy MA: *Dry skin care.* In Bulechek GM, McCloskey JC, editors: *Nursing interventions: essential nursing treatments*, ed 2, Philadelphia, 1992, WB Saunders.

Jablonski RS: Nausea: the forgotten symptom, *Holistic Nurs Pract* 7(2):64-72, 1993.

Pervan V: Understanding anti-emetics, *Nurs Times* 89(10):36-37, 1993.

Pervan V: Practical aspects of dealing with cancer therapy-induced nausea and vomiting, *Semin Oncol Nurs* 6:3-5(suppl 1), 1990.

BIBLIOGRAPHY

Fitzpatrick JE: Common inflammatory skin diseases of the elderly, *Geriatrics* 44:40, 1989.

Frantz RA, Kinney CK: Variables associated with skin dryness in the elderly, *Nurs Res* 35:98-100, 1986.

Kenny MJ: Gastrointestinal emergencies, *Br J Nurs* 2:588-590, 1993.

Impaired verbal communication

Gail Ladwig

Definition The state in which an individual experiences a decreased or absent ability to use or understand language in human interaction.

Defining Characteristics

*Inability to speak dominant language; *difficulties with speech or verbalizations; *refusal or inability to speak; stuttering; slurring; difficulty forming words or sentences; difficulty expressing thoughts verbally; inappropriate verbalizations; dyspnea; disorientation. (*Critical)

Related Factors (r/t)

Decrease in circulation to brain; brain tumor; physical barrier (e.g., tracheostomy, intubation); anatomical defect; impaired hearing; cleft palate; psychological barriers (e.g., psychosis, lack of stimuli); cultural difference; developmental- or age-related factors.

Client Outcomes/Goals

- Uses effective communication techniques.
- Uses alternate methods of communication effectively.
- Demonstrates congruency of verbal and nonverbal behavior.
- Expresses desire for social interactions.

Nursing Interventions and Rationales

- Determine language spoken; obtain language dictionary or interpreter if possible.
  For a clear understanding, the nurse and client must speak the same language or have a means of understanding the other's language.
- Listen carefully; validate verbal and nonverbal expressions.
  Client satisfaction studies have repeatedly shown that what clients want most from their nurses is common courtesy—someone who really listens to their fears and concerns and treats them like a real person, not a disease (Long, Greeneich, 1994).
- Anticipate client's needs until effective communication is possible.
  Anticipation of clients' needs increases client satisfaction (Long, Greeneich, 1994).
- Use simple communication; speak in a well-modulated voice; smile and show concern for the client.
  Such techniques have been described by clients as demonstrating caring (Clark, 1993).
- Maintain eye contact at client's level; read client's lips as able.
  Standing while the client is lying or sitting makes the nurse appear rushed and hinders communication (Bailey, Bailey, 1993).
- Use touch as appropriate.
  Physical touch reduces client anxiety (Bulechek, McCloskey, 1992).
- Spend time with client; allow time for responses; make call light readily available to client.
  Clients consider good care to include listening, helping, and being there (Murdaugh et al, 1992).
- Obtain communication equipment such as electronic devices, letterboards, picture boards, and magic slates.
  Alternative methods of communication are necessary when the client is unable to use verbal communication.
- Establish an alternative method of communication such as writing or pointing to letters, word phrases, or picture cards.
  Alternative methods of communication are necessary when the client is unable to use verbal communication.

- Obtain order for speech therapy; supplement work of speech therapist with appropriate exercises.
  Consultation and collaboration with a specialist may be necessary to provide the best approach to improving communication.
- Give praise for progress noted; ignore mistakes and watch for frustration or fatigue.
  Positive reinforcement increases confidence, which can increase communication (Boss, 1991).
- Encourage family to bring in familiar pictures or calendars.
- Establish an understanding of client's symbolic speech (especially with schizophrenic clients); ask what the client means by a particular statement.
  Clarification is a necessary communication skill and is used when there is a lack of understanding about the meaning of a client's communication (Bailey, Bailey, 1993).
- If there is a comprehension deficit, keep environment quiet when communicating and get the client's attention before attempting to communicate (e.g., touch the client's shoulder, call the client's name).
  When the client is confused, a distracting environment interferes with communication; it is necessary to get the client's full attention before any communication can take place (Boss, 1991).
- Do not raise your voice or shout at the client.
  A loud voice can be frightening to the client and decrease communication.

Geriatric

- Encourage client to wear prescribed eyeglasses and hearing aids.
  Communication is blocked if needed aids are not used.
- When communicating with client, face toward client's unaffected side or better-hearing ear.
  This position increases client's awareness of the interaction and enhances the client's ability to interact.
- Provide sufficient light and remove distractions such as glare and background noise.
  Background noise further impairs the elderly client's hearing.
- Use low voice tones and recognize that perception of *f, s, th, ch, sh, b, t, p, k,* and *d* sounds are impaired with hearing loss resulting from aging.
  Presbycusis decreases the ability to hear high-pitched sounds and consonant sounds listed in the preceding paragraph. Perception of consonants is important to understanding language.
- Allow time for thought comprehension when communicating with client.
  Older clients do not like to be rushed. They fare much better in a calm, consistent environment that functions at a moderately slow pace (Bailey, Bailey, 1993).
- Encourage the elderly client to talk about feelings, fears, and worries; allow the client to talk about old memories.
  Sometimes the elderly dwell in the past as a means of dealing with the painfulness of the present. They may also be attempting to understand their present situation by reviewing past events in their lives (Bailey, Bailey, 1993).

Client/Family Teaching

- Teach client and family techniques to increase communication.
  Alternative methods of communication are necessary when the client is unable to use verbal communication.
- Teach client how to use communication devices.

REFERENCES

Bailey DS, Bailey DR: *Therapeutic approaches to the care of the mentally ill*, ed 3, Philadelphia, 1993, FA Davis.

Boss BJ: Managing communication disorders in stroke, *Nurs Clin North Am* 26:985-995, 1991.

Bulechek G, McCloskey J: *Nursing interventions: essential nursing treatments*, ed 2, Philadelphia, 1992, WB Saunders.

Clark S: Challenges in critical care nursing: helping patients and families cope, *Crit Care Nurse (suppl)* volume 2, August 1993.

Long C, Greeneich D: Four strategies for keeping patients satisfied, *Am J Nurs* 94:27, 1994.

Murdaugh C et al: Knowledge about care and caring: state of the art and future developments. In Bulechek G, McCloskey J, editors: *Nursing interventions: essential nursing treatments,* ed 2, Philadelphia, 1992, WB Saunders.

BIBLIOGRAPHY

Buckwalter KC et al: Family involvement with communication-impaired residents in long-term care settings, *Appl Nurs Res* 4:77-84, 1991.

Ineffective community coping

Margaret Lunney

Definition A pattern of community activities for adaptation and problem solving that is unsatisfactory for meeting the demands or needs of the community.

Defining Characteristics

Community does not meet its own expectations; deficits of community participation; deficits in communication methods; excessive community conflicts; expressed difficulty in meeting demands for change; expressed vulnerability; high illness rates; stressors perceived as excessive.

Related Factors (r/t)

Deficits in social support; inadequate resources for problem solving; powerlessness.

Community Outcomes/Goals

- Improvement of communication strategies among community members.
- Demonstration of community cohesiveness in problem solving.
- Increase in participation of community members in problem solving.
- Development of new strategies for problem solving.
- Community members express power to deal with change and manage problems.

Nursing Interventions and Rationales

- Refer to **Ineffective management of therapeutic regimen (community)** and **Potential for enhanced community coping**.
  NOTE: The diagnosis of **Ineffective coping** does not apply and should not be used when stress is being imposed by external sources or circumstance. If the community is a victim of circumstances, using the nursing diagnosis **Ineffective coping** would be equivalent to blaming the victim.
- Help community identify stressors.
  Excessive stress may be prompted by the community's own behavior.
- Work with community members to increase awareness of ineffective coping behaviors (e.g., conflicts that prevent community members from working together, anger and hate that paralyzes the community).
  Problem solving is essential for effective coping. Behaviors that interfere with problem solving can be modified by community members with the assistance of nurses and other health providers (Maglacas, 1988).
- Provide support to the community and help the community identify and mobilize additional supports.
  Social support is associated with positive coping strategies (Pender, 1987).
- Work with members of the community to identify and develop coping strategies that promote a sense of power (e.g., obtaining sources of funding, collaborating with other communities).
  Power is an essential aspect of coping. A first step in attaining a sense of power is for the community to identify and develop its own strategies (Freire, 1990).
- Help community members plan for management of stress (e.g., recreational and relaxation programs).
  Strategies for stress management are as important for communities as they are for individuals and families.

Community Teaching

- Teach strategies for stress management.

REFERENCES
Freire P: *Pedagogy of the oppressed.* New York, 1990, Continuum.
Pender NJ: *Health promotion in nursing practice*, ed 2. Norwalk, 1987, Appleton & Lange.
Maglacas AM: Health for all: nursing's role, *Nurs Outlook*, 36:66-71, 1988.

Potential for enhanced community coping

Margaret Lunney

Definition A pattern of community activities for adaptation and problem solving that is satisfactory for meeting the demands or needs of the community but can be improved for management of current and future problems and stressors.

Defining Characteristics

Major Deficits in one, or a few, of the characteristics that indicate effective coping.

Minor Active planning by community for predicted stressors; active problem solving by community when faced with issues; agreement that community is responsible for stress management; positive communication among community members; positive communication between community aggregates and the larger community; programs available for recreation and relaxation; resources sufficient for managing stressors.

Community Outcomes/Goals

- Community modifies specific coping strategies.
- Community maintains effective coping.

Nursing Interventions and Rationales

NOTE: Interventions depend on the specific aspects of community coping that can be enhanced (e.g., planning for stress management, communication, development of community power, community perceptions of stress, community coping strategies).

- Help community obtain funding for additional programs.
  Vulnerable communities often need additional funding sources to strengthen coping resources.
- Encourage positive attitudes toward the community through the media and other sources.
  Negative attitudes or stigmas create additional stress and deficits in social support.
- Help community members work together to enhance power and coping skills.
  Community members may not have sufficient skills to collaborate for enhanced coping. Effective collaboration skills can be promoted by health providers (Freire, 1990).
- Encourage rational thinking.
  Rational thinking supports problem-solving ability.
- Demonstrate the optimum use of resources.
  Optimum use of resources supports community coping; community members benefit from such demonstrations (Miller, 1992).

Community Teaching

- Review coping skills, power for coping, and the use of power resources.

REFERENCES

Freire P: *Pedagogy of the oppressed.* New York, 1990, Continuum.

Miller JF: *Coping with chronic illness: overcoming powerlessness*, ed 2, Philadelphia, 1992, FA Davis.

Ineffective management of therapeutic regimen (community)

Margaret Lunney

Definition A pattern of regulating and integrating into community processes programs for the treatment of illness and the sequelae of illness that are unsatisfactory for meeting health-related goals.

Defining Characteristics

Major Number of health care resources are insufficient for the incidence or prevalence of illnesses.

Minor Expected or unexpected acceleration of illnesses; deficits in advocates for aggregates; deficits in community activities for primary, secondary, and tertiary prevention; deficits in persons and programs to be accountable for illness care of aggregates; illness symptoms above the norm; unavailable resources for illness care.

Related Factors (r/t)

Complexity of community and aggregate problems and needs; decreased communication among and between community and society; decreased valuing of community and aggregates by members of society; decreased valuing of health protection; decreased valuing of self by community and aggregates; disorganization of health care system; economic factors (e.g., poor management of available finances; excessive exposure to risk factors (e.g., toxic chemicals); local, state, or national policies.

Community Outcomes/Goals

- Persons who are accountable for illness care of specific aggregates are obtained for the community.
- Community members are involved in advocacy for illness care and prevention programs.
- Community members develop health care plans for effective prevention and treatment of illnesses.
- Resources are made available for illness care and prevention.
- Strategies for prevention of the sequelae of illnesses are initiated or improved.

Nursing Interventions and Rationales

- Nursing interventions are conducted in collaboration with key members of the community, members of other disciplines, and community or public health nurse leaders.
- Seek community leaders who are willing to learn about community assessment data and diagnosis and who have the potential to work with interdisciplinary health providers in planning for positive changes.
  Communities need to be involved in obtaining the services and resources they need for illness care and prevention. Only services that are valued and perceived as needed by community members are used effectively. Community health interventions are complex and often require multidisciplinary strategies (Lunney et al, in press).
- Advocate for and with the community in multiple arenas (e.g., newspapers, television, legislative activities, community boards).
  The community benefits from the advocacy of nurses and other health providers, whose opinions are respected (Anderson, McFarlane, 1988; Mason, Talbott, Leavitt, 1993; Milio, 1981).
- Provide information to public and private sources about community assessment and diagnosis and the plan of care.

The commitment that is needed for improvements in health services can only be obtained when others have adequate information.

- Mobilize support for the community in obtaining the resources necessary for illness care and prevention.
  As with individuals and families, community social supports enable the community to achieve health-related goals (Anderson, McFarlane, 1988).
- Recruit additional health providers as needed.
  If health providers are aware of inadequate community services, they may be able to contribute the necessary services.
- Write grants for funding of new programs or expansion of existing programs.
  Public and private sources of funds can often supply the financial bases of health care programs when they become aware of community problems.
- Conduct any research needed to convince others of the need for improved services or changes in policy.
  Community assessment and diagnosis may not be sufficient for change. More advanced research findings may be needed to obtain broad support for needed change.
- With other persons and groups, obtain changes in health policy as indicated.
  Health policies set the stage for effective health programs (Milio, 1981; Mason, Talbott, Leavitt, 1993).

REFERENCES

Anderson ET, McFarlane JM: *Community as client: application of the nursing process*, Philadelphia, 1988, JB Lippincott.

Mason DJ, Talbott SW, Leavitt JK: *Policy and politics for nurses: Action and change in the workplace, government, organizations and community*, ed 2, Philadelphia, 1993, WB Saunders.

Milio N: *Promoting health through public policy*, Philadelphia, 1981, FA Davis.

BIBLIOGRAPHY

Lunney M et al: Community diagnosis: analysis and synthesis of the literature. In *Proceedings of the 1994 Spring Institute, Association for Community Health Nursing Educators (ACHNE)*, Chicago, Ill, In press, ACHNE.

Acute confusion

Gail Ladwig

Definition The abrupt onset of a cluster of global, transient changes and disturbances in attention, cognition, psychomotor activity level of consciousness, or the sleep/wake cycle.

Defining Characteristics

Major Fluctuations in cognition; fluctuations in the sleep-wake cycle; fluctuations in levels of consciousness; fluctuations in psychomotor activity; increased agitation or restlessness; misperceptions; lack of motivation to initiate or follow through with goal-directed or purposeful behavior.

Minor Hallucinations.

Related Factors (r/t)

Over 60 years of age; dementia; alcohol abuse; abuse; delirium.

Client Outcomes/Goals

- Obtains optimal cognitive functioning.
- Maintains adequate sleep.
- Maintains an optimal level of consciousness.
- Demonstrates normal motor behavior.
- Demonstrates decreased agitation and restlessness.
- Initiates and follows through with goal-directed or purposeful behavior.
- Maintains optimal orientation.

Nursing Interventions and Rationales

- Refer to care plan for **Chronic confusion**.
- Assess client's behavior at least once daily, preferably at the completion of the day shift. Also assess client after any episodes of confusion.
  Delirious clients have higher fatality rates than demented, depressed, or cognitively intact persons. Nurses play a vital role in identifying the signs of delirium and can thus affect patient prognosis and outcome through early assessment and intervention (Rabins, Folstein, 1992).
- Obtain a baseline history that includes the recent mental status change (months, years), onset of any symptoms of confusion, time of day of confusional episodes, sleep patterns, medical illnesses, medication use, education level of client.
  The client's history is the most important aspect of assessing the confused older client (Matzo, 1990).
- Perform an accurate cognitive mental status exam that includes the following:
  1. Overall appearance, manner, and attitude
  2. Behavior observations and level of psychomotor agitation
  3. Mood and affect (observed and self-report by client; presence of suicidal or homicidal ideation)
  4. Insight and judgment
  5. Cognition as evidenced by level of consciousness, orientation (to time, place, and person), attention, concentration, memory (recent and remote), fund of knowledge, thought process and content (perceptual disturbances such as illusions and hallucinations, paranoia, delusions, abstract thinking)

  Identifying delirium in the hospitalized client depends on the performance of an accurate cognitive mental status examination as part of the routine clinical assessment (Inaba-Roland, Maricle, 1992).

- Assess for physiological alterations (e.g., sepsis, hypoglycemia, hypotension, infection, changes in temperature, fluid and electrolyte imbalances, medications with known cognitive and psychotropic side effects).
  Such alterations may be contributing to confusion and must be corrected (Matthiesen et al, 1994).
- Use orientation techniques; have client identify self and repeat the place and time of day, use wall calendars, have family bring in familiar items for bedside, and have family identify selves; offer reassurance.
  These orientation techniques help the client differentiate between reality and unreality. Confusion associated with delirium is treatable, reversible, and short term (Inaba-Roland, Maricle, 1992).
- Use restraints as infrequently as possible.
  Restraints have been shown to increase agitation, and they have even led to death (Dube, Mitchell, 1986).

Geriatric

- Mobilize client as soon as possible, provide active and passive range of motion.
  Older clients who had a low level of physical activity before injury are at a particular risk for acute confusion (Matthiesen et al, 1994).
- Provide sufficient medication to relieve pain.
  Older clients may give inaccurate pain histories, underreport symptoms, not want to bother the nurse, and exhibit restlessness, agitation, or increased confusion (Matthiesen et al, 1994).
- Non-narcotic analgesics should be substituted for narcotics.
  Oversedation poses risks for confusion and postoperative complications such as falls (Matthiesen et al, 1994).
- Urinary catheters should be removed as soon as possible.
  Elderly clients are at a great risk for urinary tract infections and urosepsis (Matthiesen et al, 1994).
- Call older clients by the name they prefer.
  Such steps help decrease the strangeness of the health care environment (Campbell, Williams, Mynarczyx, 1986).
- Explain hospital routines and procedures slowly and in simple terms; repeat information as necessary.
  Anxiety and sensory impairment decreases the older client's ability to integrate new information (Matthiesen et al, 1994).
- Give choices regarding hospital routines, but do not give too many options at once. Allow client time to respond.
  Loss of control or independence is difficult for older clients; they need as much control as possible and may need more time to process information (Matthiesen et al, 1994).
- Provide continuity of care when possible (e.g., provide the same caregivers, avoid room changes).
  Continuity of care helps decrease the disorienting effects of hospitalization (Matthiesen et al, 1994).
- If client knows that he or she is not thinking clearly, acknowledge the concern.
  Confusion is very frightening (Matthiesen et al, 1994).
- Correctly interpret environmental stimuli for the client.
  Acutely confused older clients may misperceive sensory input and experience illusions, delusions, or hallucinations (Campbell, Williams, Mynarczyx, 1986).

- Do not use the intercom to answer a call light.
  The intercom may be frightening to the older confused client (Matthiesen et al, 1994).
- Keep client's sleep-wake cycle as normal as possible (e.g., no daytime naps, avoid waking clients at night, give sedatives but not diuretics at bedtime, provide pain relief and backrubs).
  Acute confusion is accompanied by disruption of the sleep-wake cycle (Matthiesen et al, 1994).

Client/Family Teaching

- Teach family to recognize signs of early confusion and seek medical help.
  Early intervention prevents long-term complications.
- Have family stay with client in the evening; leave on night light; have call light within reach; turn off television.
  A secure feeling in the evening helps to decrease sundowning phenomenon (Matthiesen et al, 1994).
- Have familiar people or objects present. Encourage family members and friends to visit as often as possible.
  Familiar persons help keep the older client oriented (Matthiesen et al, 1994).

REFERENCES

Campbell E, Williams M, Mynarczyx S: After the fall—confusion, *AJN* 86(2):151-154, 1986.

Dube C, Mitchell E: Accidental strangulation from vest restraints. *JAMA*, 256:2725-2726, 1986.

Inaba-Roland K, Maricle R: Assessing delirium in the acute care setting, *Heart Lung*, 21:49, 1992.

Matthiesen V et al: Acute confusion: nursing intervention in older patients, *Orthop Nurs* 13:25, 1994.

Matzo M: Confusion in older adults: assessment and differential diagnosis, *Nurse Pract*, 15:32-44, 1990.

Rabins P, Folstein M: Delirium and dementia: diagnostic criteria and fatality rates, *Br J Psychiatry* 140:149-153, 1992.

Chronic confusion

Nancy English and Betty Ackley

Definition An irreversible, long-standing, and/or progressive deterioration of intellect and personality that is characterized by a decreased ability to interpret environmental stimuli and a decreased capacity for intellectual thought processes and is manifested by disturbances of memory, orientation, and behavior.

Defining Characteristics

Major: Clinical evidence of organic impairment; altered interpretation or response to stimuli; progressive or longstanding cognitive impairment.

Minor: No change in level of consciousness; impaired socialization; impaired short-term or long-term memory; altered personality.

Related Factors (r/t)

Alzheimer's disease; Korsakoff's psychosis; multi-infarct dementia; cerebral vascular accident; head injury.

Client Outcomes/Goals

- Remains content and free from harm.
- Functions at maximum of cognitive level.
- Independently participates in activities of daily living at the maximum of functional ability.

Nursing Interventions and Rationales

- Determine client's cognitive level using a screening tool such as the Mini Mental State Exam (MMSE).
  Using an evaluation tool such as the MMSE can help determine the client's abilities and plan appropriate nursing interventions (Agostinelli et al, 1994).
- Gather information about client before the onset of confusion including social situation, physical condition, and psychological functioning.
  Knowing the client's background can help the nurse understand the client's behavior if he or she becomes delusional and hallucinates. Sharing memories helps soothe the client.
- Ensure that client is in a safe environment by removing potential hazards such as sharp objects and harmful liquids.
  Clients with dementia lose the ability to make good judgments and can easily harm self or others.
- Place an identification bracelet on client.
  Clients with dementia wander and can become lost; identification bracelets increase their safety.
- Avoid unfamiliar situations and people as much as possible. Maintain continuity of caregivers; maintain routines of care through established mealtimes, bathing, and sleeping schedules; and send familiar person with client when he or she goes for diagnostic testing.
  Situational anxiety associated with environmental, interpersonal, or structural change can escalate into agitated behavior (Gerdner, Buckwalter, 1994).
- Keep environment quiet and nonstimulating; avoid using buzzers and alarms if possible.
- Begin each interaction with the client by identifying self and calling the client by name.
- Approach client with a caring, loving, and accepting attitude and speak in a calm, slow manner.
  Dementia clients can sense feelings of compassion; a calm, slow manner projects a feeling of comfort to the client (Stolley, 1994).

- Touch client gently, stroking hand or arm in a soothing fashion.
- Give one simple direction at a time and repeat it as necessary; use verbal and physical prompts, and model the desired action if needed and possible.
  "People with dementia need time to assimilate and interpret your directions, if you rephrase your question, you give them something new to process, increasing their confusion" (Stolley, 1994 p. 40).
- Break down self-care tasks into simple steps (e.g., instead of saying "Take a shower," say to client, "Please follow me. Sit down on the bed. Take off your shoes. Now take off your socks. . . ."
  Dementia clients are unable to follow complex commands; breaking down the activity into simple steps makes the activity more feasible (Agnostinelli et al, 1994).
- Keep questions simple; yes or no questions are often preferable. Use positive statements and actions and avoid negative communication (e.g., if client is trying to crawl out of bed, help him or her find hand holds to get out; lead back to bed later as necessary).
  Negative feedback leads to increased confusion and agitation; it is more effective to go along with the client and then redirect as necessary.
- Recognize that clients have good and bad days; provide decreased activity on bad days.
- Provide boundaries by placing red or yellow tape on the floor or by using a stop sign.
  Boundaries help the client identify safe areas; older clients can more easily see red and yellow colors.
- Write client's name in large block letters in the room and on client's clothing and possessions.
- Use symbols rather than words to identify areas such as the bathroom, kitchen, or dresser.
- Keep family pictures that are labeled with names in client's room.
- Limit to two visitors and provide them with guidelines on appropriate topics to discuss with client.
- Set up scheduled quiet periods. Avoid prolonged naps during the day.
  Fatigue has been associated with the onset of increased confusion and agitation (Stolley, 1994).
- Provide quiet activities such as classical or religious music in the afternoon or early evening.
  An increase in confusion and agitation may occur in the late afternoon and early evening and is referred to as sundowning syndrome. *Quiet activities can provide a calming environment.*
- Consider using doll therapy. Ask family members to bring a large, safe doll or stuffed animal such as a teddy bear.
  Doll therapy can be soothing to some dementia clients (Bailey, 1992; Paulanka, Griffin, 1993).
- If client becomes increasingly confused and agitated, perform the following steps:
  - Monitor client for physiological causes, including acute hypoxia, pain, medication effects, infection, fatigue, electrolyte disturbances, or constipation (Gerdner, Buckwalter, 1994).
  - Monitor for psychological causes, including changes in environment, caregiver, or routine; demands to perform beyond capacity; multiple competing stimuli.
  - Avoid confrontations with the client; allow client to dissipate energy by performing repetitive tasks or by pacing.

- If client is delusional or is hallucinating, do not confront him or her with reality but instead use validation therapy to verbally reflect back to the emotions that the client appears to be feeling. Use statements such as "I can see you are afraid," "I will stay with you," or "Can you tell me more about what is going on right now?"
  Orienting the client to reality can increase agitation; validation therapy conveys empathy and understanding and can help determine the internal stimulus that is creating the change in behavior (Feil, 1993).
- Decrease stimuli in the environment (e.g., turn off television, take client to a quiet place); institute activities that are associated with pleasant emotions such as playing soft music the client likes, looking through a photo album, or providing favorite food.
  Decreasing stimuli can decrease agitation; reassuring activities can help bring pleasant emotions to help soothe the client.
- Avoid using restraints if at all possible; obtain physician's order if they become necessary.
  Restrained elders often have increased incidences of falls, possibly because of muscle deconditioning or loss of coordination (Tinetti, Liu, Ginter, 1992).
- Use prn psychotropic or antianxiety drugs only as a last resort. Start with the lowest possible dose.

• For early dementia clients with memory loss only, refer to care plan for **Impaired memory**.
• For clients with self-care deficits, refer to the appropriate care plan **(Self-care deficit: feeding, Self-care deficit: dressing, Self-care deficit: toileting).**

Geriatric

NOTE: Most of the preceding interventions apply to the geriatric client.

• Use Reminiscence and Life Review therapeutic interventions, and use statements such as "Tell me about your work, years bringing up children, time in the service. What was really important to you as you look back?"
  Reminiscence and life review can help the older person to reframe and accept life events (Burnside, Haight, 1994).

Client/Family Teaching

• Recommend that the family develop a memory aid wallet or booklet for client, which contains pictures and text that chronicle the client's life.
  Using memory aids such as wallets or booklets helps dementia clients make more factual statements and stay on topic and decreases the number of confused, erroneous, and repetitive statements (Bourgeois, 1992).
• Teach family how to converse with a memory-impaired person. Guidelines include the following:
  - Ask client to have a conversation with you
  - Guide conversation onto specific, nonthreatening topics, and redirect the conversation back on topic when the client begins to ramble
  - Reassure and help out when the client gets stuck or cannot find the right words
  - Smile and act interested in what client is saying even if unsure what it means
  - Thank client for talking
  - Avoid quizzing client or asking a lot of specific questions
  - Avoid correcting or contradicting something that was stated even if it is wrong

  These guidelines can help families interact more effectively with clients and decrease frustration levels (Bourgeois, 1992).

- Teach family how to set up environment, use care techniques, and use interventions listed so that client will experience a progressively lowered stress threshold. *Alzheimer's clients are unable to deal with stress; decreasing stress can decrease confusion and changes in behavior (Hall, 1991; Stolley, 1994).*

NOTE: The nursing diagnoses **Impaired environmental interpretation syndrome** and **Chronic confusion** are very similar in definition and interventions. **Impaired environmental interpretation** must be interpreted as a syndrome where other nursing diagnoses would also apply. **Chronic confusion** may be interpreted as the human response to a situation or situations that require a level of cognition no longer available to the individual. Further research is in progress to make this distinction clear to the practicing nurse.

REFERENCES

Agostinelli B et al: Targeted interventions: use of the Mini-Mental State Exam, *J Gerontol Nurs* 20:15-23, 46-47, 1994.

Bailey J: To find a soul, *Nursing '92*:63-64, 1992.

Bouregois MS: *Conversing with memory impaired individuals using memory aids: a memory aid workbook*, Gaylord, Mich, 1992, Northern Speech Services.

Burnside I, Haight B: Reminiscence and life review: therapeutic interventions for older people, *Nurse Pract*: 55-61, 1994.

Feil N: *The validation breakthrough: simple techniques for communicating with people with Alzheimer's-type dementia,* Baltimore, 1993, Health Professions.

Gerdner LA, Buckwalter KC: A nursing challenge: assessment and management of agitation in Alzheimer's Patients, *J Gerontol Nurs* 20:11-20, 1994.

Hall GR, This hospital patient has Alzheimer's, *Am J Nurs* 91:44-50, 1991.

Paulanka, BJ, Griffin LS: Behavioral responses of memory impaired clients to selected nursing interventions, *Phys Occup Ther Geriatr* 12:65-78, 1993.

Stolley, JM: When your patient has Alzheimer's disease, *Am J Nurs*, 94:34-41, 1994.

Tinetti ME, Liu WL, Ginter SF: Mechanical restraint use and fall-related injuries among residents of skilled nursing facilities, *Ann Intern Med* 116:369-373, 1992.

Constipation

Kathie Hesnan

Definition

The state in which an individual experiences a change in normal bowel habits characterized by a decrease in frequency and/or passage of hard, dry stools.

Defining Characteristics

Decreased frequency of defecation (less than usual pattern or greater than every 3 days); hard, formed stool; straining at stool; feeling of rectal fullness and pressure; abdominal pain; palpable mass; appetite impairment; back pain; headache; interference with daily living; use of laxatives.

Related Factors (r/t)

Decreased activity level; decreased fluid intake; inadequate fiber in diet; emotional disturbances; lack of privacy; embarrassment about defecating in hospital environment; decreased peristalsis from hypokalemia or hypothyroidism; side effects from medications such as anticholinergics, antidepressants, antipsychotics, narcotics, antacids, iron, barium, and neuroleptics.

Client Outcomes/Goals

- Maintains soft, formed stool without straining every 3 days.
- States relief from discomfort of constipation.
- Identifies measures that prevent or treat constipation.

Nursing Interventions and Rationales

- Observe usual pattern or have patient keep diary of defecation, including time of day; usual stimulus; consistency, amount, and frequency of stool; type, amount, and time of food consumed; fluid intake; history of bowel habits or laxative use; diet; exercise patterns; personal remedies for constipation; OB/GYN history; medications; surgeries; alterations in perianal sensation; and present bowel regimen.
  The underlying cause determines the appropriate nursing interventions.
- Review client's current medications.
  Many medications affect normal bowel function, including antidepressants, anticholinergics, diuretics, anticonvulsants, antacids containing aluminum and calcium, muscle relaxants, and narcotics (Cameron, 1992).
- Palpate for abdominal distention and auscultate bowel sounds twice daily.
- Check for impaction; perform digital removal per physician's order.
- Assess for anxiety or embarrassment regarding defecation.
- Encourage a fluid intake of 64 ounces per day; if oral intake is low, gradually increase fluid intake. Fluid intake must be within the cardiac and renal reserve.
  Adequate fluid intake is necessary to prevent hard, dry stools.
- Encourage ambulation and/or a daily exercise program.
  Activity, even minimal activity such as waist twists, increases peristalsis, which is necessary to prevent constipation (Yakabowich, 1990).
- At each meal, sprinkle bran over client's food as allowed by client and prescribed diet.
  The number of bowel movements is increased and the use of laxatives is decreased in a client who eats more wheat bran (Schmelzer, 1990).
- If sprinkling bran over the food is not effective, use the special recipe reported by Behm (1983). Mix 3 cups of sugar-free applesauce, 2 cups of unprocessed coarse wheat bran, and 1½ cups of unsweetened prune juice. Cover and refrigerate. Give client 2 tablespoons a day with a glass of water, and titrate the dosage up to 3 tablespoons twice a day until adequate bowel function is reached.

Use of this recipe has shown to decrease laxative and enema use by 80% and allow clients to experience a regular pattern of bowel function (Smith, Newman, 1989).

- Encourage intake of foods containing fiber such as fresh fruits, vegetables, and bran cereals.
- Initiate a regular schedule for defecation, using the client's normal evacuation time whenever possible. An optimal time for many individuals is 30 minutes after breakfast because of the gastrocolic reflex.
  A schedule gives the client a sense of control, but more important, it promotes evacuation before drying of stool and constipation occur (Doughty, 1992).
- Reinforce to the client the necessary items for a normal bowel regimen (e.g., fluid, fiber, activity, and time).
- Help client onto bedside commode or toilet with client's hips flexed and feet flat. Have client deep breathe through mouth to encourage relaxation of the pelvic floor muscle, and have client use the abdominal muscles to help evacuation.
- Provide laxatives, suppositories, and enemas only as needed and as ordered; establish a goal of not needing these. Avoid soapsud enemas.
  Soapsud enemas can cause damage to the colonic mucosa (Schmelzer, Wright, 1993).
- For the stable neuro client, consider use of a bowel routine of suppositories every other day or performing digital stimulation with physician's permission.

Geriatric

- Explain the importance of fluid intake and activity for soft, formed stool.
  Activity, fiber, and fluid intake are often decreased in elderly clients.
- Determine client's perception of normal bowel elimination; promote adherence to a regular schedule.
  Misconceptions regarding how frequently bowel movements should occur can lead to anxiety and overuse of laxatives.
- Explain Valsalva's maneuver and why it should be avoided.
- Respond quickly to client's call for help with toileting.
- If there is impaction, break up the stool digitally and remove gently according to protocol and physician's order.
  Breaking up the stool promotes easier evacuation.
- Avoid regular use of enemas in the elderly.
  Enemas can cause fluid and electrolyte imbalances (Yakabowich, 1990) and cause damage to the colonic mucosa (Schmelzer, Wright, 1993).
- Use narcotics cautiously.
  Narcotics can cause constipation.
- Position client on toilet or commode and place a small footstool under the feet.
  Placing a small footstool under the feet increases intra-abdominal pressure and makes defecation easier for the elderly client with weak abdominal muscles.

Client/Family Teaching

- Instruct client on normal bowel function and how fluid, fiber, and activity are essential components of a bowel program.
- Encourage client to heed defecation warning signs and to develop a regular schedule of defecation by using a stimulus such as a warm drink or prune juice.
- Teach client the natural methods of softening stool and increasing peristalsis.
- Encourage client to avoid long-term use of laxatives or enemas and to gradually withdraw their use if they have been used regularly.
- If not contraindicated, teach client how to do bent-leg sit-ups to increase abdominal

tone; also encourage client to contract abdominal muscles frequently throughout the day.

- Teach client to increase fluids and roughage.
- Help client develop a daily exercise program to increase peristalsis.

REFERENCES

Cameron T: Constipation related to narcotic therapy, *Cancer Nurs* 15:5, 1992.

Doughty D: A step-by-step approach to bowel training, *Progressions* 4:12-23, 1992.

Schmelzer M: Effectiveness of wheat bran in prevention of constipation in hospitalized orthopaedic surgery patients, *Orthop Nurs* 15:10, 1990.

Schmelzer M, Wright K: Working smart, *Am J Nurs* 93(3):1993.

Smith D, Newman D: Beating the cycle of constipation, laxative abuse, and fecal incontinence. *TNH,* p. 12, Sept 1989.

Yakabowich M: Prescribe with care: the role of laxatives in the treatment of constipation, *J Gerontol Nurs* 16:4-11, 1990.

BIBLIOGRAPHY

Beverley L, Travis I: Constipation: proposed natural laxative mixtures, *J Gerontol Nurs* 18:5, 1992.

Doughty D: *Urinary and fecal incontinence: nursing management*, St Louis, 1991, Mosby.

Colonic constipation

Definition The state in which an individual's pattern of elimination is characterized by a hard, dry stool that results from a delay in passage of food residue.

Defining Characteristics

Major: Decreased frequency of defecation; hard, dry stool; straining at stool; abdominal distention; painful defecation; palpable mass.

Minor: Rectal pressure; headache; appetite impairment; abdominal pain.

Related Factors (r/t)

Inadequate fluid intake; inadequate fiber in diet; inadequate dietary intake; decreased activity level; immobility; emotional disturbances; stress; lack of privacy; change in daily routine; decreased peristalsis resulting from hypokalemia, hypocalcemia, or hypothyroidism; decreased gastrointestinal motility resulting from hormonal changes of pregnancy; hesitancy or reluctance to pass stool secondary to previous experience with rectal fissures or bleeding.

Client Outcomes/Goals, Nursing Interventions and Rationales, Client/Family Teaching

Refer to care plan for **Constipation**.

Perceived constipation

Kathie Hesnan

Definition The state in which an individual makes a self-diagnosis of constipation and ensures a daily bowel movement through the abuse of laxatives, enemas, and suppositories.

Defining Characteristics

Expectation of a daily bowel movement that results in an overuse of laxatives, enemas, and suppositories; expectation of a bowel movement at the same time every day.

Related Factors (r/t)

Cultural or family beliefs; faulty appraisals; impaired thought processes.

Client Outcomes/Goals

- Regularly defecates soft, formed stool without using any aids.
- Explains the need to decrease or eliminate the use of laxatives, suppositories, and enemas.
- Identifies alternatives to laxatives, enemas, and suppositories for ensuring defecation.
- Explains that defecation does not have to occur every day.

Nursing Interventions and Rationales

- Observe usual pattern of defecation (e.g., timing, consistency, amount, and frequency of stool; diet; and fluid intake).
  This bowel record provides both the client and the nurse a way to assess the present bowel program, identify areas of concern, and develop an individualized bowel program.
- Determine client's perception of an appropriate defecation pattern.
  The client may need to be taught that one bowel movement every 1 to 4 days is normal (Yakabowich, 1990).
- Monitor use of laxatives, suppositories, or enemas and offer alternatives such as natural laxatives.
  Natural laxatives have been shown to be successful in treating constipation (Beverly, Travis, 1992; Smith, Newman, 1989).
- Encourage client to promptly respond to the defecation reflex.
  Not responding to the urge to defecate can be a contributing factor to constipation (Battle, Hanna, 1989).
- Obtain a dietary referral for analysis and input on diet.
- Provide privacy for defecation and encourage client to avoid using a bedpan if possible.
  Many individuals need privacy to defecate. Using a bedpan makes it more difficult to use the abdominal muscles to help evacuate the rectum, and the client may have a feeling of incomplete emptying.
- Observe for potential body image disturbance or the use of laxatives to control or decrease weight.

Client/Family Teaching

- Explain normal bowel function and the necessary items for a regular bowel regimen.
- Work with client and family to develop a diet that fits life-style and includes increased roughage and fiber.
- Teach client that it is not necessary to have daily bowel movements and that normal people range from three stools each day to three stools each week.
- Explain to client the harmful effects of the continual use of defecation aids.
- Encourage client to gradually decrease use of usual laxatives and enemas and to set a date to be free from all defecation aids.

- Determine how to increase client's fluid intake and fit this practice into client's lifestyle.
- Explain Valsalva's maneuver and why it should be avoided.
- Work with client and family to design a bowel training routine that is based on previous patterns (before laxative or enema abuse) and incorporates warm fluids, privacy, and a predictable routine.

Additional Nursing Interventions and Rationales, Client/Family Teaching

Refer to care plan for **Constipation**

REFERENCES

Battle E, Hanna C: Evaluation of a dietary regimen for chronic constipation, *J Gerontol Nurs* 6:527-532, 1989.

Beverley L, Travis I: Constipation: proposed natural laxative mixtures, *J Gerontol Nurs* 18:5, 1992.

Smith D, Newman D: Beating the cycle of constipation, laxative abuse, and fecal incontinence. *TNH,* 1989.

Yakabowich, M: Prescribe with care: the role of laxatives in the treatment of constipation, *J Gerontol Nurs* 16:4-11, 1990.

BIBLIOGRAPHY

Doughty D: A step by step approach to bowel training, *Progressions* 4:12, 1992.

Doughty D: *Urinary and fecal incontinence: nursing management*, St Louis, 1991, Mosby.

Defensive coping

Gail Ladwig

Definition The state in which an individual repeatedly projects falsely positive self-evaluations based on a self-protective pattern that defends against underlying perceived threats to positive self-regard.

Defining Characteristics

Major Denial of obvious problems or weaknesses; projection of blame or responsibility; rationalization of failures; hypersensitivity to slight criticism; grandiosity.

Minor Superior attitude toward others; difficulty establishing or maintaining relationships; hostile laughter or ridicule of others; difficulties with reality-testing perceptions; lack of follow-through or participation in treatment or therapy.

Related Factors (r/t)

Situational crises; psychological impairment; substance abuse.

Client Outcomes/Goals

- Accepts responsibility for actions.
- Accepts constructive criticism without feeling personally rejected.
- Able to interact with others.
- Participates in therapy and establishes realistic goals.

Nursing Interventions and Rationales

- Determine client's perception of the problem.
  Each human being perceives the world in a different way, and each may cope differently with a given situation (Barry, 1994).
- Help client to identify the situations or people that trigger feelings of defensiveness; acknowledge that these are triggers, and emphasize that the client is ultimately responsible for his or her own behavior.
  Identifying exact situations and feelings helps direct interventions. A client who does not take responsibility for certain unacceptable behaviors blames persons, places, and things for these behaviors (Johnson, 1993).
- Encourage client to feel good about himself or herself; use group or individual therapy, role-playing, one-to-one interactions, and role-modeling.
  A positive attitude is the most important characteristic of healing (Criddle, 1993). These traditional interventions promote positive self-esteem.
- Teach client to use positive thinking by blocking negative thoughts with the word "stop" and inserting positive thoughts (e.g., "I'm a good person, friend, or student").
  Once a client learns to recognize negative and distorted thoughts, he or she can learn to interrupt or stop these self-defeating thoughts and replace them with realistic and positive appraisals (Norrus, 1992).
- Provide feedback regarding others' perceptions of the client's behavior through group therapy, milieu therapy, or one-to-one interactions.
  A client needs feedback to face the reality of his or her behavior. Group therapy promotes the development of appropriate social skills (Johnson, 1993).
- Encourage client to use "I" statements and to accept responsibility for actions and consequences of these actions.
  "I" statements encourage personal responsibility and help the client to overcome defensiveness. All clients have the capacity for change (Murray, 1993).

Geriatric

- Assess client for anger, and identify previous outlets for anger.
  Using previously used familiar outlets for anger, if appropriate, can help the client dissipate the emotion.

- Explore new outlets for anger, including physical activities within client's capabilities (e.g., hitting a pillow, woodworking, sanding, scrubbing floors).
  Physical activities help the client direct anger outward instead of holding it inside.
- Assess client for dementia or depression.
  Symptoms of dementia or depression may be masked by inappropriate coping techniques. Depression may be overlooked because there is a focus on the physiological problems of aging (Abraham, Neudorfer, Currie, 1992).

Client/Family Teaching

- Teach the actions and side effects of medications and the importance of taking them as prescribed, even when the client is feeling "good."
  The client needs to know that feeling "good" may result from the medications and that it is important to continue taking them.
- Refer client to appropriate therapist for grandiose and possibly harmful symptoms such as promiscuity, insomnia, euphoria, overspending, and alcohol or drug abuse.
  Harmful behaviors need appropriate intervention from a qualified professional.
- Work with client's support group to identify harmful behaviors and to seek help for client if unable to control behavior.
  The client's support group needs to be involved in the treatment plan to ensure safety and compliance.

REFERENCES

Abraham I, Neudorfer M, Currie L: Effects of group interventions on cognition and depression in nursing home residents, *Nursing Res* 41:196-202, 1992.

Barry P: *Mental health and mental illness*, ed 5, Philadelphia, 1994, JB Lippincott.

Criddle L: Healing from surgery: a phenomenological study, *Image J Nurs Sch* 25:208-213, 1993.

Johnson B: *Psychiatric mental health nursing: adaptation and growth*, ed 3, Philadelphia, 1993, JB Lippincott.

Murray RB, Bair M: Use of therapeutic mileau in a community setting, *J Psychosoc Nurs Ment Health Serv* 31:11-16, 1993.

Norris J: Nursing intervention for self-esteem disturbances, *Nurs Diag* 3:48-53, 1992.

Ineffective individual coping

Gail Ladwig

Definition

Impairment of adaptive behaviors and problem-solving abilities in meeting life's demands and roles.

Defining Characteristics

*Verbalized inability to cope or ask for help; inability to meet role expectations; inability to meet basic needs; *inability to problem solve; alteration in social participation; destructive behavior toward self or others; inappropriate use of defense mechanisms; change in usual communication patterns; verbal manipulation; high illness rate; high rate of accidents. (*Critical)

Related Factors (r/t)

Situational crises; maturational crises; personal vulnerability.

Client Outcomes/Goals

- Verbalizes ability to cope and asks for help when needed.
- Demonstrates ability to solve problems and participates at usual level in society.
- Free of destructive behavior toward self or others.
- Able to communicate needs and negotiate with others to meet needs.
- Able to discuss how recent life stressors have overwhelmed normal coping strategies.
- Illness and accident rate not excessive for age and developmental level.

Nursing Interventions and Rationales

- Observe for causes of ineffective coping such as poor self-concept, grief, lack of problem-solving skills, lack of support, or recent change in life situations.
  The problem or stressor needs to be identified to plan useful solutions and coping strategies.
- Observe for strengths such as the ability to relate facts and recognize source of stressors.
  If a client cannot find something meaningful in life that will give him or her a purpose to live, the client is at risk of focusing on the escape route of death (Buchanan, 1991).
- Monitor risk of harming self or others and intervene appropriately; refer to nursing diagnosis **Risk for violence.**
  A client with hopelessness and an inability to problem solve often runs the risk of suicide (Buchanan, 1991). In these cases immediate referral for mental health care is essential (Norris, 1992).
- Help client set realistic goals and identify personal skills and knowledge.
  Involving the client in decision-making helps him or her move toward independence (Connelly et al, 1993).
- Encourage client to verbalize fears and express emotions.
  If the client is allowed to discuss anxieties and feelings, much emotional pressure seems to be relieved (Bailey, Bailey, 1993).
- Encourage client to make choices and to participate in planning of care and scheduled activities.
  Participation gives a feeling of control and increases self-esteem.
- Provide mental and physical activities within the client's ability (e.g., reading, television, radio, crafts, outings, movies, dinners out, social gatherings, exercise, sports, or games).
  The client needs a variety of choices to enhance coping. Physical fitness enhances mental health, and as a client progresses, recreational needs become important.

Planning renewal of a previously enjoyed activity provides the client with a sense of accomplishment (Haber et al, 1992).

- Discuss changes with client before making them.
  Knowledge about changes gives a feeling of control and increases self-esteem.
- Discuss client's power to change a situation or the need to accept a situation.
  Such a discussion helps the client maintain self-esteem and look at the situation realistically with the aid of a trusted individual (Norris, 1992).
- Use active listening and acceptance to help client express emotions such as crying and anger (within appropriate limits).
  Acceptance of the client's anger, despair, or anxiety without criticism encourages the client to believe that the expression of such feelings need not be destructive or a sign of weakness. Facilitating the expression of feelings by calm acceptance leads a client out of depression because, when emotional responsiveness returns, so does a reasonable basis for hope (Haber et al, 1992).
- Avoid false reassurance; give honest answers and provide only the information requested.
  Overload needs to be avoided in stressful situations; honesty promotes trust.
- Encourage client to describe previous stressors and the coping mechanisms used.
  Describing previous experiences strengthens effective coping and helps eliminate ineffective coping mechanisms.
- Be supportive of coping behaviors; allow client time to relax.
  Such support is a positive reinforcement for success.
- Encourage use of cognitive behavioral relaxation (e.g., music therapy, imagery).
  Music is not a cure but can lift the human spirit, comfort the heart, and inspire the soul. Imagery is useful for relaxation and distraction (Fontaine, 1994).
- Refer for counseling as needed.
  Follow-up may be needed to reinforce new behaviors.

Geriatric

- Observe client's fear of illness; identify and reinforce patterns the elderly client has previously used to respond to stress.
  The elderly client has had a lifetime of experience dealing with stressful events.
- Observe any physiological imbalance as a contributor to ineffective coping; take appropriate nursing actions to correct imbalances, and notify physician of abnormal laboratory results or medication side effects or interactions.
  Physiological problems may be manifested as emotional problems.
- Increase and mobilize support available to the elderly client.
  Involvement of significant others enhances the effectiveness of interventions.
- Maintain continuity of care by keeping the number of caregivers to a minimum.
  The elderly client needs to develop trust before sharing concerns.

Client/Family Teaching

- Teach client to problem solve; teach client to define the problem and cause and list each option and its advantages and disadvantages.
  Problem-solving skills promote the client's sense of control.
- Teach relaxation techniques.
  Relaxation decreases stress and enhances coping (Fontaine, 1994).
- Teach client about available community resources (e.g., therapists, ministers, counselors, self-help groups).
  Client and family teaching that promotes the ability to understand and carry out any necessary medical, rehabilitative, or daily-living activities contributes to a sense of

mastery, competency, and control and is vital to discharge planning and community-based assessments (Norris, 1992).

REFERENCES

Bailey DS, Bailey DR: *Therapeutic approaches to the care of the mentally ill*, ed 3, Philadelphia, 1993, FA Davis.

Buchanan D: Suicide: a conceptual model for an avoidable death, *Arch Psychiatr Nurs* 5:341-347, 1991.

Connelly L et al: A place to be yourself: empowerment from the client's perspective, *Image: J Nurs Sch* 25:297-303, 1993.

Fontaine D: Recognition, assessment, and treatment of anxiety in the critical care setting, *Crit Care Nurse* (Suppl) 3:7-10, Aug 1994.

Haber J et al: *Comprehensive Psychiatric Nursing*, ed 4, St Louis, 1992, Mosby.

Norris J: Nursing interventions for self-esteem disturbances, *Nurs Diag* 3:48-53, 1992.

Decisional conflict

Gail Ladwig

Definition The state of uncertainty about the course of action to be taken when choice among competing actions involves risk, loss, or challenge to personal life values.

Defining Characteristics

Major Verbalization of uncertainty about the choices; verbalization of undesired consequences of alternatives; vacillation between alternative choices; delayed decision making.

Minor Verbalization of distress while attempting a decision; self-focusing; physical signs of distress or tension (e.g., increased heart rate, increased muscle tension, restlessness); questioning of personal values and beliefs while attempting a decision.

Related Factors (r/t)

Unclear personal values or beliefs; perceived threat to value system; lack of experience in or interference with decision making; lack of relevant information; support system deficit; multiple or divergent sources of information; impact of ethical and moral beliefs on choices and health outcomes (e.g., birth of defective child); unplanned life event (e.g., pregnancy).

Client Outcomes/Goals

- States the advantages and disadvantages of choices.
- Shares fears and concerns regarding choices and responses of others.
- Makes an informed choice.

Nursing Interventions and Rationales

- Observe for factors causing or contributing to conflict (e.g., value conflicts, fears of outcome, poor problem-solving skills).
  Baseline data are important in directing interventions; no single set of values is appropriate for all individuals. Values clarification emphasizes the client's capacity for intelligent self-directed behavior (Dossey et al, 1988).
- Give client time and permission to express feelings associated with decision making.
  Decisions become more difficult when feelings are "bottled up." Once some of this stress is removed by talking through problems or releasing pent-up emotions, the decision process often becomes easier (Burnard, 1992).
- Explore client's perception of the future in relation to different decisions.
  Perceiving the future helps the client focus on what is important. Accurate time orientation (the ability to view the future on the basis of present and past experience) indicates that the client will have better coping skills (Haber et al, 1992).
- Demonstrate unconditional respect for and acceptance of client's values, spiritual beliefs, and cultural norms.
  Using a therapeutic approach promotes trust.
- Encourage client to list the advantages and disadvantages of each alternative.
  Listing alternatives helps the client learn how to problem solve. The client might not believe he or she has alternatives and may need assistance in exploring alternatives (Chez, 1994).
- Initiate health teaching and referrals when needed.
  All interventions need to be individualized.
- Facilitate communication between family members regarding the final decision; offer support to person making the final decision.
  Family members may share in decision making with client or may be the primary decision makers when the client is incapable of making a decision as a result of extreme age or mental incapacity.

Geriatric

- Discuss with client and family the importance of discussing and recording end-of-life decisions.
  These decisions are of extreme importance to an aging client. Discussing these issues gives the client both a sense of control and the opportunity to prepare for the inevitable (Dossey et al, 1988).
- If end-of-life discussions are being avoided, describe the possible consequences.
  The reality of the situation must be confronted.
- Discuss the purpose of a living will and advance directives.
  Elderly clients and their significant others need to know how to legally make end-of-life decisions.
- Discuss choices or changes to be made (e.g., moving in with children, into a nursing home, or into an adult foster care home).
  Exploring options gives the client and family a sense of control. For a change to be effective, the client must accept and own it (Fleury, 1991).
- Teach family members how to be supportive of final decision or how to refrain from being destructive if unable to be supportive.
  It is important to support the decisions that the client makes.

Client/Family Teaching

- Instruct the client and family members to provide directives in the following areas:
  - Person to contact in an emergency
  - Preference to die at home or in the hospital or no preference
  - Desire to sign a living will
  - Desire to donate an organ
  - Funeral arrangements (e.g., burial, cremation)

  Sharing specific information makes the decision-making process easier.
- Inform family of treatment options; encourage and defend self-determination.
  Exploring options gives the client and family a sense of control.
- Identify reasons for family decisions regarding care; explore ways family decisions can be respected.
  Family issues need to be identified to provide optimal care (e.g., does the family understand the prognosis or have unresolved issues with the client, are they waiting for someone to come from out of town, must other things be resolved before final decisions can be made) (Campbell, 1994).

REFERENCES

Burnard P: *Counseling: a guide to practice in nursing*, Oxford, England, 1992, Butterworth-Heinemann.
Campbell M: Making an end-of-life difference, *Crit Care Nurse* 14:111-117, 1994.
Chez N: Helping the victim of domestic violence, *Am J Nurs* 94:33-37, 1994.
Dossey B et al: *Holistic nursing: a handbook for practice*, Rockville, Md, 1988, Aspen.
Fleury J: Empowering potential: a theory of wellness motivation, *Nurs Res* 40:286-291, 1991.
Haber J, et al: *Comprehensive Psychiatric Nursing*, ed 4, St Louis, 1992, Mosby.

Ineffective denial

Gail Ladwig

Definition The state of a conscious or unconscious attempt to disavow the knowledge or meaning of an event to reduce anxiety and fear to the detriment of health.

Defining Characteristics

Major Delays or refuses health care to the detriment of health; does not perceive personal relevance of symptoms or danger.

Minor Uses home remedies (self-treatment) to relieve symptoms; does not admit fear of death or invalidism; minimizes symptoms; displaces source of symptoms to other organs; displaces fear of impact of the condition; is unable to admit impact of disease on life pattern; makes dismissive gestures or comments when speaking of distressing events; displays inappropriate affect.

Related Factors (r/t)

Fear of consequences; chronic or terminal illness; actual or perceived fear of possible losses (e.g., job, significant other); refusal to acknowledge substance-abuse problem; fear of the social stigma of disease.

Client Outcomes/Goals

- Seeks out health care attention when needed.
- Uses home remedies only when appropriate.
- Displays appropriate affect and verbalizes fears.
- Acknowledges substance-abuse problem and seeks help.

Nursing Interventions and Rationales

- Assess client's understanding of symptoms and illness.
  Allowing a client to define his or her own reality shows regard for the client's needs and values and establishes the client as an expert (Ersek, 1992).
- Spend one-to-one time with client.
  The most critical intervention a nurse can make is to offer to spend time with the client (Harrenstein, 1992).
- Allow client to express and use denial.
  At certain stages of an illness, denial may be appropriate. Denial is common and sometimes necessary immediately following the diagnosis of cancer; denial controls the threat of that information until other coping mechanisms can be mobilized (Weisman, 1992).
- Sit at eye level.
  Eye-level communication promotes emotional comfort (Ringsven, Bond, 1991).
- Use touch if appropriate; touch client's hand or arm.
  Touch conveys empathy.
- Explain signs and symptoms of illness; reinforce use of prescribed treatment plan.
  Accurate information and encouragement to follow treatment regimen enhances compliance.
- Help client recognize existing and additional sources of support; allow time for adjustment.
  Involvement of a support system enhances compliance.
- If appropriate, refer family to a skilled mental health counselor for help in planning an intervention to confront client about the self-destructive behaviors (e.g., drinking, drugs, eating disorders).
  Specialized treatment may be required for certain potentially harmful behaviors.

- Allow client to express feelings; acknowledge client's fear (e.g., say to the client "I sense that you may be feeling afraid").
  Acceptance of the client's feelings encourages the client to believe that their expression need not be destructive or a sign of weakness (Haber et al, 1992).
- Give positive feedback when client follows the appropriate treatment plan.
  Positive feedback encourages repetition of behavior.
- Observe whether denial has been or is being used as a coping mechanism in other areas of life.
  At times denial is effective; assess if it has been used appropriately.

Geriatric

- Identify recent losses of client; grieving may prolong denial. Encourage client to take one day at a time.
  The elderly client may have experienced multiple losses and may need supportive care and extra time to adapt (Ringsven, Bond, 1991).
- Encourage client to verbalize feelings.
  Verbalization allows the client to release emotions and develop a sense of control.

Client/Family Teaching

- Teach signs and symptoms of illness and appropriate responses of client (taking medication, going to the emergency room, calling the physician).
  Accurate information and encouragement to follow treatment regimen enhances compliance.
- If problem is substance abuse, refer to an appropriate community agency (e.g., Alcoholics Anonymous).
  Specialized treatment may be required for certain potentially harmful behaviors.

REFERENCES

Ersek J: Examining the process and dilemmas of reality negotiation, *Image: J Nurs Sch* 24:19-25, 1992.

Haber J et al: *Comprehensive psychiatric nursing*, ed 4, St Louis, 1992, Mosby.

Harrenstein E: Young women and depression: origin, outcome and nursing care, *Nurs Clin North Am* 26:607-609, 1992.

Ringsven M, Bond D: *Gerontology and leadership skills for nurses*, Albany, NY, 1991, Delmar.

Weisman A: Coping with cancer, *Image: J Nurs Sch* 24:19-25, 1992.

Diarrhea

Kathie Hesnan

Definition The state in which an individual experiences a change in normal bowel habits characterized by the frequent passage of loose, fluid, and unformed stools.

Defining Characteristics

Abdominal pain and cramping; increased frequency or urgency of defecation; increased frequency of bowel sounds; loose, liquid stool with possible color change.

Related Factors (r/t)

Infection (viral, bacterial, protozoan); change in diet or food; gastrointestinal disorders; stress; medication effects; impaction.

Client Outcomes/Goals

- Formed, soft stool every day to every third day.
- Rectal area is free of irritation.
- States relief from cramping and less or no diarrhea.
- Explains cause of diarrhea and rationale for treatment.
- Good skin turgor; weight at usual level.
- Appropriate containment of stool if client has previously been incontinent.

Nursing Interventions and Rationales

- Assess pattern or have client keep a diary of defecation that includes time of day; usual stimulus; consistency, amount, and frequency of stool; type, amount, and time of food consumed; fluid intake; history of bowel habits and laxative use; diet; exercise patterns; OB/GYN, medical, and surgical history; medications; surgeries; alteration in perianal sensation; and present bowel regimen.
  The underlying cause determines the appropriate nursing interventions.
- Identify cause of diarrhea (e.g., exposure to infected person, food, medication effects, tube feeding, antibiotics, radiation therapy, protein malnutrition, laxative abuse). Refer to related factors.
  Identification of the underlying cause is imperative because the treatment and expected outcome depend on it.
- Obtain stool specimens to either rule out or diagnose an infectious process (e.g., ova and parasites, *C. Difficile*, bacterial cultures).
- If client has infectious diarrhea, avoid using medications that slow peristalsis.
  If an infectious process is occurring, medication to slow down peristalsis should generally not be given. The increase in gut motility helps eliminate the causative factor.
- Observe and record number and consistency of stools per day; if desired, use a fecal incontinence collector for accurate measurement of output.
  Documentation of output provides a baseline and helps prevent dehydration.
- Inspect, palpate, percuss, and auscultate abdomen; note if bowel sounds are frequent.
- Assess for dehydration by observing skin turgor over sternum and inspecting for longitudinal furrows of the tongue.
- Observe for symptoms of sodium and potassium loss (e.g., weakness, abdominal or leg cramping, dysrhythmias).
- Monitor and record intake and output; note oliguria.
- Weigh client daily and note decreased weight.
- Give clear fluids as tolerated (e.g., clear soda, Jell-O, Gatorade); serve fluids at lukewarm temperature.
- Encourage client to eat small, frequent meals and foods that normally cause constipation and are easy to digest (e.g., bananas, crackers, pretzels, rice, applesauce). Encourage client to avoid milk products, foods high in fiber, and caffeine.

- Provide a readily available bedpan, commode, or bathroom.
- Maintain perirectal skin integrity. The products chosen depend on the volume of diarrhea, enzymatic content of stool, incontinence, and status of perirectal skin.
  Classes of products include but are not limited to skin cleansers and remoisturizers that maintain skin hydration, skin sealants or moisture-barrier ointments that provide a protective barrier from stool, or collection devices (e.g., perianal pouch or rectal Foley catheter with physician's approval). NOTE: Rectal Foley catheters can cause rectal necrosis, sphincter damage, or rupture; and the nursing staff may not have the time to properly follow the necessary and very time-consuming steps of their care (Bosley, 1994).
- If client is receiving a tube feeding, do not assume that diarrhea is a result of the tube feeding. Perform a complete assessment to rule out other causes of diarrhea such as medication effects or an infectious state.
  Research has shown that tube feedings do not usually cause diarrhea (Campbell, 1994).
- If client is receiving a tube feeding, note amount of sorbitol in liquid medications, which causes diarrhea; dilute feeding per physician's order and suggest formulas that contain a bulking agent (Doughty, 1991). Note rate of infusion; prevent contamination of feeding by rinsing container q8h and replacing it q24h.
  Increased osmolality and rate of infusion contribute to diarrhea (Smith et al).

Geriatric

- Monitor closely to detect presence of impaction that is causing diarrhea; remove impaction as ordered.
- Seek medical attention if diarrhea is severe or persists for more than 24 hours.
- Provide emotional support for the client who is having trouble controling unpredictable episodes of diarrhea.
- Observe for signs of dehydration and electrolyte imbalances.
  Diarrhea can lead to excessive loss of fluids and electrolytes. Postural hypotension and tachycardia can develop in the elderly client.

Client/Family Teaching

- Encourage avoidance of coffee, spices, milk products, and foods that irritate or stimulate the gastrointestinal tract.
- Teach appropriate method of taking ordered antidiarrheal medications; explain their side effects.
- Explain how to prevent the spread of infectious diarrhea (e.g., careful handwashing, appropriate handling and storage of food).
- Help client to determine stressors and set up an appropriate stress-reduction plan.
- Teach signs and symptoms of dehydration and electrolyte imbalance.
- Teach perirectal skin care.

REFERENCES

Bosley C: Three methods of stool management for patients with diarrhea, *Ostomy Wound Manag* 40:52-57, 1994.

Campbell C: Research for practice: diarrhea not always linked to tube feedings, *Am J Nurs* 94(4):59-60, 1994.

Doughty D: Maintaining normal bowel function in the patient with cancer, *J ET Nurs* 18:90-94, 1991.

Smith C et al: Diarrhea associated with tube feeding in mechanically ventilated critically ill patients. *Nurs Res*, 148.

BIBLIOGRAPHY

Anastasi J: Diarrhea in acquired immune deficiency syndrome (AIDS), *Ostomy Wound Manag* 39:14-23, 1993.

Risk for disuse syndrome

Betty Ackley

Definition The state in which an individual is at risk for a deterioration of body systems as the result of prescribed or unavoidable musculoskeletal inactivity.

NOTE: Complications from immobility can include pressure ulcers, constipation, stasis of pulmonary secretions, thrombosis, urinary tract infection or retention, decreased strength and endurance, orthostatic hypotension, decreased range of joint motion, disorientation, body image disturbance, and powerlessness.

Defining Characteristics

Presence of risk factors such as *Paralysis; altered level of consciousness; mechanical immobilization; prescribed immobilization; severe pain. (*Critical)

Related Factors (r/t)

Refer to risk factors.

Client Outcomes/Goals

- Maintains full range of motion in joints.
- Maintains intact skin, good peripheral blood flow, and normal pulmonary function.
- Maintains normal bowel and bladder function.
- Expresses feelings about imposed immobility.
- Explains methods to prevent complications of immobility.

Nursing Interventions and Rationales

- Have client do exercises in bed if not contraindicated (e.g., flexing and extending feet and quadriceps, performing gluteal and abdominal sitting exercises, lifting small weights to maintain muscle strength).
  Unused muscles lose about one eighth of their strength for each week of bedrest; the muscles also atrophy, change shape, and shorten; muscle fatigue occurs more readily (Corcoran, 1991; Harper, Lyles, 1988).
- If not contraindicated by client's condition, obtain referral to physical therapy to use tilt table to provide weight bearing on long bones.
  The upright position helps maintain bone strength, increases circulation, and maintains cardiovascular reflexes. The best measure to prevent osteoporosis is to begin weight-bearing exercises as soon as possible (Jiricka, 1994).
- Perform range of motion for all possible joints at least twice daily; perform passive or active range of motion as appropriate.
  If not used, muscles weaken and shorten and are predisposed to contractures; if nonuse continues, the contracture eventually involves the tendons, ligaments, and joint capsules and limits the range of motion (Jiricka, 1994).
- Use high-top sneakers or specialized boots from the Occupational Therapy Department to prevent foot-drop; remove shoes twice daily to provide foot care.
  Such shoes help keep the foot in normal anatomical alignment; foot-drop can make it difficult or impossible to walk after bedrest.
- Position client so that joints are in normal anatomical alignment at all times.
  This positioning prevents joint deformities.
- Get client up in chair as soon as appropriate; use a "stretcher chair" if necessary.
- When getting client up after bedrest, do so slowly and watch for signs of postural hypotension, tachycardia, nausea, diaphoresis, or syncope.
  Sitting or standing after 3 or 4 days of bedrest results in postural hypotension because of cardiovascular reflex dysfunction (Jiricka, 1994).
- Obtain assistive devices to help client reach and maintain as much mobility as possible.

- Turn client at least every 2 hours and carefully observe skin condition, especially bony prominences.
  Systematic inspection can identify impending problems early (Bryant, 1993).
- Provide client with a pressure-relieving mattress.
  Pressure-relieving mattresses prevent pressure ulcers.
- Apply antiembolism stockings or a sequential compression system to legs as ordered.
  Such procedures help decrease the formation of deep vein thrombosis.
- Monitor peripheral circulation and especially note color, pulse, and calf or thigh swelling, check Homan's sign.
  Bedrest predisposes the client to deep vein thrombosis because of venous stasis, pressure of mattress against veins, and hypercoagulability of blood (Harper, Lyles, 1988).
- Have client cough and deep breathe or use incentive spirometry q2h while awake.
  Bedrest compromises breathing because of decreased chest expansion and decreased size of thoracic compartment; deep breathing helps prevent complications (Jiricka, 1994).
- Monitor respiratory functions, noting breath sounds and respiratory rate; percuss for new onset of dullness in lungs.
  Immobility predisposes the client to atelectasis and the pooling of respiratory secretions and thus pneumonia (Corcoran, 1991).
- Note bowel function daily. Provide increased fluids, fiber, and natural laxatives such as prune juice as needed.
  Constipation is common in immobilized clients because of decreased activity and food intake (Rubin, 1988).
- Increase fluid intake to 2500 ml per day, within the client's cardiac and renal reserve.
  Adequate fluids help prevent kidney stones and constipation and help counteract dehydration associated with bedrest (Rubin, 1988).
- Encourage intake of a balanced diet with adequate amounts of fiber and protein.
  Reduced muscular activity and lowered metabolism generally reduce the appetite of the client on bedrest (Rubin, 1988).

Geriatric

- Recognize the importance of keeping the elderly client active if possible.
  Ten to fifteen percent of muscle strength can be lost for every week that muscles are resting completely (Mobily, Kelley, 1991).
- Keep careful track of bowel function in the elderly; do not allow client to become constipated.
  The elderly can easily develop impactions as a result of immobility.

Client/Family Teaching

- Teach how to perform range-of-motion exercises in bed if not contraindicated.
- Teach family how to turn and position client.

NOTE: Nursing diagnoses that are commonly relevant when the client is on bedrest include **Constipation, Risk for impaired skin integrity**, **Sensory perceptual alterations**, **Sleep pattern disturbance**, and **Powerlessness**.

REFERENCES

Bryant R, editor: *Acute and chronic wounds*, St Louis, 1993, Mosby.

Corcoran PJ: Use it or lose it: the hazards of bed rest and inactivity, *West J Med* 154:536-538, 1991.

Harper CM, Lyles YM: Physiology and complications of bedrest, *J Am Geriatr Soc* 36:1047-1054, 1988.

Jiricka MK: Alterations in activity intolerance. In Porth CM, editor: *Pathophysiology: concepts of altered health states*, Philadelphia, 1994, JB Lippincott.

Mobily PR, Kelley LS: Iatrogenesis in the elderly: factors of immobility, *J of Gerontol Nurs* 17:5-12, 1991.

Olson EV et al: The hazards of immobility, *Am J Nurs* 67(4):780-797, 1967.

Rubin M: The physiology of bed rest, *Am J Nurs* 88:50-58, 1988.

Diversional activity deficit

Betty Ackley

Definition

The state in which an individual experiences decreased stimulation from or interest or engagement in recreational or leisure activities.

Defining Characteristics

*Verbalization of boredom; verbalization of desire to do something; inability to undertake usual hobbies in hospital. (*Critical)

Related Factors (r/t)

Environmental lack of diversional activity as a result of long-term hospitalization or frequent or lengthy treatments.

Client Outcomes/Goals

- Engages in personally satisfying diversional activities.

Nursing Interventions and Rationales

- Observe ability to engage in activities that require good vision and use of hands.
  Diversional activities must be tailored to the client's capabilities.
- Discuss with client activities that are interesting and feasible in the present environment.
- Encourage client to share feelings about situation of inactivity away from usual life activities.
  Work and hobbies provide structure and continuity to life; the client can feel a sense of loss when unable to engage in usual activities.
- Encourage a mix of physical and mental activities (e.g., crafts, videotapes).
- Encourage client to schedule visitors so that not all are present at once or at inconvenient times.
  A schedule prevents the client from becoming exhausted from frequent company.
- Provide reading material, television, radio, and books on tape.
- If client is able to write, have him or her keep a journal; if client is unable to write, have him or her record thoughts on tape.
  Keeping a journal is diversional and can also help the client deal with the many feelings that result from hospitalization or confinement; a journal can also help the client gain perspective on the situation.
- Request an occupational therapy referral to assist with providing diversional activities.
- Provide a change in scenery; get client out of room as much as possible.
  A lack of sensory stimulation and diversity has a significantly adverse affect on clients (Hamilton, 1992).
- Provide "environmental structuring" to modify environment as needed to promote optimal comfort and sensory diversity (e.g., have family bring in posters, banners, or a sound system; change lighting or direction in which bed faces).
  Modification of the environment is sometimes necessary for the well-being of the client (Williams, 1988).
- Recommend activities in which the client can watch movement of animals and develop involvement (e.g., birdwatching, keeping a fishtank).
- Work with family to provide music enjoyable to the client.
  Music can help catalyze the client's own self-healing capacity (Guzzeta, 1987).
- Structure client's schedule around personal wishes for care and relaxing and fun activities.
  Increased client control fosters increased self-esteem.

- Spend time with the client when possible, or arrange for a friendly visitor.
  Simply being there for the client as a fellow human being is important and helpful (Gardner, 1992).

Geriatric

- Encourage involvement in senior citizen activities (e.g., AARP, YMCA, church groups, Gray Panthers).
- Arrange transportation to activities.
- Encourage client to use his or her ability to help others by volunteering.
  Helping others can help the client grow as a generative human being.
- Provide an environment that promotes activity (e.g., adequate lighting for crafts, large-print books); allow periods of solitude and privacy.
  Periods of solitude are important for emotional well-being in the elderly.
- Use reminiscence therapy and pet therapy, either individually or in groups.
  Reminiscence therapy can increase social interaction, self-esteem, and self-care activities (Hamilton, 1992). Elderly individuals who have or can interact with pets are healthier and live longer.

Client/Family Teaching

- Work with client and family to learn diversional activities that client desires (e.g., knitting, hooking rugs, writing memoirs).

REFERENCES

Gardner DL: Presence. In Bulechek GM, McCloskey JC, editors: *Nursing interventions: essential nursing treatments*, Philadelphia, 1992, WB Saunders.

Guzzetta, CE: Effects of relaxation and music therapy on coronary care patients admitted with presumptive acute myocardial infarction, Grant NU-00824, Rockville, Md, August 1987, Department of Health and Human Services Division of Nursing.

Hamilton DB: Reminiscence therapy. In Bulechek GM, McCloskey JC, editors: *Nursing interventions: essential nursing treatments*, Philadelphia, 1992, WB Saunders.

Radziewicz RM: Using diversional activity to enhance coping, *Cancer Nurs* 15:293-298, 1992.

Williams MA: The physical environment and patient care, *Ann Rev Nurs Res*, 6:61-84, 1988.

BIBLIOGRAPHY

Friedland J: Diversional activity: does it deserve its bad name? *Am J Occup Ther* 42:603-607, 1988.

Dysreflexia

Betty Ackley

Definition The state in which an individual with a spinal cord injury at T7 or above experiences a life-threatening and uninhibited sympathetic nervous system response to a noxious stimulus.

Defining Characteristics

Individual with spinal cord injury (T7 or above) with the following symptoms:

Major Paroxysmal hypertension (sudden periodic elevated blood pressure >140/90 mm Hg); bradycardia or tachycardia (pulse rate <60 or >100); diaphoresis above the injury; red splotches on skin above the injury; pallor on skin below the injury; headache (diffuse pain in different parts of the head and not confined to any nerve distribution area).

Minor Chilling; conjunctival congestion; Horner's syndrome (contraction of pupil on one side, partial ptosis of the eyelid, recession of eyeball into the head, occasional loss of sweating over the affected side of the face); paresthesia; pilomotor reflex (gooseflesh formation when skin is cooled); blurred vision; chest pain; metallic taste in mouth; nasal congestion.

Related Factors (r/t)

Bladder distention; bowel distention; skin irritation; sexual stimulation; lack of client and caregiver knowledge.

Client Outcomes/Goals

- Vital signs normal; free of symptoms of dysreflexia.
- Explains symptoms, prevention, and treatment of dysreflexia.

Nursing Interventions and Rationales

- Monitor for symptoms of dysreflexia. Refer to defining characteristics.
- Observe with physician the cause of dysreflexia (e.g., distended bladder, impaction, pressure sore, urinary calculi, bladder infection, acute abdomen, penile pressure, ingrown toenail, or other source of noxious stimuli).
  Noxious stimuli cause exaggerated sympathetic nervous system responses.
- Use the following interventions to prevent dysreflexia:
  - Ensure good drainage from Foley catheter and ensure that bladder is not distended.
  - Ensure a regular pattern of defecation to prevent fecal impaction.
    Bladder distention and bowel impaction are the most common causes of dysreflexia (Laskowski-Jones, 1993).
  - Frequently change position of client to prevent unrelieved pressure and the formation of pressure ulcers.
  - If ordered, apply an anesthetic agent to any wound below level of injury before performing wound care.
- If symptoms of dysreflexia are present, notify physician, place client in high Fowler's position, and remove all support hose or binders.
  These steps promote venous pooling, decrease venous return, and decrease blood pressure.
- If ordered, initiate antihypertensive therapy.
- Be careful not to increase noxious sensory stimuli; if ordered, use a numbing agent on anus and 1 inch into rectum before attempting to remove a fecal impaction; spray pressure sore with a numbing agent; also use an agent instilled into bladder.
  Increased noxious sensory stimuli can exacerbate the abnormal response and worsen the client's prognosis.
- Monitor vital signs q_______h/min.

- Watch for complications of dysreflexia, including signs of cerebral hemorrhage, seizures, myocardial infarction, or intraocular hemorrhage.
  Extremely high blood pressure can cause rupture of cerebral vessels, myocardial damage, and bleeding within the eye.
- Notify all health care team members of the dysreflexia, because episodes can reoccur.
  All health care personnel working with the client should be aware of the dysreflexia because symptoms could begin while the client is away from the nursing unit.

NOTE: Recognize that dysreflexia happens when spinal shock has worn off and client is in spastic paralysis.

Client/Family Teaching

- Teach recognition of the earliest symptoms of dysreflexia, the actions that should be taken, and the need to summon help immediately.
- Teach steps to take to prevent dysreflexia episodes.

REFERENCES Laskowski-Jones, L: Acute sci: how to minimize the damage, *Am J Nurs* 93(2):22-32, 1993.

BIBLIOGRAPHY Braddom RL, Rocco JF: Autonomic dysreflexia: a survey of current treatment, *Am J Phys Med Rehabil* 70:234-240, 1991.

Dunn KL: Autonomic dysreflexia: a nursing challenge in the care of the patient with a spinal cord injury, *J Cardiovasc Nurs* 5:57-64.

Finocchiaro DN, Herzfeld ST: Understanding autonomic dysreflexia, *Am J Nurs* 90:56-59, 1990.

Trop CS, Bennett CJ: Autonomic dysreflexia and its urological implications: a review, *J Urol* 146:1461-1469, 1991.

Energy field disturbance

Helen Kelley and Gail Ladwig

Definition

A disruption of the flow of energy surrounding a person's being, which results in a disharmony of mind and spirit.

Defining Characteristics

Temperature change (warmth/coolness); visual changes (image/color); disruption of the field (vacant/hold/spike/bulge); movement (wave/spike/tingling/dense/flowing); sounds (tone/words)

Client Outcome/Goals

- States a sense of well-being.
- States feels relaxed.
- Verbalizes decreased pain.
- Verbalizes decreased tension.
- Demonstrates evidence of physical relaxation (e.g., decreased blood pressure, pulse, respiration, muscle tension).

Nursing Interventions and Rationales

Refer to care plans for **Anxiety** and **Pain.**

- Administer therapeutic touch.
  Facilitates energy flow to restore the balance of the recipient's energy field and generalized relaxation (Benson, 1975).
  NOTE: There are two general guidelines in training for the use of therapeutic touch. It is recommended by Krieger that nurses who use therapeutic touch should have had at least 6 month's experience in an acute-care setting. Learning should be guided by a nurse who has at least 2 year's experience with therapeutic touch, preferably a master's degree in nursing, and conforms to the practice guidelines of 30 hours of instruction in theory, 30 hours of supervised practice with relatively healthy individuals, and successful completion of written and practice evaluations (Kunz, Krieger, 1975-1990). It is recommended by the Nurse Healers–Professional Associates that practitioners should have a beginning workshop addressing the cognitive and therapeutic aspects of therapeutic touch. A minimum of 12 hours of instruction with a certificate of training is recommended. Family members can be instructed on basic soothing and comforting measures in less time.
- Administer therapeutic touch by performing the following steps:
  1. Center in the present moment. Shift awareness from the physical environment to an inner focus on the center within self, which is a center of calm and balance through which the nurse perceives himself or herself and the client as a unitary whole.
     The nurse's attitude becomes clear, and gentle and compassionate attention to the client and focused intent help the client. There is awareness of the physical environment, but this is not the primary focus (Meehan, 1992).
  2. Assessment. Pass palmar surface of hands 2 to 4 inches over the client's body from head-to-toe.
     Through the natural sensitivity of hands, the nurse perceives the state of energy flow as differences in subtle sensations (e.g., congestion, pressure, warmth, coolness, or tingling). During assessment the nurse also perceives information about the client through intuitive and somatic clues (Jurgens, Meehan, Wilson, 1987).

3. Treatment (unruffling). Use hands to brush or smooth out the energy flow. Sweep the hands downward and out of the field from head-to-toe, and concentrate on those areas of disturbance that were identified during the assessment.
   Areas of static congestion in the energy flow are relieved, and the field is prepared for the reception of healing energy. The client mobilizes his or her own resources for self-healing, and pain, anxiety, and discomfort are diminished (Jurgens, Meehan, Wilson, 1987).
4. Direction and modulation of energy. Rest hands on or near the body area where the block of congestion was detected or in other areas of energy imbalance; facilitate energy to these areas.
   This step balances or corrects energy imbalances (Krieger, 1979).
5. Stop. Stop procedure when there are no longer any clues or when client indicates it is time to stop. Place hands over the solar plexus (just above the waist), and focus specifically on facilitating the flow of healing energy to the client.
   This final phase allows for rest and evaluation (Jurgens, Meehan, Wilson, 1987).

Client/Family Teaching

- Teach the therapeutic touch process to family members.
  Family members can use this skill to assist with care and comfort of the client.
- Teach that therapeutic touch should be done gently and only for short periods of time in the head area or when working with the very young, the very old, or the very ill.
  In these circumstances the client is particularly sensitive to therapeutic touch (Boguslawski, 1980; Borelli, Heidt, 1981).
- Teach guided imagery to the client.
  The nurse can facilitate healing by helping the client recontact and reclaim parts of the self (energy disturbance) through guided imagery (Rancour, 1994).
- Teach the client to relax by deep breathing; ask client to have the disease, affected organ, or symptom assume an image. After the image has been identified, ask the client to speak with the image to obtain the meaning of an unmet need.
  By describing a previously unacknowledged part of the self, the liberated energy can transform resistance, defense, and disease into self-acceptance, peace, and wholeness (Remen, 1994).

REFERENCES

Benson H: *The relaxation response*, New York, Avon, 1975.

Boguslawski M: Therapeutic touch: a facilitator of pain relief, *Top Clin Nurs* 2:27-37, 1980.

Borelli M, Heidt P: *Therapeutic touch: a book of readings*, New York, 1981, Springer.

Jurgens A, Meehan T, Wilson H: Therapeutic touch as a nursing intervention, *Holistic Nurs Pract* 2:1-13, 1987.

Krieger D: *The therapeutic touch, how to use your hands to heal*, Englewood Cliffs, NJ, Prentice Hall, 1979.

Kunz D, Krieger D: *Annual Invitational Workshops on Therapeutic Touch*, Pumpkin Hollow Foundation, 1975-1990, Graysville, NY.

Meehan T: Therapeutic touch. In Bulechek G, McCloskey J, *Nursing interventions: essential nursing treatments*, Philadelphia, 1992, JB Lippincott.

Rancour P: Interactive guided imagery with oncology patients, *J Holistic Nurs* 12:149, 1994.

Remen N: Psychosynthesis and healing. In Rancour P, editor: *J Holistic Nurs* 12:150, 1994.

Impaired environmental interpretation syndrome

Nancy English and Betty Ackley

Definition Consistent lack of orientation to person, place, time, or circumstances for longer than 3 to 6 months, which necessitates a protective environment.

Defining Characteristics

Major Consistent disorientation in known and unknown environments; chronic confusional states.

Minor Loss of occupation or social functioning from memory decline; inability to follow simple directions or instructions; inability to reason; inability to concentrate; slow in responding to questions.

Related Factors (r/t)

Dementia (e.g., Alzheimer's disease, multi-infarct dementia, Pick's disease, AIDS dementia); Parkinson's disease; Huntington's disease; depression; alcoholism.

Client/Outcomes/Goals

- Remains content and free from harm.
- Functions at the maximum of cognitive level.
- Independently participates in activities of daily living at the maximum of functional ability.

Nursing Interventions and Rationales

- Determine client's cognitive level using a screening tool such as the Mini Mental State Exam (MMSE).
  An evaluation tool such as the MMSE can help determine the client's cognitive abilities and plan appropriate nursing interventions (Agostinelli et al, 1994).
- Determine client's background information before the onset of confusion, including social situation, physical condition, psychological functioning.
  Knowing the client's background can help the nurse understand the client's behavior if he or she becomes delusional or hallucinates; sharing memories can help soothe the client.
- Determine client's independent abilities of self-care.
  Assessment of independent self-care activities relating to hygiene, feeding, and toileting can help the nurse plan care to support and maintain the client's independence in self-care.
- Determine the client's daily routine before the onset of confusion, including sleep/awake cycle, elimination patterns, and morning and evening routines.
  Habitual patterns of behavior are maintained even though the client's cognition is impaired. The knowledge of these usual patterns of daily activity can help the nurse plan individualized care.
- Determine the client's special interests and hobbies before the onset of confusion.
  Knowledge of the client's interests and hobbies can help the nurse distract the client when he or she becomes fearful and agitated.
- Ensure that client is in a safe environment by removing potential hazards such as sharp objects and harmful liquids.
  Clients with dementia lose their ability to make good judgments and can easily harm themselves or others.
- Place an identification bracelet on client.
  Clients with dementia wander and may become lost; identification bracelets help increase safety.

- Help client avoid unfamiliar situations and people as much as possible by maintaining continuity of caregivers, maintaining routines of care with established meal times and activities, and by sending familiar person with client when he or she goes for diagnostic testing.
  Situational anxiety that is associated with environmental, interpersonal, or structural change can escalate into agitated behavior (Gerdner, Buckwalter, 1994).
- To keep the environment less stressful, avoid the use of buzzers and alarms around the client if possible.
- Begin each interaction with the client by identifying self and by calling the client by name.
- Approach client with a caring, loving, and accepting attitude, and speak in a calm, slow manner.
  Dementia clients can sense feelings of compassion; a calm, slow manner projects a feeling of comfort to the client (Stolley, 1994).
- Touch client gently by stroking hand or arm in a soothing manner.
- Give one simple direction at a time and repeat it exactly as said if necessary. Use verbal and physical prompts, and model the desired actions if needed and possible.
  "People with dementia need time to assimilate and interpret your directions, if you rephrase your question, you give them something new to process, increasing their confusion" (Stolley, 1994, p. 40).
- Break down self-care tasks into simple steps. Instead of "Take a shower" say to client, "Please follow me. Sit down on bed. Take off your shoes. Now take off your socks. . . ."
  Dementia clients are unable to follow complex commands, breaking down the activity into simple steps makes the activity more feasible (Agostinelli et al, 1994).
- Keep questions simple; yes or no questions are often preferable. Use positive statements and actions and avoid negative communication (e.g., if client is trying to crawl out of bed, help client find hand holds to get out and lead back to bed later as necessary).
  Negative feedback leads to increased confusion and agitation; it is more effective to go along with the client and redirect as necessary.
- Recognize that clients have good and bad days; provide decreased activity on bad days.
- Provide boundaries by placing red or yellow tape on the floor or by using a stop sign.
  Such boundaries help the client identify safe areas; red and yellow colors are more easily seen by the elderly client.
- Write client's name in large block letters in the room and on clothing and possessions.
- Use symbols rather than words to identify areas such as the bathroom, kitchen, or dresser.
- Keep pictures that have been labeled with names in client's room.
- Limit visitors to two, and provide visitors with guidelines on appropriate topics to discuss with client.
- Set up scheduled quiet periods; have client avoid prolonged naps during the day.
  Fatigue has been associated with the onset of increased confusion and agitation (Stolley, 1994).
- In the afternoon or early evening, provide client with quiet activities such as classical or religious music.
  An increase in confusion and agitation may occur in the late afternoon and early evening, which is referred to as sundowning syndrome. Quiet activities can provide a calming environment.

- Provide open and safe areas for movement.
  Freedom in movement can help relieve the anxiety and agitation that often accompanies the experience of confusion in the client.
- Recognize that sudden changes of behavior may indicate the need for prompt attention to another underlying condition (e.g., infection, pain, change in cardiac status or respiratory status).
  In the Alzheimer's client the new onset of agitated behavior can many times be associated with a change in physical condition (Gerdner, Buckwalter, 1994).
- Use validation techniques when client experiences an increase in fear and anxiety. Say to the client, "I can see you are afraid," "I will stay with you," or "Can you tell me more about what is going on right now?"
  Such statements convey empathy and understanding and can help determine the internal stimulus that is creating the change in behavior (Feil, 1993).
- Consider the use of doll therapy. Ask family members to bring a large safe doll or stuffed animal such as teddy bear.
  The use of doll therapy can be soothing to some dementia clients (Bailey, 1992; Paulanka, Griffin, 1993).
- For early dementia clients with memory loss only, refer to care plan for **Impaired memory**.
- For clients with agitation, refer to nursing interventions for **Chronic confusion**.
- For guidelines on teaching families to talk with the confused client, refer to nursing interventions for **Chronic confusion**.
- For clients with self-care deficits, refer to **Self-care deficit: feeding**, **Self-care deficit: dressing**, or **Self-care deficit: toileting** as appropriate.

Geriatric

NOTE: Most of the above interventions apply to the geriatric client.

- Use reminiscence and life review therapeutic interventions; use such statements as "Tell me about your favorite Christmas or birthday" or "What dance or music was your favorite?"
  Long-term memory is often preserved, even though the client may be unable to remember current events. Reminiscence and life review can help enhance the life of the older person by decreasing depression, resocializing, and building relationships (Burnside, Haight, 1994).

Client/Family Teaching

- Recommend that family members develop a memory aid wallet or booklet for client, which has pictures and text that chronicle the client's life.
  Memory aids such as wallets or booklets help dementia clients make more factual statements and stay on topic, and they decrease the number of confused, erroneous, and repetitive statements (Bourgeois, 1992).
- Using interventions listed above, teach family how to set up the environment and use care techniques to progressively lower the stress threshold that client will experience.
  Clients with Alzheimer's disease are unable to deal with stress; decreasing stress can decrease confusion and changes in behavior (Hall, 1991; Stolley, 1994).

NOTE: The nursing diagnoses **Impaired environmental interpretation syndrome** and **Chronic confusion** are very similar in definition and the nursing interventions. **Impaired environmental interpretation** must be interpreted as a syndrome to which other nursing diagnoses would also apply. **Chronic confusion** may be interpreted as the human response to situations that require a level of cognition that is no longer available to the individual. Further research is in progress to make this distinction clear to the practicing nurse.

REFERENCES

Agostinelli B et al: Targeted interventions: use of the Mini-Mental State Exam, *J Gerontol Nurs* 20:15-23, 46-47, 1994.

Bailey J: To find a soul, *Nursing '92*:63-64, 1992.

Bourgeois MS: *Conversing with memory impaired individuals using memory aids: a memory aid workbook*, Gaylord, Mich, 1992, Northern Speech Services.

Burnside I, Haight B: Reminiscence and life review: therapeutic interventions for older people, *Nurse Pract* :55-61, 1994.

Feil N: *The validation breakthrough: simple techniques for communicating with people with Alzheimer's-type dementia*, Baltimore, 1993, Health Professions Press.

Gerdner LA, Buckwalter KC: A nursing challenge: assessment and management of agitation in Alzheimer's patients, *J Gerontol Nurs* 20(4):11-20, 1994.

Hall GR: This hospital patient has Alzheimer's, *Am J Nurs* 91:44-50, 1991.

Paulanka BJ, Griffin LS: Behavioral responses of memory impaired clients to selected nursing interventions, *Phys Occup Ther Geriatr* 12:65-78, 1993.

Stolley JM: When your patient has Alzheimer's disease, *Am J Nurs* 94(8):34-41, 1994.

Ineffective family coping, compromised

Beverly Pickett

Definition A usually supportive primary person (family member or close friend) is providing insufficient, ineffective, or compromised support, comfort, assistance, or encouragement, which may be needed by the client to manage or master adaptive tasks related to his or her health challenge.

Defining Characteristics

Subjective Client expresses or confirms a concern or complaint about significant person's response to his or her health problem; significant person describes preoccupation with personal reaction (e.g., fear, anticipatory grief, guilt, or anxiety about client's illness, disability, or other situational or developmental crises); significant person describes or confirms an inadequate understanding or knowledge base that interferes with effective assistance or support.

Objective Significant person attempts to assist or support client with less than satisfactory results; significant person either withdraws or enters into limited or temporary personal communication with the client at time of need; significant person displays protective behavior disproportionate to the client's abilities or need for autonomy.

Related Factors (r/t)

Lack of adequate or correct information or understanding by a significant person; temporary preoccupation by a significant person who is trying to manage emotional conflicts and personal suffering and cannot perceive or act effectively in regard to client's needs; temporary family disorganization and role changes; situational or developmental crises or problems the significant person may be facing; lack of support given by the client to the significant person; prolonged disease or disability progression that exhausts the supportive capacity of significant people.

Client Outcomes/Goals

- Family or significant person verbalizes internal resources to help deal with the situation.
- Family or significant person verbalizes knowledge and understanding of illness, disability, or disease.
- Family or significant person provides support and assistance as needed.
- Family or significant person identifies need for and seeks outside support.

Nursing Interventions and Rationales

- Observe for cause of family problems.
  Ongoing assessment provides clues that include underlying feelings (Barry, 1989).
- Help significant person expand repertoire of coping skills.
  Coping skills can decrease the family's vulnerability to stress and strengthen and maintain family resources that protect the family.
- Assess how family members interact with each other.
  Understanding how families cope with stress is important. An individual's problems affect the entire family (Mears, 1990).
- Help family identify strengths and make a list that each member can refer to for positive feedback.
  Positive feedback from one family member reinforces a particular action or behavior of another member.
- Encourage family members to verbalize feelings; spend time with family members, sit down and make eye contact, and offer coffee and other nourishment.
  Acceptance of nourishment indicates a beginning acceptance of the situation.

- Talk with family about the importance of sharing feelings and ways to do this (e.g., role playing, writing a letter to significant other).
  Sharing feelings allows the family an opportunity to communicate in an effective yet nonthreatening manner.
- Involve client and family in planning of care as much as possible.
  Involving the client and family in the planned care or treatment regimen encourages compliance with treatment and enhances the client's feeling of control (Barry, 1989).
- Provide privacy during family visits; if possible, maintain flexible visiting hours to accommodate more frequent family visits.
- If possible, arrange staff assignments so the same staff members have contact with the family; familiarize other staff members with the situation in the absence of the usual staff spokesperson.
- Determine whether or not family is suffering from additional stressors (e.g., child care, financial problems).
- Refer family to appropriate resources for assistance as indicated, (e.g., counseling, psychotherapy, financial or spiritual support).
  If family members do not know who to contact, these services can be underused (Mears, 1990).

Geriatric

- Assess needs of significant person; assist in meeting needs while visiting (e.g., ensure that person who has diabetes eats meals).
- Assist in finding transportation to enable family members to visit.
- If family member is homebound and unable to visit, encourage phone contact to provide ongoing scheduled progress reports.

Client/Family Teaching

- Provide information for family and significant people regarding client's specific illness or condition.
- Involve client and family in planning of care as often as possible.
- Refer to appropriate resources for assistance as indicated (e.g., counseling, psychotherapy, financial, spiritual).

REFERENCES

Barry P: *Psychosocial nursing assessment and intervention*, Philadelphia, 1989, JB Lippincott.

Mears D: Enhancing family coping skills, *Nurs Homes*, 39(2):32-33, 1990.

BIBLIOGRAPHY

Marsden A, Dracup K: Different perspectives: the effect of heart disease on patients and spouses, *AACN Clin Issues Crit Care Nurs* 2:285-291, 1991.

Perry A, Potter P: *Fundamentals of nursing: concepts, process and practice*, St Louis, 1993, Mosby.

Watson P: Family issues in rehabilitation, *Holistic Nurs Pract* 6:51-59, 1992.

Ineffective family coping, disabling

Beverly Pickett

Definition The state in which behavior of a significant person (family member or other primary person) disables his or her own capacities and the client's capacities to effectively address tasks essential for adaptation to the health challenge.

Defining Characteristics

Neglectful care of the client in regard to basic human needs or illness; distortion of reality regarding client's health problem, including extreme denial about its existence or severity; intolerance; rejection; abandonment; desertion; continuation of usual routines and disregard for client's needs; psychosomaticism; adoption of client's symptoms; family decisions and actions that are detrimental to economic or social well-being; agitation; depression; aggression; hostility; impaired restructuring of a meaningful life for self; impaired individualization; prolonged overconcern for client; neglectful relationships with other family members; client's development of helpless, inactive dependence.

Related Factors (r/t)

Chronically unexpressed feelings of guilt, anxiety, hostility, or despair in the significant person; discrepancy between the significant person and client or among significant people regarding ways to cope with adaptive tasks; highly ambivalent family relationships; arbitrary handling of family's resistance to treatment, which tends to solidify defensiveness because it deals inadequately with underlying anxiety.

Client Outcomes/Goals

- Family or significant person expresses realistic understanding and expectations of the client.
- Family participates positively in client's care within the limits of their abilities.
- Significant person expresses feelings openly, honestly, and appropriately.

Nursing Interventions and Rationales

- Observe for causative and contributing factors.
  Ongoing assessment provides clues that include underlying feelings (Barry, 1989).
- Identify family behaviors and interactions before the illness.
  Most family members have certain roles that are disrupted by illnesses and hospitalizations; this disruption results in shifts in family functioning.
- Identify current behaviors of family members such as withdrawal (e.g., not visiting, briefly visiting, ignoring client when visiting), anger and hostility toward client and others, or expressions of guilt.
  Many of these behaviors are defense mechanisms used by the ego to protect itself until it can fully accept the implications of the illness.
- Note other stressors in family (e.g., financial, job-related).
  These facts allow the nurse to develop an appropriate plan of care.
- Encourage family to verbalize feelings.
  Many families find it difficult to maintain open and empathic communication during times of acute stress.
- Provide a role model for interpersonal skills that will help the family improve their verbal interactions.
  Interpersonal skills such as warmth, friendliness, empathy, consideration, and competence are essential in promoting a therapeutic relationship.

- Provide structure for family interactions (e.g., length of visiting time, number of visitors, content of interactions).
  Structure provides stability during times of stress and crisis.
- Help family identify its personal strengths.
  Individual coping skills assist in adjusting to life crises.
- Provide continuity of care by maintaining effective communication between staff members; initiate a multidisciplinary client-care conference that involves the client and family in problem-solving.
- Explore available hospital and community resources with the family.
  Resources will provide the family with information and assistance if necessary and appropriate.
- Observe for any symptoms of elder or child abuse or neglect.
  Abuse can take several forms such as physical assaults that may or may not result in injury; verbal attacks; isolation; social and emotional neglect.

Geriatric

- Refer family to appropriate community resources (e.g., senior centers, Medicare assistance, meal programs).
- If abuse or neglect is an issue, report to Social Services.
  The purpose of protective services is to preserve the family.
- Encourage family members to participate in appropriate support groups (e.g., COPD, Arthritis, I Can Cope, or Alzheimer's support groups).
  Support groups provide people with a setting in which they can discuss their illness-related problems with other people who have the same illness.
- Teach family ways to manage common problems related to normal aging.

Client/Family Teaching

- Discuss with family appropriate ways to demonstrate feelings.
- Teach family the skills required for client care.
- Help family identify the health care needs of the client and family unit.

REFERENCES

Barry P: *Psychosocial nursing assessment and intervention*, Philadelphia, 1989, JB Lippincott.

BIBLIOGRAPHY

Ducharme F, Rowat K: Conjugal support, family coping behaviors and the well-being of elderly couples, *Can J Nurs Res* 24(1):5-22, 1992.

Kupferschmid B et al: Families: a link or a liability, *Families* 2:252-257, 1991.

Perry A, Potter P: *Fundamentals of nursing: concepts, process and practice*, St Louis, 1993, Mosby.

Watson P: Family issues in rehabilitation, *Holistic Nurs Pract* 6:51-59, 1992.

Family coping: potential for growth

Beverly Pickett

Definition Effective managing of adaptive tasks by family member who is involved with the client's health challenge and is now exhibiting desire and readiness for enhanced health and growth in relation to self and the client.

Defining Characteristics

Family member attempts to describe growth aspect of crisis according to his or her own values, priorities, goals or relationships; family member moves in direction of a health-promoting and enriching life-style that supports and monitors maturational processes, audits and negotiates treatment programs, and generally chooses experiences that optimize wellness; individual expresses interest in making contact either with another person who has experienced a similar situation, either on a one-to-one basis or in a group setting.

Related Factors (r/t)

Needs are sufficiently gratified, and adaptive tasks are effectively addressed to enable goals of self-actualization to surface.

Client Outcomes/Goals

- Family states a plan for its growth.
- Family is able to perform tasks needed for change.
- Family states positive effects of changes made.

Nursing Interventions and Rationales

- Observe skills that the family possesses to initiate change such as a positive attitude or a statement of hope that change is possible.
  The nurse can then identify strengths on which the family may rely and weaknesses from which the family needs protection.
- Allow family time to verbalize their concerns; provide one-to-one interaction with the family.
  Interactions allow family to gather and impart information, decrease anxiety, and provide input for plan of care.
- Have family share responsibilities for change and encourage all members to have input.
  It is important to view the entire family as a system when trying to promote positive change.
- Encourage family members to write down their goals.
  The more involved the family is in goal development, the greater the probability that their goals will be achieved.
- Explore with family ways to attain their goals (e.g., adult education classes, enrichment courses, family activities such as sports, cooking, or reading, sharing time together).
- Encourage "fun-time"—a time with no tasks, just time to enjoy each other's company; family members might need to set up a schedule to do this since everyone is busy.
- Help family members communicate with each other, using techniques they are comfortable with such as role-playing, letter writing, or tape recording messages.
  These techniques give the family an opportunity to communicate in an effective yet nonthreatening manner.

Geriatric

- Encourage family members to reminisce with the older family member.
- Start and maintain a log of anecdotal stories about the older family member.
- Encourage children in family to spend time with and share activities with the older family member.
  These activities allow for knowledge of and respect for one another.

Client/Family Teaching

- Teach that it is normal for changes in families and family relationships to occur.
- Refer to parenting classes and classes for coping with older parents.
- Identify groups with similar problems and concerns (e.g., Al-Anon, I Can Cope).

BIBLIOGRAPHY
Kupferschmid B et al: Families: a link or a liability, *Families* 2:252-257, 1991.
Mears D: Enhancing family coping skills, *Nurs Homes*, p. 32-33, July 1990.
Perry A, Potter P: *Fundamentals of nursing: concepts, process and practice*, St Louis, 1993, Mosby.
Watson P: Family issues in rehabilitation, *Holistic Nurs Pract* 6:51-59, 1992.

Altered family processes

Beverly Pickett

Definition The state in which a family that normally functions effectively experiences a dysfunction.

Defining Characteristics

Family system unable to meet physical, emotional, or spiritual needs of its members; parents do not demonstrate respect for each other's views on child-rearing practices; family unable to express or accept a wide range of feelings; family unable to express or accept feelings of its members; family unable to meet security needs of its members; family members unable to relate to each other for mutual growth and maturation; family uninvolved in community activities; family unable to appropriately accept or receive help; family maintains rigidity in function and roles; family does not demonstrate respect for individuality and autonomy of its members; family unable to adapt to change or deal constructively with traumatic experiences; family unable to accomplish current or past developmental tasks; family has an unhealthy decision-making process; family unable to send and receive clear messages; family maintains boundaries inappropriately; family inappropriately or poorly communicates rules, rituals, and symbols; family has unexamined myths; family maintains inappropriate level and direction of energy.

Related Factors (r/t)

Situational transition or crisis; developmental transition or crisis.

Client Outcomes/Goals

- Family members are able to express feelings.
- Family identifies ways to cope effectively and uses appropriate support systems.
- Family treats impaired family member as normally as possible to avoid overdependence.
- Family is able to meet physical needs of members or seek appropriate assistance.
- Family demonstrates knowledge of illness or injury, treatment modalities, and prognosis.
- Impaired family member participates in the development of the plan of care to the best of his or her ability.
- Family is able to define boundaries, rules, and appropriate rituals.

Nursing Interventions and Rationales

- Observe for cause of change in family's normal pattern of functioning.
  Ongoing assessment of family members can provide important clues that indicate a possible family disruption.
- Spend time with family members; sit down and allow them to verbalize their feelings.
  Interactions help the client and family feel relieved and allow anxiety levels to decrease.
- Acknowledge the stages of grief when there is a change of health status in a family member and accept the present stage of the family; tell family members it is "normal" to be angry.
  It is important to understand the wide range of behaviors experienced during normal grief and to reassure those experiencing such behaviors.
- Encourage family members to list their personal strengths.
  A list of strengths provides information that family members can refer to for positive feedback.
- Discuss with family how they handled previous crises.
  Such a discussion gives the nurse clues and information that can help in plan of care.

- Encourage family to visit client; adjust visiting hours to accommodate family's schedule (e.g., work, school, babysitting needs).
- Assist with sleeping arrangements if family is spending the night; provide a place to lie down, pillows, and blankets.
- Allow and encourage family to assist in the client's care.
  Assisting with client's care helps maintain family's "connectedness."
- Have family participate in client conferences that involve all members of the health care team.
  Conferences allow for distribution of information, input by all members at one time, and a decrease in anxiety of family members.
- Refer to appropriate support groups if needed (e.g., counseling, social services, self-help groups, pastoral care).

Geriatric

- Teach family members about impact of developmental events (e.g., retirement, death, change in health status and household composition).
- Support group problem solving among family members, including the older or ill member.
- Refer family to counseling with a psychotherapist who is knowledgeable about gerontology.

Client/Family Teaching

- Identify community agencies that might be helpful such as Meals on Wheels, Respite Care (agency that provides care for the caregiver), and I Can Cope (group for clients diagnosed with cancer).
- Teach family how to care for client and give medications and treatments.

BIBLIOGRAPHY

Barry P: *Psychosocial nursing assessment and intervention*, Philadelphia, 1984, JB Lippincott.

Kupferschmid B et al: Families: a link or a liability: *Families* 2:252-257, 1991.

Lipkin GB, Cohen RG: *Effective approaches to patients' behavior*, New York, 1992, Springer.

Marsden A, Dracup K: Different perspectives: the effect of heart disease on patients and spouses, *AACN Clin Issues Crit Care Nurs* 2:285-291, 1991.

Mears D: Enhancing family coping skills, *Nurs Homes*, p. 32-33, July 1990.

Watson P: Family issues in rehabilitation, *Holistic Nurs Pract,* 6:51-59, 1992.

Fatigue

Betty Ackley

Definition An overwhelming, sustained sense of exhaustion and decreased capacity for physical and mental work.

Defining Characteristics

Major Verbalization of an unremitting and overwhelming lack of energy; inability to maintain usual routines.

Minor Perceived need for additional energy to accomplish routine tasks; increase in physical complaints; emotional lability or irritability; impaired ability to concentrate; decreased performance; lethargy or listlessness; disinterest in surroundings; introspection; decreased libido; accident prone.

Related Factors (r/t)

Decreased or increased metabolic energy production; overwhelming psychological or emotional demands; increased energy requirements to perform activities of daily living; excessive social or role demands; discomfort; altered body chemistry (e.g., medications, drug withdrawal, chemotherapy).

Client Outcomes/Goals

- Verbalizes increased energy and improved well-being.
- Explains energy conservation plan to offset fatigue.

Nursing Interventions and Rationales

- Assess severity of fatigue on a scale of 0 to 10; assess frequency of fatigue, activities associated with increased fatigue, times of increased energy, and usual pattern of activity.
  Such assessments establish a baseline for symptoms of fatigue.
- Evaluate adequacy of nutrition and sleep. Refer to **Altered nutrition: less than body requirements** or **Sleep pattern disturbance** if appropriate.
  Inadequate nutrition or poor sleep can contribute to fatigue.
- Schedule rest periods for at least 30 minutes after strenuous activity.
  Clients with fatigue need rest to recover for the next activity.
- Encourage client to express feelings about fatigue; use active listening techniques; help identify sources of hope.
  Fatigue has been associated with depression, anxiety, anger, and mood disturbances (Potempa, 1993).
- Encourage client to keep a journal of activities, symptoms of fatigue, and feelings.
  The journal helps the client to monitor progress toward resolving or coping with fatigue and to express feelings, which helps with adjustment (Jones, 1992).
- Assist client with activities of daily living as necessary; encourage independence without causing exhaustion.
- Help client set small, easily achieved short-term goals such as writing two sentences in a journal daily or walking to the end of the hallway twice daily.
- With physician's approval, refer to physical therapy for aerobic exercise program.
  Aerobic exercise and physical therapy can reduce fatigue (MacVicar, 1989).
- Refer client to diagnosis-appropriate support groups such as National Chronic Fatigue Syndrome Association or Multiple Sclerosis Association.
  Support groups can help clients deal with bodily changes and cope with the frequent depression that accompanies fatigue (Jones, 1992).

- Help client identify essential and nonessential tasks and determine what can be delegated. Give client permission to limit social and role demands if needed (e.g., switch to part-time employment, hire cleaning service).
  The nurse can help the client look at life realistically to balance available energy and energy demands.

Geriatric

- Identify recent losses; monitor for depression as a possible contributing factor to fatigue.
  Depression and fatigue are closely correlated; the elderly are more prone to depression because they frequently experience significant losses as they age.
- Review medications for side effects of fatigue.
  Medications may cause fatigue in the elderly (e.g., beta blockers, antihistamines, pain medications).

Client/Family Teaching

- Teach strategies for energy conservation (e.g., sitting instead of standing during showering, storing items at waist level).
- Teach client to carry a pocket calendar, make lists of required activities, and post reminders around the house.
  Chronic fatigue is often associated with memory loss and sometimes with mild confusion (Jones, 1992).
- Teach the importance of following a healthy life-style to decrease fatigue; teach the importance of adequate nutrition and rest, pain relief, and appropriate exercise.
- Teach stress reduction techniques such as controlled breathing, imagery, use of music. Refer to **Anxiety** care plan if appropriate.
  Stress is correlated with increased fatigue.

REFERENCES

Jones CA: These patients truly need our help, *RN* 55:46-54, 1992.

MacVicar M: Effects of aerobic interval training on cancer patient's functional capacity, *Nurs Res* 38:348-351, 1989.

Potempa KM: Chronic fatigue, *Annu Rev Nurs Res* 11:57-76, 1993.

BIBLIOGRAPHY

Belza BL et al: Correlates of fatigue in older adults with rheumatoid arthritis, *Nurs Res* 42:93-99, 1993.

Gift AG, Pugh LC: Dyspnea and fatigue, *Nurs Clin North Am* 28:373-384, 1993.

Reeves N et al: Fatigue in early pregnancy: an exploratory study, *J Nurse Midwife* 36:303-309, 1991.

Fear

Pam Bifano Schweitzer

Definition Feeling of dread related to an identifiable source that the person validates.

Defining Characteristics

Subjective Able to identify object of fear; scared; rattled; wired; jittery; shaky; nervous; worried; anxious; experiencing acute feelings of helplessness or dread of specific consequences.

Objective Sympathetic stimulation (e.g., cardiovascular excitation, superficial vasoconstriction, pupil dilation, increased perspiration); hyperventilation, muscular tension; vocal and hand tremors; wide-eyed appearance; darting glances; tearfulness; insomnia; restlessness; excessive reassurance-seeking; excessive self-focus; avoidance behavior.

Related Factors (r/t)

Environmental stressors; hospitalization; treatments; pain; powerlessness; separation from support system; language barrier; sensory impairment; real or imagined threat to own well-being; knowledge deficit; vicarious learning; conditioned response.

Client Outcomes/Goals

- Client verbalizes fears that are known.
- Client states accurate information about the situation.
- Client identifies, verbalizes, and demonstrates those coping behaviors that reduce own fear.
- Client reports and demonstrates reduced fear.

Nursing Interventions and Rationales

- Assess source of the fear with client.
  Fear is a normal response to actual or perceived danger and helps mobilize protective defenses.
- Discuss situation with client and help distinguish between real and imagined threats to well-being.
  The first step in helping the client deal with fear is to collect information about the situation and its effect on the client and significant others (Bailey, Bailey, 1993).
- If irrational fears are present, offer accurate information.
  Correcting mistaken beliefs reduces anxiety (Beck, Emery, 1985).
- If client's fear is a reasonable response, empathize with client. Avoid false reassurances; be truthful.
  Reassure clients that seeking help is both a sign of strength and a step toward resolution of the problem (Bailey, Bailey, 1993).
- If possible, remove the source of the client's fear.
  Fear is a normal response to actual or perceived danger; if the threat is removed, the response will stop.
- If possible, help the client confront the fear.
  Self-discovery enhances feelings of control.
- Stay with the client when he or she expresses fear; provide verbal and nonverbal (touch and hug with permission) reassurances of safety if it is within control.
  The nurse's presence and touch demonstrates caring and diminishes the intensity of feelings such as fear (Bulechek, McCloskey, 1992).
- Explain all activities, procedures, and issues that involve the client; use nonmedical terms and calm, slow speech, explain procedures in advance when possible, and validate client's understanding.
  Knowledge deficit or unfamiliarity is one factor associated with fear (Whitney, 1992).

- Explore coping skills used previously by client to deal with fear; reinforce these skills and explore other outlets.
  Methods of coping with anxiety that have previously been successful are likely to be helpful again (Clunn, Payne, 1982).

Geriatric

- Establish a trusting relationship so all fears can be identified.
  An elderly client's response to a real fear may be immobilizing.
- Monitor for dementia and use appropriate interventions.
  Fear may be an early indicator of disorientation or impaired reality testing in elderly clients.
- Provide a protective and safe environment; use consistent caregivers; maintain the accustomed environmental structure.
  Elderly clients tend to have more perceptual impairments and adapt to changes with more difficulty, especially during an illness.
- Observe for untoward changes if antianxiety drugs are taken.
  Age renders clients more sensitive to both the clinical and the toxic effects of many agents.

Client/Family Teaching

- Teach client the difference between warranted and excessive fear.
  Different interventions are indicated for rational and irrational fears.
- Teach client that fear itself is not dangerous and that avoidance increases fear.
- Teach client to visualize or fantasize absence of the fear or threat, successful experience of the situation, resolution of the conflict, or outcome of the procedure.
- Teach client to identify and use distraction or diversion tactics when possible.
  Early interruption of the anxious response prevents escalation.
- Teach client to allow fearful thoughts and feelings to be present until they dissipate.
  Purposefully and repetitively allowing and even devoting time and energy to a thought reduces associated anxiety (Beck, Emery, 1985).
- Teach use of appropriate community resources in emergency situations (e.g., hotlines, emergency rooms, law enforcement, and judicial systems).
  Serious emergencies need immediate assistance to ensure the client's safety.
- Encourage use of appropriate community resources in nonemergency situations (e.g., family, friends, neighbors, self-help and support groups, volunteer agencies, churches, clubs and centers for recreation, seniors, youths, others with similar interests).
- If medications are ordered, teach client their appropriate use.

REFERENCES

Bailey DS, Bailey DR: *Therapeutic approaches to the care of the mentally ill*, ed 3, Philadelphia, 1993, FA Davis.

Beck AT, Emery G: *Anxiety disorder and phobias: a cognitive perspective*, New York, 1985, Basic Books.

Bulechek G, McCloskey J: *Nursing interventions: essential nursing treatments,* ed 2, Philadelphia, 1992, WB Saunders.

Clunn PA, Payne DB: *Psychiatric mental health nursing*, Garden City, NJ, 1982, Medical Examination.

Whitney G: Concept analysis of fear, *Nurs Diag* 3:159, 1992.

BIBLIOGRAPHY

Peplau H: A working definition of anxiety. In Burd S, Marshall M, editors: *Some clinical approaches to psychiatric nursing*, New York, 1963, Macmillan.

Fluid volume deficit

J. Keith Hampton

Definition

The state in which an individual experiences vascular, cellular, or intracellular dehydration.

Defining Characteristics

Change in urine output; change in urine concentration; sudden weight loss or gain; decreased venous filling; hemoconcentration; increased serum sodium; increased serum and urine osmolality; increased blood urea nitrogen; hypotension; thirst; increased pulse rate; decreased skin turgor; decreased pulse volume or pressure; change in mental state; increased body temperature; dry skin; dry mucous membranes; weakness; increased urine specific gravity.

Related Factors (r/t)

Active fluid volume loss; loss of gastrointestinal fluids (e.g., vomiting, diarrhea, gastric suction); polyuria; loss of fluids through fistulas; diaphoresis; third spaced fluids; decreased fluid intake; hyperosmolar imbalances (e.g., hyperglycemia, hypernatremia).

Client Outcomes/Goals

- Intake equals output.
- Blood pressure, pulse, central venous pressure, pulmonary wedge pressure are within normal range.
- Good skin turgor, moist mucous membranes, +1200 ml urine output daily.
- Explains measures that can be taken to treat or prevent fluid volume loss.
- Laboratory values are within normal limits.
- Free of dizziness during position change.

Nursing Interventions and Rationales

- Observe for cause of fluid deficit (e.g., vomiting, nausea, diarrhea, difficulty swallowing or feeding self, active blood loss, high osmotic tube feeding, depression, fatigue, extreme heat, enemas, diuretics).
  Cause of the deficit directs clinical interventions.
- Check vital signs frequently if they are unstable, especially pulse rate and blood pressure; take blood pressure lying and standing if client is not too dizzy or weak.
  Blood pressure and pulse changes indicate systemic fluid volumes.
- Check peripheral pulses; note their quality and presence.
  Alterations in peripheral pulses can reflect alterations in fluid volume status (e.g., fluid volume deficit leading to decreased peripheral pulses).
- Keep accurate intake and output records.
- Check daily weight at same time of day; note pattern of decreasing weight with intake less than output.
  For weight to be accurate, client must be weighed at same time of day and with the same amount of clothing, bedding, or therapeutic equipment. An accurate daily weight is an excellent reflection of fluid balance.
- Note amount, color, and specific gravity of urine; if fluid loss is acute, do hourly urine measurements.
  These indicators help gain an overall measure of renal filtration and reabsorption abilities.
- Monitor mental status and note any confusion, restlessness, anxiety, or syncope.
  Mental status changes can indicate a decrease in cerebral water stores.

- Encourage a daily fluid intake of 2000 to 3000 ml if not contraindicated; note taste preferences.
  Fluid intake should meet minimal body requirements and accommodate for insensible loss (Metheny, 1992).
- Monitor lab values (sodium, potassium, hematocrit, serum and urine osmolarity, blood urea nitrogen, creatinine).
  All of these laboratory values will be elevated as long as the fluid volume deficit exists. When the deficit is corrected, the values will normalize.
- Check skin turgor, color, and warmth.
  Skin turgor, color, and warmth indicate subcutaneous fat water stores.
- Administer prescribed intravenous fluids and closely monitor client's response.
- Check for dryness in mouth and especially for longitudinal furrows on the tongue.
  Mouth dryness indicates that water stores from the mucous membranes have been diverted to the central circulation.
- Medicate for nausea, vomiting, and diarrhea promptly as ordered by physician.
  Providing antiemetics and antidiarrheal medications can help decrease fluid loss from the body.
- If client is receiving intravenous fluids at a rapid rate, monitor carefully for onset of fluid overload as evidenced by crackles in lungs, dyspnea, and a bounding pulse.
- Document hydration status at regular intervals.
  Documentation helps demonstrate the client's response to therapeutic interventions.

Nursing Interventions for Client in Hypovolemic Shock

- If blood pressure is very low, position client flat in bed with legs elevated.
  This position enhances venous return.
- Monitor vital signs frequently (every 15 to 60 minutes as needed).
  Frequent vital signs document the client's response to treatment and the evolving clinical picture.
- Monitor hemodynamic parameters (central venous pressure, right atrial pressure, pulmonary wedge pressure).
  Hemodynamic parameters indicate fluid volume status within the central circulation.
- Use pulse oximeter and note oxygen saturation continuously; administer oxygen as ordered.
  An O_2 saturation <90% (normal 95% to 100%) or a Po_2 <80 (Normal 80 to 100) indicates significant oxygen problems.
- Do hourly urine checks; report if urine output is less than 30 ml/hour or greater than 200 ml/hour.
  The average kidney filters enough blood to generate more than 30 ml/hour of urine.
- Watch continuously for any further fluid loss from any source.
- Monitor continuously for signs of worsening shock (e.g., cold and clammy skin, confusion, absence of peripheral pulses).
  Such assessments document client clinical evolution.
- Administer fluids at a rapid rate as ordered. Remember to gain a positive clinical response to administer first volume replacement and then vasoconstrictive medications such as dopamine.
  Vasoconstrictive medications work poorly with shock if there is systemic fluid volume deficit.

Geriatric

- Use a direct approach to offer fluid regularly to cognitively impaired clients.
  The elderly have decreased thirst sensation; short-term memory loss may impede the client's memory of fluid intake.
- Incorporate regular hydration into daily routines (e.g., extra glass of fluid with medication, social activities).
  Integration of hydration into regular routines increases the chance that the client will meet the daily fluid requirements.
- Recognize that the elderly can easily go from a fluid deficit to a fluid overload.
  The elderly client has a decreased compensatory mechanism to regulate fluid balance.

Client/Family Teaching

- Teach importance of regular fluid intake.
- Teach symptoms of fluid volume deficit and steps to take if symptoms appear.

REFERENCES Metheny NM: *Fluid and electrolyte balance: nursing considerations*, ed 2, Philadelphia, 1992, JB Lippincott.

BIBLIOGRAPHY Bulechek GM, McCloskey JC: *Nursing interventions: essential nursing treatments*, ed 2, Philadelphia, 1992, WB Saunders.

Cullen L: Interventions related to fluid and electrolyte balance, *Nurs Clin North Am* 27:569-597.

Rogers-Seidl, FF: *Geriatric nursing care plans*, St Louis, 1991, Mosby.

Risk for fluid volume deficit

Definition The state in which an individual is at risk of experiencing vascular, cellular, or intracellular dehydration.

Defining Characteristics

Presence of risk factors such as extremes of age; extremes of weight; excessive losses through normal routes (e.g., diarrhea); loss of fluids through abnormal routes (e.g., indwelling tubes); deviations affecting access to or intake or absorption of fluids (e.g., physical immobility); factors influencing fluid needs (e.g., hypermetabolic state); knowledge deficit regarding fluid volume; medication effects (e.g., diuretics).

Related Factors (r/t)

Refer to risk factors.

Client Outcomes/Goals, Nursing Interventions and Rationales, Client/Family Teaching

Refer to nursing diagnosis for **Fluid volume deficit**.

Fluid volume excess

J. Keith Hampton

Definition The state in which an individual experiences increased fluid retention and edema.

Defining Characteristics

Edema; effusion; anasarca; weight gain; dyspnea; orthopnea; crackles in lungs; S_3 heart sounds; signs of pulmonary congestion on chest x-ray film; intake greater than output; jugular vein distention; positive hepatojugular reflex; decreased hemoglobin, hematocrit, or serum osmolarity; specific gravity changes; altered electrolytes; oliguria; azotemia; restlessness; anxiety.

Related Factors (r/t)

Compromised regulatory mechanism; excess fluid intake; excess sodium intake.

Client Outcomes/Goals

- Clear breath sounds; vital signs within normal range.
- Free of edema and effusion; weight appropriate for client; intake equals output.
- Explains ways to prevent fluid volume excess.

Nursing Interventions and Rationales

- Determine cause of fluid volume excess (e.g., excessive fluid or sodium intake, renal dysfunction, cardiac dysfunction, hepatic cirrhosis).
  Cause of the excess directs clinical interventions (Metheny, 1992).
- Observe daily weight and intake and output; note any pattern of increased intake and decreased output or increasing weight.
  Daily measurements develop a clinical picture of patterns and trends.
- Take vital signs, noting especially increasing or decreasing blood pressure.
  Vital signs indicate systemic circulating fluid volume.
- Evaluate hemodynamic parameters; note especially increasing central venous pressure, renal artery pressure, pulmonary wedge pressure, and any changes in cardiac output.
  Hemodynamic measurements indicate central circulation fluid volumes and cardiac function (Cullen, 1992).
- Monitor for edema in feet, shins, eyelids, or sacral area if client is on bedrest.
  Edema indicates an alteration in hydrostatic pressure and the overall effect of gravity on the body.
- Observe for heart failure as evidenced by crackles in lungs, gallop rhythm, neck vein distention, dyspnea. If signs of heart failure are present refer to nursing diagnosis for **Decreased cardiac output**.
- Monitor for ascites; note any abdominal distention, presence of shifting dullness on percussion, or fluid wave with palpation.
  Ascites indicates a source of excess fluid outside of the central or systemic circulation (Metheny, 1992).
- Observe for confusion and restlessness from decreased sodium; use safety precautions if symptoms are present.
  Alterations in level of consciousness indicate that the overall fluid level in the brain has increased and that the brain is being compressed within the cranium (Cullen, 1992).
- Note laboratory results (sodium, potassium, hemoglobin, hematocrit, blood urea nitrogen, creatinine, serum albumin, total protein, serum osmolarity, urine osmolarity).
  All of these values will be diluted or decreased until the fluid volume excess is resolved.
- Assess breath sounds; monitor for distention of peripheral veins.

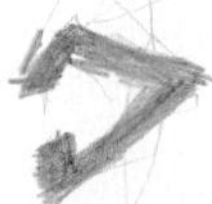

- Ensure that client receives a low-sodium diet; encourage protein intake.
- Maintain ordered fluid restriction; have client help determine how restricted fluids can best be allotted during the 24 hours.
  Client involvement will enhance compliance with fluid restrictions.

Geriatric

- Monitor for presence of edema; if edema is present, evaluate dietary intake and note serum protein and albumin levels.
  Edema in the elderly can result from malnutrition, and serum protein levels give an indication of nutrition.
- Encourage rest periods.
  Lying down favors diuresis of edematous fluid (Metheny, 1992).
- If the client with edematous tissue is on bedrest, turn and position client frequently and handle skin with care.
  Edematous tissue is more prone to skin breakdown than normal tissue (Metheny, 1992).

Client/Family Teaching

- Teach importance of fluid and sodium restrictions and how to live with the restrictions.
- Explain symptoms of fluid overload and actions to take if they occur.
- Teach family how to incorporate a low-salt diet into family food preferences.

REFERENCES Cullen L: Interventions related to fluid and electrolyte balance, *Nurs Clin North Am* 27:569-597, 1992.
Metheny NM: *Fluid and electrolyte balance: nursing considerations*, ed 2, Philadelphia, 1992, JB Lippincott.

BIBLIOGRAPHY Bulechek GM, McCloskey JC: *Nursing interventions: essential nursing treatments*, ed 2, Philadelphia, 1992, WB Saunders.

Impaired gas exchange

Betty Ackley

Definition

The state in which an individual experiences a decreased passage of oxygen and/or carbon dioxide between the alveoli of the lungs and the vascular system.

Defining Characteristics

Confusion; somnolence; restlessness; irritability; inability to move secretions; hypercapnea; hypoxia.

Related Factors (r/t)

Ventilation perfusion imbalance.

Client Outcomes/Goals

- Maintains a patent airway at all times.
- Demonstrates improved ventilation and adequate oxygenation as evidenced by blood gases within client's normal parameters.
- Maintains clear lung fields and remains free of signs of respiratory distress.
- Verbalizes understanding of oxygen and other therapeutic interventions.

Nursing Interventions and Rationales

- Monitor respiratory rate, depth, and effort, including use of accessory muscles, nasal flaring, and thoracic or abdominal breathing.
- Auscultate breath sounds q________h.
- Monitor client's behavior and mental status for onset of restlessness, agitation, confusion, and in the late stages, extreme lethargy.
  Changes in behavior and mental status can be early signs of impaired gas exchange.
- Monitor oxygen saturation continuously, using pulse oximeter; note blood gas results as available.
  An O_2 saturation <90% (normal 95% to 100%) or a Po_2 <80 (normal 80 to 100) indicates significant oxygenation problems.
- Observe for cyanosis in skin; note especially color of tongue and oral mucous membranes.
  Central cyanosis in tongue and oral mucosa is indicative of serious hypoxia and is a medical emergency; peripheral cyanosis seen in extremities may or may not be serious (Carpenter, 1993).
- If client has unilateral lung disease, alternate semi-Fowler's position with lateral position (with a 10 to 15 degree elevation and "good lung down") for 60 to 90 minutes; this method is contraindicated for the client with a pulmonary abscess or hemorrhage or interstitial emphysema.
  Gravity and hydrostatic pressure cause the dependent lung to become better ventilated and perfused, which increases oxygenation (Yeaw, 1992).
- If client has a bilateral lung disease, position client in either semi-Fowler's or side-lying positions that increase oxygenation as indicated by pulse oximetry. Turn client every 2 hours.
- Administer appropriate medications (e.g., bronchodilators, diuretics, steroids, antibiotics, anticoagulants as ordered).
- Administer intravenous fluids as indicated.
- Encourage deep breathing and coughing or use of incentive spirometry every q________h.
- Monitor the effects of sedation, narcotics, and analgesics on client's respiratory pattern.
- Schedule nursing care to provide rest and minimize fatigue.

- Administer humidified oxygen through appropriate device (e.g., nasal cannula or face mask per physician's order); watch for onset of hypoventilation as evidenced by increased somnolence after initiating or increasing oxygen therapy.
  A chronic lung client may need a hypoxic drive to breathe and may hypoventilate during oxygen therapy.
- Provide adequate fluids to liquefy secretions within the client's cardiac and renal reserve.
- Refer to Pulmonary Rehabilitation Team.
  This team is multidisciplinary, and working together can help make the client's life more livable (Tiep, 1993).
  NOTE: If client becomes ventilator dependent, refer to nursing interventions and rationales for **Inability to maintain spontaneous ventilation.**

Geriatric

- Use central nervous system depressants carefully to avoid decreasing respirations.
  An elderly client is more prone to respiratory depression.
- Maintain low-flow oxygen therapy.
  An elderly client is more susceptible to oxygen-induced respiratory depression.
- Encourage client to stop smoking.
  There are substantial health benefits for the elderly client who stops smoking (Foyt, 1992).
- To maximize oxygen exchange, encourage client to sit or stand in the most upright position possible.
  The size of the chest cavity is decreased with aging.

Client/Family Teaching

- Teach client energy conservation techniques and the importance of alternating rest periods with activity.
- Teach importance of not smoking; refer to smoking cessation programs.
- Instruct client and family on home care regimen; refer to social services for special home therapy if necessary.
- Instruct family regarding home oxygen therapy (e.g., delivery system, liter flow, safety precautions).
- Teach client relaxation therapy techniques to help reduce stress responses and panic attacks resulting from dyspnea.
  Relaxation therapy includes progressive muscle relaxation, autogenic techniques, visualization, and diaphragmatic breathing. This therapy can help modify the symptoms of dyspnea and help the client deal with feelings associated with the chronic disease (Jerman, Haggerty, 1993).

REFERENCES

Carpenter KD: A comprehensive review of cyanosis, *Crit Care Nurse* 13:66-72, 1993.

Foyt MM: Impaired gas exchange in the elderly, *Geriatr Nurs* 13:262-268, 1992.

Jerman A, Haggerty MC: Relaxation and biofeedback: coping skills training. In Casaburi R, Petty L, editors: *Principles and practice of pulmonary rehabilitation,* Philadelphia, 1993, WB Saunders.

Tiep BL: Pulmonary rehabilitation program organization. In Casaburi R, Petty L, editors: *Principles and practice of pulmonary rehabilitation,* Philadelphia, 1993, WB Saunders.

Yeaw P: Good lung down, *Am J Nurs* 92:27-32, 1992.

BIBLIOGRAPHY

Ahrens R: Changing perspectives in the assessment of oxygenation, *Crit Care Nurse* 13:78-83, 1993.

Epstein CD, Henning RJ: Oxygen transport variables in the identification and treatment of tissue hypoxia, *Heart Lung* 22:328-348, 1993.

Grieving

Betty Ackley

Definition

The state in which an individual or group of individuals reacts to an actual or perceived loss. This loss may be a person, object, function, status, relationship, or body part.

Defining Characteristics

Verbal expression of distress at loss; anger; sadness; crying; difficulty in expressing loss; alterations in eating habits, sleep patterns, dream patterns, activity levels, or libido; reliving of past experiences; interference with life function; alterations in concentration or pursuit of tasks.

Related Factors (r/t)

Actual or perceived object loss; objects may include people, possessions, job, status, home, ideals, or parts and processes of the body.

Client Outcomes/Goals

- Expresses feelings of guilt, fear, anger, or sadness.
- Identifies problems associated with grief (e.g., changes in appetite, insomnia, loss of libido, decreased energy, alteration in activity level).
- Plans for future 1 day at a time; identifies personal strengths.
- Functions at normal developmental level and performs activities of daily living.

Nursing Interventions and Rationales

- Allow family members to participate in care of the body if desired; help survivors say good-bye in the most loving and caring way possible.
- Allow family to do "holding" behaviors, including taking photographs of the deceased, or clipping a piece of hair.
  Holding behaviors can help the family preserve the fact and meaning of the loved one's existence (Carter, 1989).
- Help the bereaved client to survive during times of acute grief; ensure that the client maintains proper nutrition; help the client determine a routine to make it through the day.
  The newly bereaved can be stunned and helpless (Gifford, Cleary, 1990).
- Encourage client to share memories of the person or loss; to get client to open up, say "Tell me about your wife (husband, parent)."
  The bereaved client needs someone to listen while he or she sorts out the complex emotional reactions to the new reality of the situation.
- Actively listen to the client's grief; do not interrupt, do not tell own story, and do not offer meaningless platitudes such as, "It will be better this way."
  These behaviors do not help and can often hurt (Gifford, Cleary, 1990).
- Encourage client to "cry out" their grief and to express feelings, including sadness or anger.
  Grief work IS work and is best done as an active process in which the grieving client expresses and feels the grief.
- Help client identify previous personal coping strategies.
  Coping strategies used previously are helpful in dealing with loss.
- Refer client to spiritual counseling if desired.
  Spiritual counseling can help the client gain perspective about the loss and can give comfort.

- Provide information about the grief process, including the stages of grieving (denial, anger, bargaining, and acceptance); help client realize that the grieving process takes time and is painful.
  This information helps normalize the grief experience and provides the client with hope that he or she can survive (Gifford, Cleary, 1990).
- Help client determine how best to obtain support from others and where to find social support.
  Social support has been identified as the most important predictor of positive bereavement (Cooley, 1992).
- Assess for cases of dysfunctional grieving (e.g., sudden death, highly dependent or ambivalent relationship with deceased, lack of coping skills, lack of social support, previous physical or mental health problems).
  Life circumstances can interfere with normal grieving (Cooley, 1992).
  Refer to nursing interventions and rationales for **Dysfunctional grieving** if appropriate.
- Encourage family members to set aside time to talk with each other about the loss without criticizing each other or belittling others' feelings.
  Once these feelings are shared, family members can begin to accept the unacceptable (Gifford, Cleary, 1990).
- Identify available community resources, including bereavement groups from local hospitals and hospice.
  Mutual support groups can have positive effects on bereavement outcomes (Cooley, 1992).

NOTE: **Grieving** is not an official NANDA nursing diagnosis but is included because the authors believe that grieving is part of the normal human response to loss and that nurses can use interventions to help the client grieve. **Grieving** is a wellness-oriented nursing diagnosis.

REFERENCES

Carter SL: Themes of grief, *Nurs Res* 38:354-358, 1989.
Cooley ME: Bereavement care: a role for nurses, *Cancer Nurs* 15:125-129, 1992.
Gifford BJ, Cleary BB: Supporting the bereaved, *Am J Nurs* 90(9):49-55, 1990.

BIBLIOGRAPHY

Grainger RD: Successful grieving, *Am J Nurs* 90:12-15, 1990.
Herth K: Relationship of hope, coping styles, concurrent losses, and setting to grief resolution in the elderly widow(er), *Res Nurs Health* 13:109-117, 1990.

Anticipatory grieving

Betty Ackley

Definition Intellectual and emotional responses and behaviors by which an individual works through the process of modifying the self-concept based on the perception of potential loss.

Defining Characteristics

Potential loss of significant object; expression of distress at potential loss; denial of potential loss; guilt; anger; sorrow; choked feelings; changes in eating habits; alterations in sleep patterns; alterations in activity level; altered libido; altered communication patterns.

Related Factors (r/t)

Perceived or actual impending loss of people, objects, possessions, job, status, home, ideals, or parts and processes of the body (adapted from Carpenito).

Client Outcomes/Goals

- Expresses feelings of guilt, anger, or sorrow.
- Identifies problems associated with anticipatory grief (e.g., changes in activity, eating, libido).
- Seeks help in dealing with anticipated problems.
- Plans for the future 1 day at a time.

Nursing Interventions and Rationales

- If grief results from impending death of a loved one, help family members to stay with loved one during the dying process if desired, and help them determine appropriate times to take breaks.
  Families need nursing support during this time of great stress.
- Encourage family members to listen carefully to messages given by the dying loved one; they may hear symbolic or obscure language referring to the dying process.
  As people approach death, they develop an understanding of how their death will unfold, and they communicate this awareness in symbolic language (Callanan, 1994).
- Help family members let the loved one go as appropriate; give the loved one permission to die.
  Sometimes dying people wait until they know their family members are strong enough to accept the loss, before they allow themselves to die (Callanan, 1994).
- Use therapeutic communication; use open-ended questions such as, "What are your thoughts and fears?"
  Nurses need to give the grieving client permission and opportunity to talk about the anticipated loss.
- Actively listen to client's grief; do not interrupt, do not tell own story, and do not offer meaningless platitudes such as, "It will be better this way."
  These behaviors do not help and can often hurt (Gifford, Cleary, 1990).
- Encourage client to "cry out" his or her grief and to express feelings, including sadness or anger.
  Grief work IS work and is best done as an active process in which the grieving client expresses and feels the grief.
- Encourage the client to take care of any unfinished business if appropriate; the client can talk to the dying person or use simulated conversations to resolve issues.
  Unfinished business must be resolved before the grieving client can heal and move on (Grainger, 1990).

- Refer to spiritual counseling if desired and appropriate.
  Spiritual counseling can help the client gain perspective about the loss and can give comfort.
- Help client determine how best to obtain support from others and where to find social support.
  Social support has been identified as the most important predictor of positive bereavement (Cooley, 1992).
- Be honest; do not give false reassurances.
- Identify problems with eating or sleeping, and intervene with suggestions as appropriate.
  The grieving client can be stunned and helpless (Gifford, Cleary, 1990).
- Encourage the caregiver of a dying person to live "1 day at a time"; help the caregiver recognize that he or she is mourning while caring for the loved one. Help the caregiver express feelings of loss; encourage the caregiver to take care of himself or herself.
  Caregivers grieve as they give care to the dying person and can develop an increased intimacy and involvement in the relationship, which can help them obtain a positive bereavement outcome (Brown, Powell-Cope, 1993).

REFERENCES

Brown MA, Powell-Cope G: Themes of loss and dying in caring for a family member with AIDS, *Res Nurs Health* 16:179-191, 1993.

Callanan M: Farewell messages: dealing with death, *Am J Nurs* 94(5):19-20, 1994.

Carpenito JL: *Nursing diagnosis: application to clinical practice,* ed 5, Philadelphia, 1993, JB Lippincott.

Gifford BJ, Cleary BB: Supporting the bereaved, *Am J Nurs* 90(2):49-55, 1990.

Grainger RD: Successful grieving, *Am J Nurs* 90(9):12-15, 1990.

BIBLIOGRAPHY

Cooley ME: Bereavement care: a role for nurses, *Cancer Nurs* 15:125-129, 1992.

Dysfunctional grieving

Betty Ackley

Definition Extended, unsuccessful use of intellectual and emotional responses by which individuals attempt to work through the process of modifying self-concepts on the basis of the perception of loss.

Defining Characteristics

Verbal expression of distress at loss; denial of loss; excessive expression of guilt or unresolved issues; excessive anger, sadness, or crying; difficulty in expressing loss; alterations in eating habits, sleep patterns, dream patterns, activity levels, or libido; idealization of lost object; reliving of past experiences; interference with life function; developmental regression; labile affect; alterations in concentration or pursuit of tasks.

Client Outcomes/Goals

- Expresses appropriate feelings of guilt, fear, anger, or sadness.
- Identifies problems associated with grief (e.g., changes in appetite, insomnia, nightmares, loss of libido, decreased energy, alteration in activity levels).
- Seeks help in dealing with grief-associated problems.
- Plans for future 1 day at a time; identifies personal strengths.
- Functions at a normal developmental level and performs activities of daily living after an appropriate length of time.

Nursing Interventions and Rationales

- Assess for causes of dysfunctional grieving (e.g., sudden bereavement [less than 2 weeks to prepare for the oncoming loss], highly dependent or ambivalent relationship with the deceased, inadequate coping skills, lack of social support, previous physical or mental health problems).
  Life circumstances can interfere with normal grieving and can be risk factors for dysfunctional grieving (Cooley, 1992, Steele, 1992).
- Observe for the following reactions to loss, which predispose a client to dysfunctional grieving:
  - Delayed grieving: the bereaved exhibits little emotion and continues with a busy life.
  - Inhibited grieving: the bereaved exhibits various physical conditions and does not feel grief.
  - Chronic grieving: the behaviors of the normal grief periods continue beyond a reasonable time.

  These maladaptive grief reactions indicate that the client needs help with grief work (Gifford, Cleary, 1990).
- Identify problems of eating and sleeping; ensure that basic human needs are being met.
  Losses often interrupt appetite and sleep (Gifford, Cleary, 1990).
- Develop a trusting relationship with client by using therapeutic communication techniques.
- Establish a defined time to meet and discuss feelings about the loss and to perform grief work.
- Encourage client to "cry out" grief and to talk about feelings of anger and sadness.
  Grief work IS work and is best done as an active process where the bereaved expresses and feels the grief.
- Help client recognize that sadness will occur at intervals for the rest of his or her life but will become bearable.
  The sadness associated with chronic sorrow is permanent, but as the grief resolves there can be times of satisfaction and even happiness (Teel, 1991; Grainger, 1990).

- Help the client complete the following "guilt work" exercises:
  - Identifying "if onlys" and putting them into perspective.
  - Dealing with "I didn't do" by looking at what was accomplished.
  - Forgiving himself or herself; say to the client, "You are being awfully hard on yourself; try not to hurt yourself over something you could not have controlled."

  The client may need to resolve guilt before successfully grieving and moving on in life.
- Review past experiences, role changes, and coping skills.
- Help client to identify own strengths to use in dealing with loss; reinforce these strengths.
- Expect client to meet responsibilities; give positive reinforcement.
- Do not give false reassurances; discuss issues honestly.
- Help client identify areas of hope in life.

  A significant positive relationship has been found between the level of grief resolution and the level of hope (Herth, 1990).
- Encourage client to make time to talk to family members about the loss with the help of professional support as needed and without criticizing or belittling each others' feelings about the loss.

  Once these feelings are shared, family members can begin to accept the unacceptable (Gifford, Cleary, 1990).
- Identify available community resources, including bereavement groups from local hospitals and hospice.

  Mutual support groups can have positive effects on bereavement (Cooley, 1992).
- Identify if client is experiencing depression or another emotional disorder; determine if suicidal and refer to counseling as appropriate.

  Depression and the risk of suicide can accompany dysfunctional grieving.

Geriatric

- Use reminiscent therapy in conjunction with the expression of emotions.
- Identify previous losses and assess client for depression.

  Losses and changes in older age often occur in rapid succession without adequate recovery time.
- Evaluate the social support system of the elderly client, if support system is minimal, help the client determine how to increase available support.

  The elderly who have poor outcomes with grieving often do not live with family members and have a minimal support system.

REFERENCES

Cooley ME: Bereavement care: a role for nurses, *Cancer Nurs* 15:125-129, 1992.

Gifford BJ, Cleary BB: Supporting the bereaved, *Am J Nurs* 90(2):49-55, 1990.

Grainger RD: Successful grieving, *Am J Nurs* 90(9):12-15, 1990.

Herth K: Relationship of hope, coping styles, concurrent losses, and setting to grief resolution in the elderly widow(er), *Res Nurs Health* 13:109-117, 1990.

Steele L: Risk factor profile for bereaved spouses, *Death Stud* 16:387-399, 1992.

Teel CS: Chronic sorrow: analysis of the concept, *J Adv Nurs* 16:1311-1319, 1991.

Altered growth and development

Catherine Vincent

Definition The state in which an individual demonstrates deviations from the norms of his or her own age group.

Defining Characteristics

Major Delay or difficulty in performing skills (motor, social, or expressive) typical of age group; altered physical growth; inability to perform age-appropriate self-care or self-control activities.

Minor Flat affect; listlessness; decreased responses.

Related factors (r/t)

Inadequate caretaking; indifferent, inconsistently responsive, or multiple caretakers; separation from significant others; environmental and stimulative deficiencies; physical disability; prescribed dependence.

Client Outcomes/Goals

- Caregiver(s) identify normal patterns of growth and development.
- Caregiver(s) provide child with activities that support age-related developmental tasks.
- Child demonstrates an increase in age-appropriate behaviors (social, interpersonal, cognitive) and motor activities.

Nursing Interventions and Rationales

- Use developmental screening tests and developmental surveillance to assess growth and development.
  Developmental surveillance is a flexible and ongoing process that uses both skilled observation of the child and concerns of parents, health professionals, teachers, and others to identify children at risk for variation in normal growth and development (Curry, Duby, 1994).
- Use some type of developmental interview during health assessment.
  Developmental surveillance and the developmental interview can provide an efficient method for early identification of children at risk. Early intervention into developmental issues is beneficial to both parents and children, and it leads to improved outcomes (Curry, Duby, 1994).
- Assess caregiver concerns, understanding of normal development, and responses to illness and hospitalization.
  The primary caregiver best knows the child and his or her needs. The nurse works in collaboration with the family to develop a plan of care.
- Provide adequate nutrition.
  Nutritional needs of children vary with developmental age, metabolism, and illness. Most children who are ill have diminished appetites.
- Provide an environment that promotes sleep and rest.
  A balance of rest and activity is essential for optimal growth and development.
- Maintain a routine as close to the home routine as possible in relation to nutrition, sleep, rest, activity, and toileting.
  A homelike routine allows the child to feel maximum comfort, makes the hospital setting less stressful, and interferes less with growth and development.
- Encourage and facilitate frequent caregiver contact, especially for the infant, toddler, preschooler, or young school-age child.
  Particularly in younger children, frequent caregiver contact diminishes normal separation anxiety. Most infants and toddlers find their caregivers' presence comforting and are thus better able to cope with stress.

- Communicate with children at an appropriate cognitive level of development.
  A young child's ability to comprehend information is quite limited but increases with age. A developmentally disabled child may have unique communication needs.
- Refer to a play or recreational therapist, if available.
  The play or recreational therapist specializes in developing and providing individual and group interventions that meet growth and development needs.
- Facilitate coping strategies for the hospitalized child.
  Strategies used by the nurse to help the child cope with hospitalization usually affect the physical, cognitive, and psychosocial aspects of development.
- Ensure continuity of care by designating a primary nurse.
  A primary nursing system allows for a more consistent and personalized approach.

Client/Family Teaching

- Teach caregiver the expected patterns of growth and development; provide reading material or videos on the subject.
  Anticipatory guidance allows caregivers to prepare for behaviors, understand what is normal, and anticipate potential problems.
- Teach activities that are age appropriate and support growth and development, including safety considerations. Focus on the child's abilities rather than limitations.
- Help family identify normal responses to illness and hospitalization. Explain regression, magical thinking, separation anxiety, and fears.
  A child may regress to prior developmental levels while hospitalized. A child responds to hospitalization differently from adults, depending on cognitive development and prior experiences. When the caregivers understand the child's usual reactions to stress and illness, they are better able to support the child.
- Teach positive behavior modification techniques.
- Give information about community resources (e.g., support groups, parenting classes, child care professionals).
- Refer client for more in-depth screening and assessment as necessary.
  The presence of a risk factor alone does not always indicate the need for a referral. The nurse must consider the number and weight of risk factors and the normal individual differences of each child (Curry, Duby, 1994).

REFERENCES Curry DM, Duby JC: Developmental surveillance by pediatric nurses, *Pediatr Nurs* 20:40-44, 1994.

BIBLIOGRAPHY Reynolds EA, Ramenofsky ML: The emotional impact of trauma on toddlers, *MCN* 13:106-109, 1988.

Smith DP, editor: *Comprehensive child and family nursing skills,* St Louis, 1991, Mosby.

Whaley L, Wong D: *Nursing care of infants and children,* ed 4, St Louis, 1991, Mosby.

Wilson R, Broome ME: Promoting the young child's development in the intensive care unit, *Heart Lung* 18:274-281, 1989.

Altered health maintenance

Suzanne Skowronski

Definition The inability to identify, manage, or seek out help to maintain health.

Defining Characteristics

Lack of knowledge regarding basic health practices; lack of adaptive behaviors to internal and external environmental changes; inability to take responsibility for meeting basic health practices in any or all functional pattern areas; history of lack of health-seeking behavior; expressed interest in improving health behaviors; lack of equipment, finances, and other resources; impairment of personal support systems.

Related Factors (r/t)

Lack of or significant alteration in communication skills (written, verbal, or gestural); inability to make deliberate and thoughtful judgments; perceptual-cognitive impairment (complete or partial lack of gross or fine motor skills); ineffective individual coping; dysfunctional grieving; unachieved developmental tasks; ineffective family coping; disabling spiritual distress; lack of material resources.

Client Outcomes/Goals

- Discusses fears of or blocks to implementing a health regimen.
- Follows mutually agreed on health care maintenance plan.
- Meets goals for health care maintenance.

Nursing Interventions and Rationales

- Assess client's feelings, values, and reasons for not following prescribed plan of care; refer to related factors.
- Encourage client to share feelings about change in health status and its effects on life.
  Unresolved conflicts about the illness or condition may interfere with the client's self-care of illness.
- Determine what the client believes to be the most important aspect of the health care plan; start education and reinforcement in that area.
  A client engages in health behaviors that he or she finds relevant and acceptable (Pender, 1987).
- Help client determine how to arrange a daily schedule that incorporates the new health care regimen (e.g., taking pills before meals).
- Identify support groups related to the disease process (e.g., Reach to Recovery for a mastectomy client).
- Have client identify at least two significant support people and have them attend teaching sessions if possible.
- Refer client to community agencies for appropriate follow-up care (e.g., day treatment or adult day health program).
  Social support affects health by fostering meaning in life, facilitating health-promoting behaviors, and regulating thoughts toward health. Increased social support has been related to a reduction in mortality rates and incidences of physical and mental illness (Callaghan, Morrissey, 1993).
- Obtain or design educational material that is appropriate for the client, using pictures if possible.
  The three major learning styles are visual (seeing), aural (listening), and psychomotor (experiencing).
- Refer to social services for financial assistance if needed.

- Make sure follow-up appointments are scheduled before client is discharged; discuss with client how to ensure that appointments are kept.
  Social conditions can limit the client's achievement of health-promoting activity (Meleis, 1990).

Geriatric

- Assess sensory deficits and psychomotor skills in terms of client's ability to comply with a health program.
  Major changes in senses and bodily functions occur after age 40.
- Provide aids to assist with compliance (e.g., prepare medication schedules, prepare week's medications in daily containers).
- Recognize any resistance to change in lifelong patterns of personal health care.
  Change in one aspect of life can precipitate adjustment in all other aspects.
- Discuss with client realistic goals for changes in health maintenance.
  The focus of a chronic illness may be care rather than cure.

Client/Family Teaching

- Teach client and family prescribed health care treatments (e.g., medications, treatments, diet, activities of daily living, methods of coping, seek help when necessary).
  Compliance is enhanced through social support. Changes in life-style affect each relationship.
- Have client and family perform a return demonstration, at least twice, of any procedures to be done at home.
  Practice of a procedure brings up problems, enhances skill levels, and promotes confidence in new behaviors.
- Teach nonthreatening material before more anxiety-producing information is given.
  Anxiety focuses attention, and details may then be perceived as more important than the overall health-maintenance program.
- Establish a written contract with client to follow the agreed-on health care regimen.
  Written agreements reinforce the verbal agreement and serve as a reference.

REFERENCES

Callaghan P, Morrissey G: Social support and health: a review, *J Adv Nurs* 203:18, 1993.

Meleis A: Being and becoming healthy: the core of nursing knowledge, *Nurs Sci Q* 1:15, 1990.

Pender N: *Health promotion in nursing practice,* ed 2, Norwalk, Conn, 1987, Appleton & Lange.

BIBLIOGRAPHY

Leininger M, editor: *Culture care diversity and universality: a theory of nursing,* New York, 1991, National League for Nursing Press.

Potter P, Perr A: *Fundamentals of nursing: concepts, processes, and practices,* ed 3, St Louis, 1993, Mosby.

Wenger F: Cultural meaning of symptoms, *Holistic Nurs Pract* 22:7, 1993.

Health-seeking behaviors

Suzanne Skowronski

Definition The state in which an individual in stable health actively seeks ways to alter personal health habits or the environment to move toward a higher level of health.

NOTE: Stable health status is defined as the achievement of age-appropriate illness prevention measures, a client's report of good or excellent health, and the control of any signs and symptoms of disease.

Defining Characteristics

Major Expressed or observed desire to seek a higher level of wellness for self or family.

Minor Expressed or observed desire for increased control of health practice; expressed concern about the effect of current environmental conditions on health status; stated or observed unfamiliarity with wellness community resources; demonstrated or observed lack of knowledge regarding health-promoting behaviors.

Related Factors (r/t)

Role change; change in developmental level (e.g., marriage, parenthood, "empty-nest" syndrome, retirement); lack of knowledge regarding the need for preventive health behaviors, appropriate health screenings, optimal nutrition, weight control, regular exercise programs, stress management, supportive social networks, and responsible role participation.

Client Outcomes/Goals

- Maintains ideal weight and is knowledgeable about nutritious diet.
- Explains how to fit newly prescribed change in health habits into life-style.
- Lists community resources available for assistance in achieving wellness.
- Explains how to include wellness behaviors in current life-style.

Nursing Interventions and Rationales

- Determine health habits of client and family (e.g., diet, exercise, sleep, smoking, alcohol intake, stress levels).
  "Holistic health integrates body-mind-spirit lived within a supportive environmental system" (Edelman, Mandle, 1990, p. 8).
- Determine with client the most important wellness behavior to work on.
  The client is individually responsible for coping and maintaining health (Jones, Meleis, 1990).
- Identify environmental and social factors that the client perceives as health promoting.
  Social and political issues such as adequate housing and clean air and water promote high-level wellness. Health itself has social ramifications.

Nutrition

- Determine client's height and weight; compare with recommended weight for age or height.
- Encourage a diet low in salt, fat, sugar, and preservatives; encourage an appropriate intake of complex carbohydrates, fruits, vegetables, protein, and fat.
  Dietary intake provides nutrients that promote wellness, prevent illness, and enhance the social quality of life (Edelman, Mandle, 1990).
- Refer to dietician or weight-loss program for further assessment of diet and help with compliance.

Exercise

- Determine amount of exercise client needs per week and ability to tolerate exercise; refer to physician for testing to determine ability to tolerate exercise.

- Encourage aerobic exercise that increases heart rate within the prescribed limit; encourage client to exercise at least 3 times per week for 20 or more minutes, using exercises that the client prefers (e.g., walking, jogging, aerobics, swimming, bicycling, yoga, Tai Chi).
- Explore with client weightlifting options to increase muscle strength and stamina.
- Help client to focus on the enjoyment of exercise; set up a support and reward system.
  Exercise should involve large-muscle groups for about 20 minutes 3 times a week and use 60% of a client's cardiorespiratory capacity (Emmunds, 1991).

Stress Management

- Ask client to define stress in terms of life-style events and assign them a value on a scale from 1 to 5.
  This exercise helps distinguish between anxiety as a personality trait and anxiety as a coping response toward threatening events.
- Determine usual ways in which the client relieves stress; identify their effectiveness.
- Determine client's social support network.
- Determine amount of personal time client has; if necessary, decide how this amount can be increased.
- Teach stress-relieving techniques (e.g., deep and slow breathing, progressive muscle relaxation, exercise, meditation, power strategies, problem solving, imagery, verbalization of feelings, spiritual practices [prayer]).
  Stress management addresses the sources of tension in physical performance, emotional expression, transcendent spiritual experiences, social relationships, and the surrounding environment.

Smoking, Drinking, Self-Medication

- Determine the frequency of risk-taking habits.
- Refer the smoker to "Smoke Enders" or a similar community-based program; discuss how client can deal with loss of the behavioral habit or addiction.
- Refer the excessive drinker to Alcoholics Anonymous; identify a support person to help client into the organization.
- Discuss whether another person's excessive alcohol consumption is a family- or work-related problem; refer client to Al-Anon.
- Identify patterns of self-medication (e.g., antibiotics, mood-altering drugs).
  Excessive alcohol intake, cigarette smoking, and self-administered use of mood-altering drugs affects major body organs and predisposes the client to a chronic or life-threatening illness.

Health Screening, Appropriate Health Care

- Assess frequency of illness-preventing practices such as yearly physical examinations, dental examinations, flu shots, monthly breast self-examinations (and mammograms as recommended) for women, testicular self-examinations and prostate examinations for men, screenings for familial diseases such as glaucoma and elevated cholesterol.
  Refer to **Altered health maintenance**.

Geriatric

- Assess client's awareness of deficits that may result from normal aging (e.g., changes in sleep patterns or in frequency of urination, loss of visual acuity in night driving, loss of hearing, dietary changes, memory changes, loss of significant others).
- Identify coping mechanisms that promote wellness and place control of life choices back with the client; stress early retirement planning.

- Find suitable housing that provides support, safety, protection, meals, and social events.
- Give client information about community resources for the elderly (e.g., transportation to appointments, Meals-on-Wheels, home visitors, pets, American Association of Retired Persons).
  The aging process occurs throughout the lifespan. The elderly client hopes to remain independent and useful as long as possible without being a burden to others.
- Provide information about pneumococcal vaccinations for those over 65.
  Pneumococcal vaccines are given only once and recommended for those over 65.

Client/Family Teaching

- Provide and review pamphlets about health-seeking opportunities and wellness resources in the community.
- Discuss the role of environmental and social factors to support a healthy family life.
- Identify physical and emotional threats to family security (e.g., domestic violence, child abuse, school violence).
  Wellness and health-promoting behaviors can only be met when safety and security issues are solved personally and socially.

REFERENCES

Edelman C, Mandle C: *Health promotion throughout the lifespan,* St Louis, 1990, Mosby.

Emmunds M: Strategies for promoting physical fitness, *Nurs Clin North Am* 26:4, 1991.

Jones P, Meleis A: Health is empowerment, *Adv Nurs Sci* 1:15, 1990.

BIBLIOGRAPHY

Pender N: *Health promotion in nursing practice,* ed 2, Norwalk, Conn, 1987, Appleton & Lange.

Walker S: Wellness for elders, *Holistic Nurs Pract,* 38:7, 1993.

Impaired home maintenance management

Suzanne Skowronski

Definition The inability to independently maintain a safe, growth-promoting immediate environment.

Defining Characteristics

Subjective *Household members express difficulty in maintaining their home in a comfortable fashion; *household members request assistance with home maintenance; *household members describe outstanding debts or financial crises.

Objective Disorderly environment; *unwashed or unavailable cooking equipment, clothes, or linens; *accumulation of dirt, food wastes, or hygienic wastes; offensive odors; inappropriate household temperature; *overtaxed family members (e.g., exhausted, anxious); lack of necessary equipment or aids; presence of vermin or rodents; *repeated hygienic disorders, infestations, or infections. (*Critical)

Related Factors (r/t)

Client or family member disease or injury; insufficient family organization or planning; insufficient finances; unfamiliarity with neighborhood resources; impaired cognitive or emotional functioning; lack of knowledge; lack of role-modeling; inadequate support systems.

Client Outcomes/Goals

- Family members have clean clothing, nutritious meals, and a sanitary and safe home.
- Family members have the resources to cope physically and emotionally with the chronic illness process.
- Client and family use community resources to assist with treatment needs.

Nursing Interventions and Rationales

- Help client and family to identify what they need to provide care in a home environment.
  Continuity of care from hospital to home may require adjustment of equipment and supplies and rearrangement of the environment to promote safety.
- Assess family members' concerns, especially those of the primary caregiver, about long-term home-care issues.
  Usually one family member becomes the primary caregiver of a relative with a long-term chronic illness.
- Set up a system of relief for the main caregiver in the home and a plan for sharing household duties.
  The caregiving career does not have a specific endpoint; it lasts as long as the chronically ill person is cared for at home (Lindgren, 1993).
- Ask family to identify support people who can help with home maintenance.
- Initiate a referral to community agencies as needed, including housekeeping aides, Meals-on-Wheels, wheelchair-compatible transportation, and oxygen therapy.
  Community-based agencies provide financial help, education, and emotional support for in-home care, which reduces the burden for families coping with chronic sickness.
- Obtain adaptive equipment as appropriate to help family members continue to maintain home.
- Refer client to social services to help with debt consolidation or financial concerns.
  Financial help ranges from Medicaid and private insurance to foundations specific to an illness such as Shriner's Burn Center for Children. Hospital discharge planners are an important resource for coordinating agencies.

Geriatric

- Explore community resources to assist with home care (e.g., senior centers, Department of Aging, hospital discharge planners, churches).
  People over age 65 have difficulty paying for goods and services on a fixed retirement income. Persons who are age 85 or older are most likely to have incomes at or below the poverty level (Edelman, Mandle, 1990).
- Visit client's home to assess safety features (e.g., absence of throw rugs, safety bars in the bathroom, stair borders that distinguish each step, adequate nonglare light).
  Advancing age and the physiological changes that accompany it predispose older adults to falls and other accidents (Potter, Perry, 1993).
- Be alert to signs of elder abuse during the home visit such as unattended medical problems; poor hygiene; dehydration; substandard housing; verbal abuse from family, neighbors, or professional caregivers.
  About 3% to 4% of the nation's elderly are victims of elder mistreatment (Edelman, Mandle, 1990).

Client/Family Teaching

- Teach family members how to perform activities that maintain the home (e.g., cooking, cleaning, fire prevention).
  When one family member becomes ill and requires home care, the role of other family members may change.
- Teach caregiver the need to set aside some personal time every day to meet own needs.
- Encourage social relationships with family and friends, even if only by phone.

REFERENCES

Edelman C, Mandle C: *Health promotion throughout the lifespan,* ed 3, St Louis, 1990, Mosby.
Lindgren C: The caregiver career, *Image* 214:25, 1993.
Potter P, Perry A: *Fundamentals of nursing: concepts, processes, and practices,* ed 3, St Louis, 1993, Mosby.

BIBLIOGRAPHY

Donnelly G: Chronicity, concept and reality, *Holistic Nurs Pract* 1:8, 1993.
Hinton-Walker P: Care of the chronically ill, *Holistic Nurs Pract* 59:8, 1993.

Hopelessness

Gail Ladwig

Definition The subjective state in which an individual sees limited or unavailable alternatives or personal choices and is unable to mobilize energy on own behalf.

Defining Characteristics

Major Passivity; decreased verbalization; decreased affect; verbal cues (e.g., despondent content, saying "I can't," sighing).

Minor Lack of initiative; decreased response to stimuli; decreased affect; turning away from speaker; closing of eyes; shrugging responses; decreased appetite; increased or decreased sleep; lack of involvement in care; passively allowing care.

Related Factors (r/t)

Prolonged activity restriction that creates isolation; failing or deteriorating physiological condition; long-term stress; abandonment; lost beliefs in transcendent values or in God.

Client Outcomes/Goals

- Able to verbalize feelings; participates in care.
- Makes positive statements (e.g., "I can," "I will try").
- Makes eye contact; focuses on speaker.
- Appetite is appropriate for age and physical health.
- Sleep time is appropriate for age and physical health.

Nursing Interventions and Rationales

- Monitor and document potential for suicide; refer to **Risk for violence: self-directed** for specific interventions.
  Hopelessness is correlated with an increased risk of suicide (Buchanan, 1991).
- Spend one-to-one time with client.
  One-to-one time is an important component of the nurse-patient relationship (Bulechek, McCloskey, 1992).
- Encourage expression of feelings and acknowledge acceptance of them.
  A client's ability to express a negative emotion can be a very healthy sign; strong emotions are potentially dangerous if not expressed (Barry, 1994).
- Give client time to initiate interactions; after time is allowed, approach client in an accepting and nonjudgmental manner.
  Clients who have feelings of hopelessness need extra time to initiate relationships, but sometimes they cannot. When the client cannot initiate a relationship, to instill feelings of worth, the caregiver then needs to approach the client.
- Encourage client to participate in group activities.
  Group activities provide social support and help identify alternative ways to problem solve.
- Review with the client his or her strengths; have client list strengths on a 3 x 5 card and carry it for future reference.
  Listing strengths provides positive reinforcement of positive self-regard.
- Use humor as appropriate.
  Humor is an effective intervention for hopelessness (Hunt, 1993).
- Involve family and significant others in plan of care.
- Encourage family and significant others to express care and love for client.
- Use touch to demonstrate caring, and encourage family to use touch.

Geriatric

- Assess for clinical signs and symptoms of depression; differentiate depression from functional or organic dementia.
  It can be difficult to distinguish depression from dementia in those over age 65 because some symptoms (e.g., disorientation, memory loss, and distractibility) may suggest dementia. Concurrent medical illnesses, prescription medications, and concealed alcohol or substance abuse can also appear to be dementia (AHCPR Guideline, 1993).
- Take threats of self-harm or suicide seriously.
  Elders who are depressed or who have experienced recent losses and live alone are at the highest risk.
- Identify with client significant losses that might be leading to feelings of hopelessness.
- Discuss stages of emotional responses to multiple losses.
- Use reminiscence and life review to identify past coping skills.
  Such a review gives significance and meaning to life for the elderly client who is questioning his or her self-worth (Ringsven, Bond, 1991).
- Express hope to client and give positive feedback whenever appropriate.
- Identify client's past sources of spirituality; help client explore his or her life and identify those experiences that are noteworthy.

Client/Family Teaching

- Teach stress reduction, relaxation, and imagery.
  Anxiety cannot exist if the muscles are truly relaxed (Bulechek, McCloskey, 1992).
- Refer to self-help groups such as "I Can Cope" and "Make Today Count."
  These groups allow the client to recognize the love and care of others, and they promote a sense of belonging (Bulechek, McCloskey, 1992).
- Supply a crisis-line number and secure contract with client to use the number if thoughts of self-harm occur.
  A no-suicide contract is one type of intervention used with clients who have suicidal thoughts (Valente, 1989).

REFERENCES

Barry P: *Mental health and mental illness,* ed 5, Philadelphia, 1994, JB Lippincott.

Buchanan DM: Suicide: a conceptual model for an avoidable death, *Arch Psychiatr Nurs* 5:341-349, 1991.

Bulechek G, McCloskey J: *Nursing interventions: essential nursing treatments,* ed 2, Philadelphia, 1992, JB Lippincott.

Clinical Practice Guideline: *Depression in primary care. Volume 1: Detection and diagnosis,* Rockville, Md, 1993, US Department of Health and Human Services (AHCPR Publication 93-0550).

Hunt AH: Humor as a nursing intervention, *Cancer Nurs* 16:34-39, 1993.

Ringsven M, Bond D: *Gerontology and leadership skills for nurses,* 1991, Delmar.

Valente SM: Adolescent suicide: assessment and intervention, *J Child Adol Psychiatr Ment Health Nurs* 2:34-39, 1989.

BIBLIOGRAPHY

Abraham I, Neundorfer M, Currie L: Effect of group interventions on cognition and depression in nursing home residents, *Nurs Res* 41:196-202, 1992.

Clemons S, Cummings S: Helplessness and powerlessness: caring for clients in pain, *Holistic Nurs Pract* 6:76-85, 1991.

Hyperthermia

Marcia LaHaie and Terry VandenBosch

Definition The state in which an individual's body temperature is elevated above his or her normal range.

NOTE: Body temperature is controlled by the hypothalamus and increases in response to internal and external factors such as infection, tissue injury, and hypothalamus dysfunction. Fever is present whenever a person's temperature elevates above his or her normal daily range or above 100°F. Normally there is a proportional increase in immune system enhancement for every degree of temperature rise up to 104°F. Fever is believed to be adaptive at levels below 104°F (Kluger, 1991). Hyperthermia is a significant elevation in body temperature, usually above 104°F, and it occurs in the presence of hypothalamic dysfunction. Hyperthermia is not considered adaptive (Holtzclaw, 1992).

Defining Characteristics

Major Increase in body temperature above normal range.

NOTE: Temperature greater than 104°F.

Minor Flushed or hot skin; increased respiratory rate; tachycardia; seizures; convulsions.

Related Factors (r/t)

Exposure to hot environment; vigorous activity; medications or anesthestic; inappropriate clothing; increased metabolic rate; illness or trauma; dehydration; inability or decreased ability to perspire.

Client Outcomes/Goals

- Oral temperature is within adaptive levels (below 104°F). A lower temperature may be necessary, depending on the presence of cardiopulmonary disease or on the client's neurological status.
- Free of problems of dehydration.
- Free of seizure activity; febrile seizure activity is rare in adults.

Nursing Interventions and Rationales

- Take client's temperature at least once a day between 3 PM and 7 PM or according to institutional standards.
  Temperature screening for afebrile patients can be based on daily circadian rhythm patterns. Take client's temperature at the peak of the circadian rhythm (Samples, 1985; Angerami, 1980).
- Once a temperature elevation has been detected, retake temperature if client experiences chills or states that he or she feels warmer and after instituting interventions.
  Shivering indicates a rising body temperature.
- Notify physician of temperature according to institutional standards or written orders.
- Administer antipyretic medications on the basis of physician's order, client comfort level, and/or a temperature greater than 102.5°F.
  NOTE: This method represents conservative management of fever.
  Fever is a symptom used to diagnose, monitor a disease process, and determine the effectiveness of a treatment. Fever is adaptive. For every degree of temperature rise up to 104°F, there is a proportional increase in immune system enhancement (Kluger, 1991).
- Assess client for a history of febrile seizures; give antipyretics more aggressively only in clients with a positive history.
  In adults there is very little evidence of an association between fever and seizures and neurological damage (Styrt, Sugarman, 1990). Children who have a high fever (over

104°F) at the time of an initial febrile seizure are less likely to have a recurrence of such seizures than children who have more moderate fevers at the time of an initial seizure (El-Radhi, Withana, Banajeh, 1986).

- Assess fluid loss and administer intravenous fluids or facilitate oral intake to promote fluid replacement.
  Increased metabolic rate and diaphoresis causes a loss of body fluids.
- Notify physician of changes in client's mental status.
  A change in mental status may indicate the onset of septic shock.
- When diaphoresis is present, maintain client's comfort by assisting with clothing changes and bathing.
  Clothing changes and bathing increase comfort and decrease the possibility of continued shivering resulting from water evaporation from the skin.
- Do not use external cooling measures such as ice packs, tepid water baths, or the removal of blankets and clothing for fever management unless temperature is greater than 104°F; these measures cause shivering.
  Shivering results in significantly increased oxygen consumption (Holtzclaw, 1993). If the client's temperature drops as a result of external cooling measures, the hypothalamus resets the body temperature at a higher level, which results in more shivering (Enright, Hill, 1989).
- Use a cooling blanket if client's fever is higher than 105°F or if a high body temperature is related to hypothalamus dysfunction.
  Cooling blankets are used when the client's oral temperature exceeds 105°F and cannot be controlled by antipyretics (Styrt, Sugarman, 1990) or when the fever is caused by a heat-related illness or is neurologically related (Morgan, 1990).

Geriatric

- In hot weather encourage client to drink 8 to 10 glasses of fluids per day in spite of thirst and within the cardiac and renal reserve; encourage the use of fans or air conditioning.
  The elderly are more susceptible to heat because sweat gland function decreases and causes heat intolerance. The elderly also have decreased thirst.

Client/Family Teaching

- Teach that fever enhances the immune system response in the presence of infection; the peak of beneficial effects occurs at an oral temperature of 104°F.
  Fevers under 104°F enhance immune system functioning (Roberts, 1991).
- Recommend a liberal intake of nonalcoholic and noncaffeinated fluids.
  Liberal fluid intake replaces fluid lost through perspiration and respiration. The presence of alcohol and caffeine in fluids can promote diuresis.
- Teach client the detrimental effects of shivering; teach client to avoid activities that can cause shivering (e.g., blanket removal, lower room temperature, tepid water bath, ice packs).
  External cooling measures result in shivering and discomfort (Styrt, Sugarman, 1990).
- Teach that the use of antipyretics is the most effective way to reduce an infection-related fever below 104°F if the client is uncomfortable.
  Antipyretics effectively reduce infection-related fevers (Clark, 1991).
- Teach client to avoid vigorous physical activity, wear light clothing, and wear a hat to minimize sun exposure during periods of excessive outdoor heat.
  Such methods reduce exposure to high environmental temperatures, which can cause heat stroke.

REFERENCES

Angerami ES: Epidemiological study of body temperature in patients in a teaching hospital, *Int J Nurs Stud* 17:91-99, 1980.

Clark WG: *Antipyretics.* In Mackowiak P editor: *Fever: basic mechanisms and management,* New York, 1991, Raven Press.

El-Radhi AS et al: Recurrence rate of febrile convulsions related to the degree of pyrexia during the first attack, *Clin Pediatr* 25:311-313, 1986.

Enright T, Hill MG: Treatment of fever, *Focus Crit Care* 16:96-102, 1989.

Holtzclaw BJ: *Clinical predictors and metabolic consequences of postoperative shivering after cardiac surgery.* Presented at the Fifth National Conference on Research for Clinical Practice, Key Aspects of Caring for the Acutely Ill: Technological Aspects, Patient Education, and Quality of Life, Chapel Hill, NC, April 23, 1993.

Holtzclaw BJ: The febrile response in critical care: state of the science, *Heart Lung* 21:482-501, 1992.

Kluger MJ: The adaptive value of fever. In Mackowiak PA, editor, *Fever: basic mechanisms and management,* New York, 1991, Raven Press.

Morgan, SP: A comparison of three methods of managing fever in the neurologic patient, *J Neurosci Nurs* 22:19-24, 1990.

Roberts NJ: The immunological consequences of fever. In Mackowiak PA, editor: *Fever: basic mechanisms and management,* New York, 1991, Raven Press.

Samples JF et al: Circadian rhythms: basis for screening for fever, *Nurs Res* 34:377-379, 1985.

Styrt B, Sugarman B: Antipyresis and fever, *Arch Intern Med,* 150:1589-1597, 1990.

BIBLIOGRAPHY

Bruce J, Grove SK: Fever: pathology and treatment, *Crit Care Nurse* 12:40-48, 1992.

Cunha BA: Clinical implications of fever, *Postgrad Med* 85:188-200, 1989.

Mackowiak PA: A critical appraisal of 98.6°F, the upper limit of the normal body temperature and other legacies of Carl Reinhold August Wunderlich, *JAMA* 268:1578-1580, 1992.

Mackowiak PA, editor, *Fever: basic mechanisms and management,* New York, 1991, Raven Press.

May A, Bauchner H: Fever phobia: the pediatrician's contribution, *Pediatr* 90:851-854, 1992.

Hypothermia

Sandra Cunningham

Definition The state in which an individual's body temperature is reduced below his or her normal range.

Defining Characteristics

Major Reduction in body temperature below normal range; mild shivering; cool skin; moderate pallor.

Minor Slow capillary refill; piloerection; cyanotic nail beds; bradycardia; bradypnea; decreased mentation; drowsiness; confusion (adapted from Carpenito).

Related Factors (r/t)

Exposure to cool or cold environment; illness; trauma; damage to hypothalamus; inability or decreased ability to shiver; malnutrition; inadequate clothing; alcohol consumption; medications that cause vasodilation; evaporation of perspiration from skin in cool environment; decreased metabolic rate; inactivity; aging.

Client Outcomes/Goals

- Body temperature within normal range.
- Identifies risk factors of hypothermia.
- States measures to prevent hypothermia.
- Identifies symptoms of hypothermia and the actions to take when hypothermia is present.

Nursing Interventions and Rationales

- Determine factors leading to hypothermic episode; refer to related factors.
  It is important to assess risk factors and precipitating events.
- Remove client from cause(s) of hypothermic episode (e.g., cold environment, cold or wet clothing).
  These steps eliminate causative or contributing factors.
- Institute a low-reading, continuous core-temperature monitoring device as appropriate.
  This device monitors client's response to interventions. The normal range is 96.8°F to 100.4°F (Black, Matassarin-Jacobs, 1993).
- Monitor client's vital signs every hour and as appropriate; note changes associated with hypothermia such as decreased pulse, irregular pulse rhythm, decreased respiratory rate, or initially increased, then decreased blood pressure.
  Decreased circulating volume during hypothermia results in decreased cardiac output and depressed oxygen delivery. Hypoxia, metabolic acidosis, and intrinsic irritability of a cold myocardium result in various dysrhythmias.
- Monitor for signs of hypothermia (e.g., shivering, cool skin, piloerection, pallor, slow capillary refill, cyanotic nail beds, decreased mentation, coma).
- Monitor client for response to interventions and evidence of persistent hypothermia.
- Rewarm passively (e.g., set room temperature at 70° to 75°F, layer clothing and blankets, cover client's head, offer warm fluid with physician's order); allow client to rewarm at own pace.
  Passive rewarming prevents heat loss via radiation and evaporation. A client's response relies on his or her ability to generate heat (Dexter, 1990). Gradual rewarming limits complications associated with hypothermia.
- Rewarm actively (e.g., cover client with warmed cotton blankets or a forced warm air blanket, use radiant heat lights as available). With physician's order apply hydrothermic

blankets, administer heated and humidified oxygen, and carefully administer heated intravenous fluids at prescribed temperature.
Active rewarming increases heat gain via the four major mechanisms of heat transfer—radiation, conduction, convection, and evaporation (Stevens, 1993).

- Rewarm client using active core rewarming techniques (e.g., colonic lavage, hemodialysis, peritoneal lavage, extracorporeal blood rewarming, bladder irrigations). Follow physician's order carefully.
  Active core rewarming increases heat gain via conduction.
- Request a social service referral to help client obtain the heat, shelter, and food needed to maintain body temperature.
  A preventive approach that includes adequate food and fluid intake, shelter, heat, and clothing decreases the risk of hypothermia.
- Encourage proper nutrition and hydration. Request a dietician referral to identify minimum dietary needs.
  Insufficient calorie and fluid intake predisposes the client to hypothermia.

Geriatric

- Assess neurological signs frequently.
  Older adults are less likely to shiver or complain of feeling cold. Early signs of hypothermia are subtle (Miller, 1990).
- Assess client's heat source and refer for assistance if heat is inadequate.
  Public utilities ensure that elders have adequate heat.

Client/Family Teaching

- If age appropriate, teach how to take a temperature and monitor for signs of hypothermia.
- Teach client how to prevent hypothermia by wearing adequate clothing, heating environment to a minimum of 68°F, and ingesting adequate food and fluid.
  Simple measures such as layering clothes, wearing a hat, and avoiding extremes in temperature prevent significant heat loss.

REFERENCES

Black JM, Matassarin-Jacobs E: *Luckmann and Sorenson's medical-surgical nursing: a psychophysiologic approach,* Philadelphia, 1993, WB Saunders.

Carpenito JL: *Nursing diagnosis: application to clinical practice,* ed 5, Philadelphia, 1993, JB Lippincott.

Dexter WW: Hypothermia: safe and efficient methods of rewarming, *Postgrad Med* 88:55-58, 1990.

Miller CA: Nursing care of older adults: theory and practice, Glenview, Ill, 1990, Foresman & Little.

Stevens T: Managing postoperative hypothermia, rewarming, and its complications, *Crit Care Nurse* 16:60-77, 1993.

BIBLIOGRAPHY

Danzl DF, Ghezzi KT: Hot tips on handling hypothermia, *Patient Care* 25:89-92, 1991.

Giuffre M et al: Rewarming postoperative patients: lights, blankets, or forced warm air, *J Post Anesth Nurs* 6:387-393, 1991.

Hortzclaw BJ: Monitoring body temperature, *AACN Clin Issues Crit Care Nurs* 4:44-55, 1993.

Summers S: Inadvertent hypothermia: clinical validation in postanesthesia patients, *Nurs Diag* 3:54-64, 1992.

Bowel incontinence

Kathie Hesnan

Definition The state in which an individual experiences a change in normal bowel habits characterized by involuntary passage of stool.

Defining Characteristics

*Involuntary passage of stool. (*Critical)

Related Factors (r/t)

Loss of control of rectal sphincter; neurological dysfunction; dementia; severe regression; gastrointestinal disorders (e.g., inflammatory bowel syndrome); colonic or rectal surgery; anorectal trauma; diarrhea (adapted from Carpenito).

Client Outcomes/Goals

- Continent of formed stool at least every day to every third day.
- Intact skin in rectal-sacral area.
- Decreased incidence of incontinence.
- Able to use commode or toilet at regular intervals (once per day) without experiencing intervening episodes of incontinence.
- Increased pelvic strength and endurance (if incontinence is related to pelvic muscle weakness).

Nursing Interventions and Rationales

- Complete a focused nursing history that includes previous and present bowel routines, diet history, functional status, and neurological and rectal examinations.
  A nursing history is needed to develop an individualized and appropriate plan of care.
- Document or have the client complete a bowel record that can include frequency and timing of incontinence, diet, fluid intake, and activities that correlate with incontinent episodes.
  This record confirms the verbal history and provides a method for evaluating treatment success.
- Identify the underlying cause of incontinence (e.g., impaction, stool consistency, altered sensation, altered cognitive status, poor rectal accommodation, decreased pelvic muscle strength, medication, diet, disease process).
  Multiple factors may result in fecal incontinence (Doughty, 1991).
- Provide easy access to bedpan, commode, or bathroom.
- Respond immediately to client's call for bedpan or commode.
- Provide privacy; give nonjudgmental and accepting care.
- Assist client daily with use of commode or bedpan at usual time of defecation.
- Cleanse skin thoroughly after each incontinent stool; use spray cleansers designed for this purpose.
  Do not use soap and water frequently because soap can be very harsh on skin.
- Apply petroleum-based ointment to perirectal skin after each cleaning.
- If incontinence is frequent, use an absorbent product or external collection device.
- If client is obtunded or comatose and stool is liquid, ask for physician's order to apply fecal incontinence pouch.
- For a neurologically altered but stable client, establish a bowel routine with suppository every other day or digital stimulation with physician's order.
- For the client with a decrease in pelvic muscle strength, instruct in Kegel's exercises with or without biofeedback.
  Kegel's exercises have been proven to decrease fecal incontinence (Doughty, 1991).

Geriatric

- Observe etiology of incontinence and treat appropriately, (e.g., modify environment for ease of toileting, toilet regularly after meals, modify diet, provide medications as prescribed).
- Check for impaction as ordered.
- Teach muscle-strengthening exercises and use behavior modification to help control bowel function.

Client/Family Teaching

- Establish a bowel training program that includes using warm fluids in the morning and a private place for defecation.
- Teach how to deal with incontinence to decrease embarrassment of client or family.

NOTE: If constipation or diarrhea is the underlying cause of fecal incontinence, refer to the specific care plan.

REFERENCES

Carpenito JL: *Nursing diagnosis: application to clinical practice,* ed 5, Philadelphia, 1993, JB Lippincott.

Doughty D: *Urinary and fecal incontinence: nursing management,* St Louis, 1991, Mosby.

BIBLIOGRAPHY

Alterescu V: Theoretical foundations for an approach to fecal incontinence. *J Enterostom Ther* 13:44, 1986.

Dodge J et al: Fecal incontinence in elderly patients, *Postgrad Med* 83:258, 1988.

Doughty D: A step-by-step approach to bowel training, *Progressions* 4:12, 1992.

Functional incontinence

Kathie Hesnan

Definition The state in which an individual finds it difficult or is unable to reach the toilet in time as a result of environmental barriers, cognitive changes, or physical limitations (adapted from Carpenito).

Defining Characteristics

Major Voiding urges or bladder contractions are strong enough to result in a loss of urine before reaching an appropriate receptacle.

Related Factors (r/t)

Altered environment; sensory, cognitive, or mobility deficits.

Client Outcomes/Goals

- Elimination or reduced incidents of urinary incontinence.
- Environmental barriers to using the bathroom are removed or minimized.
- Adaptive equipment is used to enhance the client's ability to toilet.
- If incontinent episodes can only be reduced, skin integrity is maintained with appropriate containment options.

Nursing Interventions and Rationales

- Assess client for acute causes of incontinence (e.g., urinary tract infections; abnormal urinalysis results; atrophic changes; constipation or impaction; bladder irritants such as caffeinated or citrus beverages; poor fluid intake; polyuria; retention; medication).
  These factors can increase the severity of incontinence or be the underlying cause (Urinary Incontinence Guideline Panel, 1992; Doughty, 1991).
- Assess client for other type(s) of incontinence; if other types are present, institute appropriate interventions for them.
  The treatment for urinary incontinence is specific to the type.
- Assess client for clothing that limits easy access to toileting such as girdles, snaps, buttons, diapers, pantyhose, or multiple layers of clothing.
  For the client with a decreased functional or cognitive status, certain items of clothing may be too difficult to rapidly remove to facilitate toileting or may result in dependency on a caregiver to enable toileting.
- Assess for obstacles to reaching an appropriate receptacle such as poor lighting, lack of siderails, lack of privacy, frequently occupied bathrooms, toilet or commode height, lack of assistive devices.
- Using a bladder record or diary, monitor frequency of toileting, incontinent episodes, and fluid intake; have client or caregiver keep record.
  A voiding record can help identify an appropriate voiding schedule. The complexity and amount of information recorded should match the client's or caregiver's ability.
- Initiate a voiding schedule according to the results of the bladder record.
  An individualized toileting schedule effectively reduces urinary incontinence (Colling et al, 1992).
- If a voiding record cannot be completed, have client initially void every 2 hours; also have client void on awakening and before going to sleep.
- Provide an appropriate and safe urinary receptacle such as a 3-in-1 commode, female or male urinal, or no-spill urinal.
  These receptacles provide access to a toilet substitute and enhance the potential for continence (Wells, 1992).

- Ensure that client has ready access to a call light or other mechanism to get assistance (e.g., bell) at all times; answer lights immediately.
  Answering the light rapidly can result in continence and is a positive reinforcement that provides encouragement to the client.
- Obtain a consultation for physical therapy if ambulation problems inhibit toileting.
  A physical therapist can institute an exercise regimen to increase strength and endurance, which results in easier access to toileting.
- Obtain a consultation for occupational therapy to acquire assistive devices for increased access to toileting.

Geriatric

- Provide reality orientation when needed to increase client's awareness of time, place, and environment.
  Clients with dementia may forget when they last toileted.
- If client's clothing is a barrier to urination, modify it with velcro fasteners.
- Use prompted voiding techniques (e.g., check client regularly, provide positive reinforcement if dry, prompt client to toilet, praise client after toileting, return client to toilet in a specified time).
  Prompted voiding techniques have proven to reduce the number of incontinent episodes in nursing home patients (Hu et al, 1989; Urinary Incontinence Guideline Panel, 1992).

Client/Family Teaching

- Work with client and family to set up schedule of voiding using environmental and behavioral cues such as meals, bedtime, and television shows.
- Teach the client and family how to keep a record of voiding; teach them that the record helps determine a voiding schedule and shows progress.
- Discuss with client and family how to obtain and use devices that increase accessibility to toileting.

REFERENCES

Carpenito JL: *Nursing diagnosis: application to clinical practice,* ed 5, Philadelphia, 1993, JB Lippincott.

Colling J et al: The effects of patterned urge-response toileting (PURT) on urinary incontinence among nursing home residents, *J Am Geriatr Soc* 40:135-141, 1992.

Doughty, D: *Urinary and fecal incontinence: nursing management,* St Louis, 1991, Mosby.

Hu T et al: A clinical trial of a behavioral therapy program to reduce urinary incontinence in nursing homes, *JAMA* 261:2656, 1989.

Urinary Incontinence Guideline Panel: *Urinary incontinence in adults: clinical practice guideline.* Rockville, Md, March 1992, Agency for Health Care Policy and Research, Public Health Service, US Department of Health and Human Services (AHCPR Publication 92-0038).

Wells T: Managing incontinence through managing the environment, *Urol* 12:48, 1992.

BIBLIOGRAPHY

Heller B et al: Incontinence, *J Gerontol Nurs* 15:16, 1989.

McCormick K et al: Nursing management of urinary incontinence in geriatric inpatients. *Nurs Clin North Am* 23:231, 1988.

Reflex incontinence

Kathie Hesnan

Definition The state in which an individual experiences an involuntary loss of urine as a result of a lesion in the spinal cord.

Defining Characteristics

Major No awareness of bladder filling; no urge to void; no feelings of bladder fullness; uninhibited bladder contraction.

Related Factors (r/t)

Neurological impairment (e.g., spinal cord lesion that interferes with conduction of cerebral messages above the level of the reflex arc).

Client Outcomes/Goals

- Follows prescribed voiding schedule; urine is clear.
- Able to perform and be compliant with catheterization schedule.
- Demonstrates successful use of triggering techniques to stimulate voiding.
- Perineal area is free from irritation or breakdown.
- Identifies types of containment devices that maintain skin integrity and prevent embarrassing accidents.

  NOTE: A client who is acutely ill with flaccid paralysis (lower motor neuron involvement) will generally need a Foley catheter or intermittent catheterization. When client is experiencing spastic paralysis and is stable, voiding techniques can be used. It is very important that the bladder be regularly and adequately emptied to prevent urinary tract infections and hydronephrosis.

Nursing Interventions and Rationales

- Monitor client's patterns of urination, fluid intake, ability to urinate voluntarily, clarity of urine, incidence of incontinence of urine, bladder distention, and amount of residual urine after urination.

  This basic evaluation is necessary to develop an individualized plan of care.
- Explain treatment options such as triggered voiding, clean intermittent catheterization, external collection, and medication.

  The client must have a good understanding of available and manageable options.
- If clean, intermittent catheterization is to be used, teach client care of the catheter and other supplies.

  Proper care of supplies decreases the chance of clinical bacteriuria or infection. Plastic urethral catheters may be used, but the ability of the client and the environment must be taken into consideration (Moore et al, 1993).
- Do not routinely teach Crede's procedures.

  A urological evaluation must be done to make sure sphincter and bladder are coordinated so that reflux does not occur.
- Regulate client's fluid intake if dependent on catheterization schedule.

  A large volume of fluid consumed before bedtime may cause the client to get up during the night to catheterize.
- A client who is not in retention may be a candidate for a bladder training program. The following is an example of a bladder training program:
  - Indwelling catheter removed at 7 AM
  - Glass of fluid—240 ml q hour
  - After 2 or 3 hours, attempt to void by using triggering mechanisms (Upper Motor Neuron Bladder)

- If client voids, BladderScan or catheterize for residual (physician's order); if client is unable to void and a BladderScan is available, check bladder volume; if volume is greater than 400 ml, perform intermittent catheterization
- Continue with program

- Have client keep a written record of fluid intake, voiding pattern, and catheterization schedule.
- If self-catheterization is not feasible, bladder training is ineffective, and client is not retaining urine, use an external drainage device for a male. Try using an external female incontinence device for an ambulatory female.
  These methods of maintaining skin integrity can be very effective if the client is correctly measured for the device (Rousseau, 1991).
- Refer to continence nurse or rehabilitation nurse for further help in establishing an appropriate urination schedule.

Geriatric

- Instruct client in clean, intermittent catheterization.
  Intermittent catheterization can be an effective treatment for the elderly client (Whitelaw et al, 1987).
- If difficulties arise in teaching client, refer to a nurse who specializes in the elderly and incontinence.

Client/Family Teaching

- Teach signs of a full bladder (e.g., sweating, restlessness, abdominal discomfort).
- Teach techniques to trigger voiding—Upper Motor Neuron Bladder (e.g., tapping suprapubic area; stroking penis, inner thigh, or abdomen; pulling pubic hair; stretching anal sphincter with gloved finger; doing pushups on the commode). Watch for retention because reflex incontinence can lead to dysynergia of the detrusor and urethral sphincter.
- Teach signs and symptoms of urinary tract infections.
- Teach client and family intermittent straight catheterization techniques if ordered. Teach how to determine number of times or frequency of catheterization (e.g., if volume obtained greater than 450 ml, increase frequency).

REFERENCES

Moore K et al: Bacteriuria in intermittent catheterization users: the effect of sterile versus clean reused catheters, *Rehabil Nurs* 18:306-309, 1993.

Rousseau P: Urinary collection devices in geriatric incontinence, *J Enterostom Ther* 18:26-30, 1991.

Whitelaw S et al: Clean intermittent self-catheterization in the elderly, *Br J Urol* 60:125-127, 1987.

BIBLIOGRAPHY

Doughty D: *Urinary and fecal incontinence: nursing management,* St Louis, 1991, Mosby.

Stress incontinence

Kathie Hesnan

Definition The state in which an individual experiences a urine loss of less than 50 ml accompanied by increased intra-abdominal pressure.

Defining Characteristics

Reported or observed leakage with increased intra-abdominal pressure; small amounts of leakage with coughing, sneezing, activity, or position changes.

Related Factors (r/t)

Age-related degenerative changes in pelvic muscles and structural supports; high intra-abdominal pressure (e.g., obesity, gravid uterus); incompetent bladder outlet; overdistention between voiding; weak pelvic muscles and structural supports.

Client Outcomes/Goals

- Reports a decreased incidence or cessation of stress incontinence events.
- Verbalizes the cause of and treatment options for stress incontinence.
- Identifies types of containment devices that maintain skin integrity and prevent embarrassing accidents.
- Demonstrates proper techniques of Kegel's exercise.

Nursing Interventions and Rationales

- Assess client for acute causes of incontinence (e.g., urinary tract infections; abnormal urinalysis results; atrophic changes; constipation or impaction; bladder irritants such as caffeinated or citrus beverages; poor fluid intake; polyuria; retention; medication effects).
  These factors can increase the severity of incontinence or be the underlying cause (Urinary Incontinence Guideline Panel, 1992; Doughty, 1991).
- Obtain a nursing history that focuses on incontinence (e.g., onset, duration, past treatment, type, medications, past medical history, obstetrical or gynecological history).
- Perform physical examinations as appropriate, which may include examination of abdomen, pelvis, rectum, or skin integrity.
- If other types of incontinence are present, institute interventions for each type.
- Encourage client to verbalize feelings about stress incontinence.
  Verbalizing feelings helps decrease the client's anxiety.
- Discuss use of and provide client with small adhesive peripads to wear in underclothing.
- Perform digital vaginal examination to identify pelvic muscle strength; instruct patient on proper techniques of Kegel's exercise.
  The client must be taught to isolate the pelvic muscles so that the proper exercise techniques are performed (Dougherty et al, 1986).
- Educate client on treatment options for stress incontinence (e.g., behavioral and pharmacological treatments, bulking agents, surgery).
  Behavioral techniques, medication, and surgery are options for treatment of stress incontinence (Urinary Incontinence Guideline Panel, 1992).
- Refer client to supportive and educational groups such as HIP (Help for Incontinent People) or the Simon Foundation.
- Identify local continence clinics where the client can go for additional therapy. Therapies include biofeedback, stimulation, and further testing.
  Stress incontinence can be decreased with Kegel's exercises and biofeedback treatment (Burns et al, 1990).
- Refer client to a health care provider who specializes in the treatment of incontinence.

Geriatric

- Assess client's cognitive status, using an instrument such as Folstein's mini-mental state examination.
  Behavioral treatments for incontinence are very effective in the able and willing older adult (McDowell et al, 1992).
- Refer client to a geriatric center that specializes in the elderly and the treatment of incontinence.

Client/Family Teaching

- Teach client normal anatomy, bladder function, and causes of stress incontinence.
- Teach client how to perform Kegel's exercises to increase perineal strength and endurance.
- Work with the client to incorporate Kegel's exercises into normal activities of daily living (e.g., do 10 exercises after each void).
  One of the most difficult parts of behavioral therapy is follow-through. Initiating exercises at a time that is convenient and easy to remember can enhance compliance.
- Instruct the client to do exercises 60 to 80 times daily; tell client that it may take up to 6 weeks for improvement to occur (Urinary Incontinence Guideline Panel, 1992).
- Encourage client to increase fluid intake to between 1500 and 2000 ml/day.
  Concentrated urine can irritate the urinary tract and increase the severity of leakage.
- Encourage client to avoid caffeinated fluids such as coffee, tea, and soda.
  Alcohol serves as a diuretic; caffeine irritates the urinary tract.

Geriatric

- Provide cassette tapes to reinforce appropriate way to do Kegel's exercises; talk client through the pelvic muscle exercise session.
- Encourage the postmenopausal client to have regular gynecological evaluations to assess her need for estrogen therapy.
  A decrease in estrogen causes a multitude of changes in the perineum, which can increase urinary incontinence. Some clients may benefit from estrogen replacement therapy (Urinary Incontinence Guideline Panel, 1992).

REFERENCES

Burns P et al: Treatment of stress incontinence with pelvic floor exercises and biofeedback. *J Am Geriatr Soc* 38:341, 1990.

Dougherty M et al: An instrument to assess the dynamic characteristics of the circumvaginal musculature, *Nurs Res* 35:202, 1986.

Doughty D: *Urinary and fecal incontinence: nursing management,* Philadelphia, 1991, Mosby.

McDowell B et al: An interdisciplinary approach to the assessment and behavioral treatment of urinary incontinence in geriatric outpatients, *J Am Geriatr Soc* 40:370, 1992.

Urinary Incontinence Guideline Panel. *Urinary Incontinence in Adults: Clinical Practice Guideline.* Rockville, Md, March 1992, Agency for Health Care Policy and Research, Public Health Service, US Department of Health and Human Services (AHCPR Publication No. 92-0038).

Wells T et al: Pelvic muscle exercises for stress urinary incontinence in elderly women, *J Am Geriatr Soc* 39:785, 1991.

BIBLIOGRAPHY

Baigis-Smith J et al: Managing urinary incontinence in community-residing elderly persons, *Gerontologist* 29:229, 1989.

Burgio K, Engel B: Biofeedback-assisted behavior training for elderly men and women. *J Am Geriatr Soc* 38:338, 1990.

Brink C et al: A digital test for pelvic muscle strength in older women with urinary incontinence. *Nurs Res* 38:196, 1989.

Total incontinence

Kathie Hesnan

Definition The state in which an individual experiences a continuous and unpredictable loss of urine.

Defining Characteristics

Major: Constant flow of urine occurs at unpredictable times without distention or uninhibited bladder contractions or spasms; urinary incontinence is refractory to other treatments; nocturia occurs more than two times during sleep.

Minor: Lack of perineal or bladder-filling awareness; unawareness of incontinence.

Related Factors (r/t)

Neuropathy prevents transmission of the reflex that indicates bladder fullness; neurological dysfunction triggers micturition at unpredictable times; detrusor reflex independently contracts as a result of surgery, trauma, or disease that affects spinal cord nerves; anatomic incontinence (fistula).

Client Outcomes/Goals

- Perineal area free from irritation or breakdown.
- States that dignity has been maintained.
- Identifies types of containment devices that maintain skin integrity and prevent embarrassing accidents.

Nursing Interventions and Rationales

- Assess client for acute causes of incontinence (e.g., urinary tract infections; abnormal urinalysis results; atrophic changes; constipation or impaction; bladder irritants such as caffeinated or citrus beverages; poor fluid intake; polyuria; retention; medication effects).
  These factors can increase the severity of incontinence or be the underlying cause. (Urinary Incontinence Guideline Panel, 1992; Doughty, 1991).
- Obtain a nursing history that focuses on incontinence (e.g., onset, duration, past treatment, type, medications, past medical history, obstetrical or gynecological history).
- Perform a physical examination, which may include examination of abdomen, pelvis, rectum, or skin integrity.
- Observe patterns of voiding and incontinence.
  These observations help identify total incontinence or determine the presence of another type of incontinence.
- Provide appropriate absorbent product.
  Product selection depends on volume of leakage, absorbency of product, frequency of changing absorbent product, and toileting schedule.
- Rinse perineal area with water after each attempt to void or when changing absorbent product.
  Do not rub or cleanse with soap each time because this will dry the skin and possibly cause irritation.
- If client is male, consider using an external condom catheter connected to a Foley bag; change q24 to 48h; observe for skin breakdown.
- If client is female and not bedridden, consider a female external collection device.
  This device collects the urine with a periurethral cup that drains the urine through tubing to a leg bag or overnight bag.
- If cleansing skin frequently, maintain skin hydration with skin moisturizer.
  Moisturizers reduce the chance of skin breakdown.

- Initiate use of a protective barrier or ointment if client is at risk of a pressure ulcer or if the absorbent product is being changed infrequently.
  Matching the skin-care product with the client's needs and the caregiver's ability to use the product can alleviate expense and frustration and prevent skin complications.
- A Foley catheter should only be used when client has urinary retention and clean intermittent catheterization cannot be done, for short-term monitoring of fluid balance for a terminally ill client for whom padding changes or clothing changes are painful, or for a client with a stage 3 or 4 pressure ulcer *(Urinary Incontinence Guideline Panel, 1992).*
- Decrease fluid intake in the evening.
  Decreasing fluid helps prevent or decrease nighttime incontinence.
- Offer bedpan, male or female urinal, or toileting at intervals that are based on fluid intake.

Geriatric

- If possible, assess and modify drug regimen that may be interfering with continence.
- Use meticulous infection control procedures if an indwelling catheter is used.

Client/Family Teaching

- Teach how to deal with urinary incontinence (e.g., reusable or disposable absorbent products, protective clothing, pattern of fluid intake, toileting regimen).
- Teach measures to prevent urinary tract infections.
- Refer to rehabilitation or gerontology center for help in dealing with incontinence.

REFERENCES

Doughty D: *Urinary and fecal incontinence: nursing management*, Philadelphia, 1991, Mosby.

Urinary Incontinence Guideline Panel. *Urinary Incontinence in Adults: Clinical Practice Guideline.* Rockville, Md, March 1992, Agency for Health Care Policy and Research, Public Health Service, US Department of Health and Human Services (AHCPR Publication No. 92-0038).

BIBLIOGRAPHY

Bierwirth W: Which pad is for you? *Urologic Nurs* 12:75, 1992.

Johnson D et al: An external urine collection device for incontinent women. *Geriatr Soc* 38:1016, 1990.

McCormick K et al: Nursing management of urinary incontinence in geriatric inpatients. *Nurs Clin North Am* 23:231, 1988.

Verdell L, editor: Help for incontinent people (HIP), *Resource guide of continence products and services,* ed 6, Union, SC, 1994, HIP.

Urge incontinence

Kathie Hesnan

Definition The state in which an individual experiences an involuntary passage of urine occurring with or soon after a strong sense of urgency to void.

Defining Characteristics

Urinary urgency or frequency (voiding more often than every 2 hours); uninhibited bladder contraction, which results in a large volume of leakage; nocturia (more than two times per night); voiding in small amounts (less than 100 ml); inability to reach the toilet in time.

Related Factors (r/t)

Decreased bladder capacity (e.g., history of pelvic inflammatory disease, abdominal surgeries, indwelling urinary catheter); irritation of bladder stretch receptors, which is causing spasms (e.g., bladder infection); alcohol; caffeine; increase or decrease in oral intake of fluids; urinary retention.

Client Outcomes/Goals

- Follows mutually agreed on bladder retraining program.
- Voids clear, straw-colored urine without incontinence or urgency every 3 or more hours during the day.
- Decreases or eliminates incontinent episodes.

Nursing Interventions and Rationales

- Assess client for acute causes of incontinence such as urinary tract infections, abnormal urinalysis results, atrophic changes, constipation or impaction, bladder irritants such as caffeinated or citrus beverages, poor fluid intake, polyuria, retention, or medication effects.
  These factors can increase the severity of incontinence or be the underlying cause (Urinary Incontinence Guideline Panel, 1992; Doughty, 1991).
- Perform a nursing history that focuses on incontinence (e.g., onset, duration, past treatment, type, medications, past medical history, obstetrical or gynecological history).
- Perform a physical examination, which may include examination of the abdomen, pelvis, rectum, or skin integrity.
- Review completed bladder record, which may include intervals between voids, times of accidents, events precipitating an incontinent episode, and the amount and type of fluid intake.
  The bladder record provides a tool that individualizes the client's treatment program and records the changes in incontinent episodes.
- Provide convenient access to toilet or bathroom (e.g., bedside commode, fracture bedpan, female or male urinals).
- Instruct or help client to go to the bathroom immediately before going to sleep.
  Voiding before going to sleep may help decrease nocturia.
- Refer client to a health care provider that specializes in incontinence.

Geriatric

- Check for impaction and remove according to the institution's protocol.
- Develop a regular toileting schedule for the client.
- Answer call bell as soon as client requests assistance to toilet.

Client/Family Teaching

- Teach need for fluids and avoidance of caffeine and alcohol.
- Teach bladder retraining. Have client void at predetermined times, then increase the length of time between voiding until client successfully reaches the designated time

interval. To help client control the urge, urge inhibition techniques must be taught (e.g., sphincter contraction [Kegel's exercises], relaxation breathing, counting backwards from 100 by 7s). Bladder retraining is a lot of work for the client, so provide positive reinforcement.
Bladder training reduces the number of incontinent episodes and the quantity of lost fluids (Fantl et al, 1991).

- Work with the client to incorporate Kegel's exercises into normal activities of daily living (e.g., do 10 exercises after each void).
  One of the most difficult parts of behavioral therapy is follow-through; initiating exercises at a time that is convenient and easy to remember can help with compliance.
- Instruct the client to do 60 to 80 exercises each day, and inform client that it may take up to 6 weeks for improvement (*Urinary Incontinence Guideline Panel,* 1992).
- Teach measures needed to prevent urinary tract infection.
- Teach client how to choose an absorbent product.
  Product selection depends on volume of leakage, absorbency of product, frequency of changing absorbent product, and toileting schedule.
- Rinse perineal area with water after each attempt to void or when changing an absorbent product.
  Do not rub or cleanse area with soap each time because this will dry the skin and may cause irritation.

REFERENCES

Doughty D: *Urinary and fecal incontinence: nursing management,* Philadelphia, 1991, Mosby.

Fantl JA et al: Efficacy of bladder training in older women with urinary incontinence, *JAMA* 265:609, 1991.

Urinary Incontinence Guideline Panel. *Urinary Incontinence in Adults: Clinical Practice Guideline.* Rockville, Md, March 1992, Agency for Health Care Policy and Research, Public Health Service, US Department of Health and Human Services (AHCPR Publication No 92-0038).

BIBLIOGRAPHY

Baigis-Smith J et al: Managing urinary incontinence in community-residing elderly persons, *Gerontologist* 29:229, 1989.

Burgio K, Engel B: Biofeedback-assisted behavioral training for elderly men and women, *J Am Geriatr Soc* 38:338, 1990.

McCormick K, Palmer M: Urinary incontinence in older adults, *Annu Rev Nurs Res* 10:25-53, 1994.

Disorganized infant behavior

Mary DeWys

Definition Alteration in the integration and modulation of the physiological and behavioral systems of functioning (e.g., autonomic, motor, state, organizational, self-regulatory, and attentional-interactional systems).

Defining Characteristics

Major *Physiological cues:* decreased oxygen saturation; tachycardia; bradycardia; irregular respirations (e.g., pauses, apnea, tachypnea, and yawning).

Color fluctuations: pale; mottled; red; dusky; cyanotic skin.

Visceral Cues: gagging; vomiting; feeding intolerances or difficulties; gastrointestinal reflux; bowel straining; bowel movement with stress.

Neurological/Motor Cues: tremors; startles; twitches; hyperextension of arms and legs; arching; frantic activity; finger or toe extensions; facial grimaces; hypertonicity; hypotonicity.

State Control: difficulty maintaining sleep or awake state; sleep disturbances; rapid state changes; deficient self-regulatory behaviors in one or all systems; deficient ability to orient or attend to visual or auditory stimuli; deficient ability to engage in social interactions; inability to regulate without facilitation by another.

Minor Hiccoughing; sneezing; coughing.

Related Factors (r/t)

Internal Factors

Pain; hunger; fatigue; respiratory, visceral, or neurological compromise; altered sensory integration; lack of or depletion of energy; pathological condition resulting from prematurity; prenatal exposure to alcohol; cocaine or multidrug use.

External Factors

Overstimulating environment (e.g., bright lights, visual clutter, noise levels above 60 decibels), handling when physiologically compromised; care noncontingent to infant state or behavior cues; invasive or painful procedures.

Client Outcomes/Goals

Infant

- Displays organization and integration of the neurobehavioral subsystems of functioning.
- Displays minimal maladaptive or abnormal compensatory behavioral patterns.

Parent/Significant Other

- Recognizes that behavior is an infant's unique style of communication.
- Recognizes behavior that communicates approach, self-regulation, avoidance, and stress, and demonstrates ways to respond in a contingent way.
- Recognizes how sensory stimulation affects infant behavior, and demonstrate ways to modify stimulation.

Nursing Interventions and Rationales

- Identify the infant's current level of organization in each subsystem (e.g., autonomic, motoric, state organizational, attentional-interactive, and self-regulatory systems) and at the point of threshold at which disorganization occurs.
  All behavior is meaningful, interactional, and transactional within the context of the environment. Organization and homeostasis are synonymous and reflect smooth system functioning, whereas disorganization disrupts the smooth balance of each system, causing instability as the regulatory capacity is exceeded. Cues of disorganization can be seen across subsystems of functioning. The goal of caregiving interventions is to stabilize each system (Als, 1986; Becker et al, 1993; D'Apolito, 1991).

- Correlate the level of organization and disorganization to internal and external factors.
It is essential to correlate disorganized behavior with internal factors (e.g., pain, hunger, respiratory insufficiency, infection) and external factors (e.g., lights, noise, position, handling, temperature) to modify caregiving interventions and sensory input to alleviate stress (Als, 1986; Franck, 1987; Lawhon, 1989).
- Identify behaviors used by the infant to self-regulate such as hands to face or mouth, foot or leg bracing, or grasping; assess their effectiveness, and facilitate and support them.
Helps the infant use self-regulatory behaviors in an adaptive way and reduces the incidence of developing maladaptive behavior responses to stress (Als, 1986, 1989).
- Structure and organize the environment, and modify care to minimize stress and maximize organization.
Because premature and sick infants have a lower threshold for sensory input, it is important to grade sensory stimuli and match behavioral cues and developmental readiness (Oehler, 1993; Weibley, 1989; Zwick, 1993).
- Facilitate motor organization, control, and normal sensory motor growth and experience to enhance development.
Premature infants lack the additional weeks in utero for developing physiological flexion and consequently manifest hypotonia from 24 to 30 weeks gestation. The combination of immobilization and laying on flat surfaces can interfere with developing normal posture, tone, and movement as the infant attempts to pull up against gravity, which increases the risk for developing positional disorders (e.g., neck hyperextension, shoulder elevation, shoulder retraction, decreased midline orientation, wide hip abduction, frog-leg position of lower extremities) (Fay, 1988; Semmler, 1989).
- Minimize stress, build trust, and decrease energy expenditure during care.
Trust is developed by sensitive and predictable caregiving that matches the infant's behavioral cues. Such individualized care involves slowly introducing care and signaling completion of care. (Cole, 1984; Gorski, 1983; Kenner, Hetteberg, 1994).
- Identify ways to help infant develop state organization (e.g., maintain a state for a period of time and achieve ease of transition between states).
Critical to state organization is appropriate timing, intensity, and duration of stimuli and social interactions. An infant's ability to change state (e.g., fall asleep, fuss) in response to inappropriate stimuli is the infant's first line of defense (Blackburn, Barnard, 1985; White-Traut, Pate, 1987).
- Identify infant's ability to attend to stimuli and to engage in social interactions.
An infant's ability to attend to sensory stimuli (e.g., look, listen, interact) depends on state, ability to maintain organization, and available energy to process cognitive, social, and emotional information (Korner, 1990; Newman, 1981). Infants exposed to cocaine have a lower sensory threshold and often display increased tone and jittery movements and have greater difficulty maintaining state organization (DeWys, McComish, 1992).
- Promote and support adaptive parent-infant communication patterns by reading infant cues, allowing the infant to take the lead during interactions, and modifying the parent's and infant's responses contingent to behavior cues.
A key factor to the infant's future development and communication skills is mutual coregulation of interactions in which each partner modifies and adapts his or her behavior in response to the other (Field et al, 1978; Hedlund, 1986; Rauh et al, 1987).

- Provide sensory and motor experiences contingent to behavioral cues, state, and developmental maturation, and readiness (e.g., tactile, kinesthetic, vestibular, proprioceptive, auditory, visual).
  Excessive sensory input can overload an immature nervous system, making it difficult for the infant to integrate multiple stimuli (Glass, 1994; Vergara, 1992).

Client/Family Teaching

- Teach parent to recognize the infant's behavior in terms of organization and disorganization in the subsystems of functioning (D'Apolito, 1991).
- Help parent recognize the infant's behaviors that communicate avoidance, stress, approach, and stability (Cole, 1984; Litovsky, 1990).
- Help parent recognize and support the infant's self-regulatory coping behaviors.
- Help parent recognize environmental stimuli that overstimulates the infant and ways to modify environmental factors (Blackburn, Barnard, 1985; Glass, 1994).
- Demonstrate and help parent use developmentally correct positioning and handling techniques (Fay, 1988).
- Help parent recognize and support the infant's alertness and ways to soothe the infant when distressed (White-Traut, 1987).
- Help parent recognize how interactional style affects the infant's responses and how to modify behavior (Field, 1978; Rauh, 1987).
- Support parent's strengths, competencies, level of confidence, and involvement (Minde, 1978).

REFERENCES

Als H: A synactive model of neonatal behavioral organization: framework for the assessment and support of neurobehavioral development of premature infants and their parents in the environment of the NICU, *Phys Occup Ther Pediatr* 6:3-53, 1986.

Als H: Self regulation and motor development in preterm infants. In Lockman J, Hazen N, editors: *Perspectives on early development: action in social context,* New York, 1989, Plenum Press.

Becker P, Grunwald P, Moorman T, Sturhr S: Effects of developmental care on behavioral organization in very low birth-weight infants, *Nurs Res* 42:214-220, 1993.

Blackburn S, Barnard G: Analysis of caregiving events relating to preterm infants in the special care units. In Gottfried A, Gaiter J, editors: Infant stress under intensive care, Baltimore, 1985, University Park Press.

Cole J: Infant stimulation re-examined: an environmental and behavioral-based approach, *Neonatal Network* 3:24-31, 1984.

D'Apolito K: What is an organized infant? *Neonatal Network* 10:23-29, 1991.

DeWys M, McComish J: Infant states and cues: facilitating effective parent-infant interaction. In *Caring for infants: a resource manual for caring for infant trainers* (Unit 11, pp. 1-17, Unit 12, pp. 1-17), Board of Trustees, Michigan State University, 1992, Lansing, Mich.

Fay M: The positive effects of positioning, *Neonatal Network* 6:23-28, 1988.

Field T et al: The mother's assessment of the behavior of her infant, *Infant Behavior and Development* 1:156-167, 1978.

Franck L: A national survey of the assessment and treatment of pain and agitation in the neonatal intensive care unit *JOGNN,* 387-392, 1987.

Glass P: The venerable neonate and the neonatal intensive care environment. In Avery G, Fletcher M, McDonald, editors: Neonatology: pathophysiology and management of newborn, ed 4, Philadelphia, 1994, JB Lippincott.

Gorski P: Premature infant behavioral and physiological responses to caregiving interventions in the intensive care nursery. In Call J, Galenson E, Tyson R, editors: *Frontiers of infant psychiatry,* New York, 1983, Basic Books.

Hedlund R: Fostering positive social interactions between parents and infants, *Teaching Exceptional Children* pp. 43-48, 1986.

Kenner C, Hetteberg C: Nursing challenges in the care of very low birth weight infants (<1,000 grams), *AACN Clin Issues* 5:231-241, 1994.

Korner A: Infant stimulation: issues of theory and research, *Clin Perinatol,* 17:173-185, 1990.

Lawhon G: Management of stress in premature infants. In Angelini, Whelan-Knapp, Gribbs, editors. *Perinatal/neonatal nursing: a clinical handbook,* Boston, 1989, Blackwell Scientific.

Litovsky R: Stimulus differentiation by pre-term infants can guide caregivers, *Pre Perinat Psych* 5:41-67, 1990.

Minde K et al: Mother-child relationships in the premature nursery: an observation study. *Pediatr* 61:373-379, 1978.

Newman L: Social and sensory environment of low birth weight infants in a special care nursery: an anthropological investigation, *J Nerv Ment Dis* 169:448-455, 1981.

Oehler T: Developmental care of low birth weight infants, *Nurs Clin North Am J* 28:289-301, 1993.

Rauh V et al: The mother-infant transactional program: an intervention for all mothers of low birth weight infants. In *Infant stimulation: for whom, what kind, when and how much?* Johnson & Johnson Baby Care Products, Pediatric Round Table Series 13:144-156, 1987.

Semmler C: Positioning and position: Induced deformities. In Semmler C, editor: *A guide to care and management of very low birth weight infants: a team approach,* Tucson, 1989, Therapy Skill Builders, A division of Communication Skill Builders.

Vergara E: The importance of identifying and providing for the sensory needs of preterm infants, *Sensory Integration Special Interest Section Newsletter,* pp. 2-6, September 1992.

Weibley T: Inside the incubator, *MCN* 14:96-100, 1989.

White-Traut R, Pate C: Modulating infant state in pre-mature infants, *J Pediatr Nurs* 2:96-101, 1987.

Zwick M: Decreasing environmental noise in the NICU through staff education, *Neonatal Intensive Care* 6(2):16-19, 1993.

Potential for enhanced organized infant behavior

Mary DeWys

Definition A pattern of modulation of an infant's physiological and behavioral systems of functioning (e.g., autonomic, motor, state, organizational, self-regulatory, attentional-interactional systems) that is satisfactory but can be improved and result in higher levels of integration in response to environmental stimuli.

Defining Characteristics

Stable physiological measures; ability to maintain clear, well-defined states and smooth transition between states; use of some self-regulatory behaviors; progressive development toward smooth, well-coordinated movement; minimal startles, twitches, or tremors; attempts to engage in social interactions.

Related Factors (r/t)

Internal Pain; hunger; fatigue; respiratory, visceral, or neurological compromise; altered sensory integration; lack of or depletion of energy; pathological condition resulting from prematurity or prenatal exposure to alcohol.

External Overstimulating environment (e.g., bright lights, visual clutter, noise levels above 60 decibels); handling when physiologically compromised; care noncontingent to infant state or behavior cues; invasive or painful procedures.

Client Outcomes/Goals

Infant

- Displays organization and integration of the neurobehavioral subsystems of functioning.
- Displays minimal maladaptive or abnormal compensatory behavioral patterns.

Parent/Significant Other

- Recognizes that behavior is an infant's unique style of communication.
- Recognizes behavior that communicates approach, self-regulation, avoidance, and stress and demonstrates ways to respond in a contingent way.
- Recognizes how sensory stimulation affects infant behavior, and demonstrates ways to modify stimulation.

Nursing Interventions and Rationales

- Identify the infant's current level of organization in each subsystem (e.g., autonomic, motoric, state organizational, attentional-interactive, and self-regulatory systems) and at the point of threshold at which disorganization occurs.
  All behavior is meaningful, interactional, and transactional within the context of the environment. Organization and homeostasis are synonymous and reflect smooth system functioning, whereas disorganization disrupts the smooth balance of each system, causing instability as the regulatory capacity is exceeded. Cues of disorganization can be seen across subsystems of functioning. The goal of caregiving interventions is to stabilize each system (Als, 1986; Becker et al, 1993; D'Apolito, 1991).
- Correlate the level of organization and disorganization to internal and external factors.
  It is essential to correlate disorganized behavior with internal factors (e.g., pain, hunger, respiratory insufficiency, infection) and external factors (e.g., lights, noise, position, handling, temperature) in order to modify caregiving interventions and sensory input to alleviate stress (Als, 1986; Franck, 1987; Lawhon, 1989).
- Identify behaviors used by the infant to self-regulate such as hands to face or mouth, foot or leg bracing, or grasping; assess their effectiveness, and facilitate and support them.
  Help the infant use self-regulatory behaviors in an adaptive way and reduce the incidence of developing maladaptive behavior responses to stress (Als, 1986, 1989).

- Structure and organize the environment, and modify care to minimize stress and maximize organization.
  Because premature and sick infants have a lower threshold for sensory input, it is important to grade sensory stimuli and match behavioral cues and developmental readiness (Oehler, 1993; Weibley, 1989; Zwick, 1993).
- To enhance development support infant's current level of motor organization, control, normal sensory motor growth, and experiences.
  Providing an environment that contains positive sensory motor feedback contingent to the infant's developmental level optimizes neuromotor functioning (Fay, 1988; Updike, 1986).
- Minimize stress, build trust, and decrease energy expenditure during care.
  Trust is developed by sensitive and predictable caregiving that matches the infant's behavioral cues. Such individualized care involves slowly introducing care and signaling completion of care (Cole, 1984; Kenner, Hetteberg, 1994; Yeh et al, 1984).
- Identify ways to help infant maintain state organization (e.g., maintain a state for a period of time and achieve ease of transition between states).
  Critical to state organization is appropriate timing, intensity, and duration of stimuli and social interactions. An infant's ability to change state (e.g., fall asleep, fuss) in response to inappropriate stimuli is the infant's first line of defense (Blackburn, Barnard, 1985; White-Traut, Pate, 1987).
- Support infant's ability to attend to stimuli and to engage in social interactions.
  An infant's ability to attend to sensory stimuli (e.g., look, listen, interact) depends on state, ability to maintain organization, and available energy to process cognitive, social, and emotional information (Korner, 1990; Newman, 1981).
- Promote and support adaptive parent-infant communication patterns by reading infant cues, allowing the infant to take the lead during interactions, and modifying the parent's and infant's responses contingent to behavior cues.
  A key factor to the infant's future development and communication skills is mutual coregulation of interactions in which each partner modifies and adapts his or her behavior in response to the other (Field et al, 1987; Hedlund, 1986; Rauh et al, 1987).
- Provide sensory and motor experiences contingent to behavioral cues, state and developmental maturation, and readiness (e.g., tactile, kinesthetic, vestibular, proprioceptive, auditory, visual).
  Excessive sensory input can overload an immature nervous system, making it difficult for the infant to integrate multiple stimuli. (Glass, 1994; Vergara, 1992).

Client/Family Teaching

Refer to client/family teaching for **Disorganized infant behavior**.

REFERENCES

Als H: A synactive model of neonatal behavioral organization: framework for the assessment and support of neurobehavioral development of premature infants and their parents in the environment of the NICU, *Phys Occup Ther Pediatr* 6:3-53, 1986.

Als H: Self regulation and motor development in preterm infants. In Lockman J, Hazen N, editors: *Perspectives on early development: action in social context,* New York, 1989, Plenum Press.

Becker P et al: Effects of developmental care on behavioral organization in very low birth-weight infants, *Nurs Res* 42:214-220, 1993.

Blackburn S, Barnard G: Analysis of caregiving events relating to preterm infants in the special care units. In Gottfried A, Gaiter J, editors: *Infant stress under intensive care,* Baltimore, 1985, University Park Press.

Cole J: Infant stimulation re-examined: An environmental and behavioral-based approach, *Neonatal Network* 3:24-31, 1984.

D'Apolito K: What is an organized infant? *Neonatal Network* 10:23-29, 1991.
Fay M: The positive effects of positioning, *Neonatal Network* 6:23-28, 1988.
Field T et al: The mother's assessment of the behavior of her infant, *Infant Beh Dev* 1:156-167, 1978.
Franck L: A national survey of the assessment and treatment of pain and agitation in the neonatal intensive care unit, *JOGNN* 387-392, 1987.
Glass P: The venerable neonate and the neonatal intensive care environment. In Avery G, Fletcher M, McDonald, editors: *Neonatology: pathophysiology and management of newborn,* ed 4, Philadelphia, 1994, JB Lippincott.
Hedlund R: Fostering positive social interactions between parents and infants, *Teaching Exceptional Children* 43-48, 1986.
Kenner C, Hetteberg C: Nursing challenges in the care of very low birth weight infants (<1,000 grams), *AACN Clin Issues* 5:231-241, 1994.
Korner A: Infant stimulation: issues of theory and research. *Clin Perinatol* 17:173-185, 1990.
Lawhon G: Management of stress in premature infants. In Angeli, Whelan-Knapp, Gibbs, editors: Perinatal/neonatal nursing: a clinical handbook, Boston, 1989, Blackwell Scientific.
Newman L: Social and sensory environment of low birth weight infants in a special care nursery: an anthropological investigation, *J Nerv Ment Dis* 169:448-455, 1981.
Oehler T: Developmental care of low birth weight infants, *Nurs Clin North Am J* 28:289-301, 1993.
Rauh V et al: The mother-infant transactional program: an intervention for all mothers of low birth weight infants. In *Infant stimulation: for whom, what kind, when and how much?* Johnson & Johnson Baby Care Products, Pediatric Round Table Series 13:144-156, 1987.
Updike C et al: Positional support for premature infants, *Am J Occup Ther* 40:712-715, 1986.
Vergara E: The importance of identifying and providing for the sensory needs of preterm infants, *Sensory Integration Special Interest Section Newsletter* 2-6, 1992.
Weibley T: Inside the incubator, *MCN* 14:96-100, 1989.
White-Traut R, Pate C: Modulating infant state in pre-mature infants, *J Pediat Nurs* 2:96-101, 1987.
Yeh T et al: Increased O_2 consumption and energy loss in premature infants following medical care procedures, *Biol Neonate* 46:157-162, 1984.
Zwick M: Decreasing environmental noise in the NICU through staff education, *Neonatal Intensive Care* 6(2):16-19, 1993.

Risk for disorganized infant behavior

Mary DeWys

Definition Risk for alteration in the integration and modulation of the physiological and behavioral systems of functioning (e.g., autonomic, motor, state, organizational, self-regulatory, attentional-interactional systems).

Defining Characteristics

Presence of risk factors such as

Internal: Pain; hunger; fatigue; respiratory, visceral, or neurological compromise; altered sensory integration; lack of or depletion of energy; pathological condition as a result of prematurity; prenatal exposure to alcohol, cocaine, or multidrug use.

External: Overstimulating environment (bright lights, visual clutter, noise levels above 60 decibels); handling when physiologically compromised; care noncontingent to infant state or behavior cues; invasive or painful procedures.

Related Factors (r/t)

Refer to risk factors.

Client Outcomes/Goals, Nursing Interventions and Rationales, Client/Family Teaching

Refer to nursing diagnosis for **Disorganized infant behavior.**

Ineffective infant feeding pattern

Vicki McClurg and Virginia Wall

Definition The state in which an infant demonstrates an impaired ability to suck or coordinate the suck-swallow response.

Defining Characteristics

Inability to initiate or sustain an effective suck; inability to coordinate sucking, swallowing, and breathing.

Related Factors (r/t)

Prematurity; neurological impairment or delay; oral hypersensitivity; prolonged NPO.

Client Outcomes/Goals

- Infant receives adequate nourishment without compromising autonomic stability.
- Infant progresses to a normal feeding pattern.
- Family learns successful techniques for feeding the infant.

Nursing Interventions and Rationales

- Assess infant's oral reflexes (e.g., root, gag, suck, and swallow).
  These reflexes are necessary for successful oral feedings. Feeding by nipple or breast should be encouraged because it encourages growth and maturity of the gastrointestinal tract and provides comfort for hunger and oral gratification (Dickason, Silverman, Schult, 1994; Danner, 1992b).
- Determine infant's ability to coordinate suck, swallow, and breathing reflexes.
  At approximately 37 weeks of gestation infants become better able to coordinate breathing with sucking and swallowing (Dickason, Silverman, Schult, 1994; Pickler, Higgins, Crummette, 1993).
- Collaborate with other health care providers (e.g., physician, neonatal nutritionist, physical therapist, and lactation specialist) to develop a feeding plan.
  Various health care providers contribute expertise to the care of an infant with special needs.
- Implement gavage feedings (or another alternative feeding method) before infant is ready for by-mouth feedings.
  Even after a preterm infant develops the ability to suck and swallow, too much energy may be required to do so, and gavage feedings may be necessary. "Serious illness can impair a neonate's ability to suck, and calorie and nutrient needs are increased by the stress of illness" (Mott, James, Sperhac, 1990; Kinneer, Beachy, 1994).
- Provide a pacifier for sucking during gavage feedings (or during other alternative feeding methods).
  Sucking helps calm infants, which raises the oxygen level, may aid digestion, may increase average daily weight gain, and may prepare infants for earlier nipple feedings and discharge (Mott, James, Sperhac, 1990; Dickason, Silverman, Schult, 1994).
- Evaluate the feeding environment and minimize sensory stimuli.
  Noxious stimuli must be kept to a minimum to decrease physiological stress on at-risk infants. The neonatal intensive care unit environment can interfere with normal infant development and breast-feeding success and must therefore be modified to enhance attachment and normal development (Meier et al, 1993; Dickason, Silverman, Schult, 1994).
- Position preterm infant in a flexed feeding posture that is similar for a full-term infant.
  The "total sucking pattern" of the full-term newborn combines strong physiological flexion and high rib cage position to provide support for the tongue and jaw, which is essential for effective nippling (Shaker, 1990).

- Attempt to nipple-feed baby only when infant is in a quiet-alert state.
  The infant must be able to find and grasp the nipple effectively and then be ready and eager to suck. The quiet-awake state was found to be optimal for feeding preterm infants (Kinneer, Beachy, 1994).
- Allow appropriate time for nipple feeding to ensure infant's safety without exceeding calorie expenditure.
  Nipple feeding can lead to nutritional deficits because of the increased metabolic demands placed on the at-risk infant as a result of thermoregulation, work of respiration and feeding, and decreased ability to absorb nutrients (Dickason, Silverman, Schult, 1994).
- Monitor infant's physiological condition during feeding.
  Cardiorespiratory and color stability are necessary for nipple feedings (Kinneer, Beachy, 1994).
- Determine infant's active feeding behaviors without prodding.
  Infants must be alert and eager to eat (e.g., rooting, latching on, and sucking readily) to ensure a successful feeding. Prodding compromises the infant's safety, interrupts learning, and may give an inaccurate picture of the infant's ability to take in adequate nutrients in preparation for discharge (Shaker, 1990).
- Assess infant's ability to take in enough calories to sustain temperature and growth.
  Calories are needed to sustain basal metabolic rate, activity, digestive and metabolic processes, and growth (Danner, 1992a).
- Encourage family to participate in the feeding process.
  Nurses can promote the psychosocial development of the at-risk infant and family by encouraging the caretaking ability of the parents (Cusson, Lee, 1994).
- Refer to a neonatal nutritionist, physical or occupational therapist, or lactation specialist as needed.
  Collaborative practice with others specially trained to meet the needs of this vulnerable population helps ensure feeding and parenting success (Meier et al, 1993).

Client/Family Teaching

- Provide anticipatory guidance for infant's expected feeding course.
  Knowing what to anticipate helps the family feel involved and enhances attachment.
- Teach parents infant feeding methods.
  Parents should be involved in the feeding process as soon as possible to provide positive feedback about their ability to nurture a child and enhance attachment (Dickason, Silverman, Schult, 1994).
- Teach parents how to recognize infant cues.
  The parents' understanding of the infant's cues may increase their involvement in infant care by improving their perception of the infant's abilities (Cusson, Lee, 1994).
- Provide anticipatory guidance for the infant's discharge.
  Parents need assistance in assuming responsibility for infant care as the day of discharge approaches (Cusson, Lee, 1994).

REFERENCES

Cusson RM, Lee AL: Parental interventions and the development of the preterm infant, *JOGNN* 23:60-68, 1994.

Danner SC: Breastfeeding the infant with a cleft defect, *NAACOG's Clin Issues Perinatal Women Health Nurs* 3:634-639, 1992.

Danner SC: Breastfeeding the neurologically impaired infant, *NAACOG's Clin Issues Perinatal Women Health Nurs* 3:640-646, 1992.

Dickason EJ, Silverman BL, Schult MO: *Maternal-infant nursing care,* ed 2, St Louis, 1994, Mosby.

Kinneer MD, Beachy P: Nipple feeding premature infants in the neonatal intensive-care unit: factors and decisions, *JOGNN* 23:105-112, 1994.

Meier PP et al: Breastfeeding support services in the neonatal intensive-care unit, *JOGNN* 22:338-347, 1993.

Mott SR, James SR, Spechac AM: *Nursing care of children and families,* ed 2, Redwood City, Calif, 1990, Addison-Wesley.

Pickler RH, Higgins KE, Crummette BD: The effect of nonnutritive sucking on bottle-feeding stress in preterm infants, *JOGNN* 22:230-234, 1993.

Shaker CS: Nipple feeding premature infants: a different perspective, *Neonatal Network* 8:9-17, 1990.

BIBLIOGRAPHY

Pridham KF et al: Nipple feeding for preterm infants with bronchopulmonary dysplasia, *JOGNN* 22:147-155, 1993.

Risk for infection

Gail Ladwig

Definition The state in which an individual is at an increased risk of invasion by pathogenic organisms.

Defining Characteristics

Presence of risk factors such as inadequate primary defenses (e.g., broken skin, traumatized tissue, decrease in ciliary action, stasis of body fluids, change in pH secretions, altered peristalsis); inadequate secondary defenses (e.g., decreased hemoglobin, leukopenia, suppressed inflammatory response); immunosuppression; inadequate acquired immunity; tissue destruction and increased environmental exposure; chronic disease; malnutrition; invasive procedures; pharmaceutical agents; trauma; rupture of amniotic membranes; insufficient knowledge regarding avoidance of exposure to pathogens.

Related Factors (r/t)

Refer to risk factors.

Client Outcomes/Goals

- Free from symptoms of infection.
- States symptoms of infection to observe for.
- Demonstrates appropriate care of infection-prone site.
- White blood cell count and differential are within normal limits.
- Demonstrates appropriate hygienic measures such as handwashing, oral care, and perineal care.

Nursing Interventions and Rationales

- Observe for signs of infection such as redness, warmth, discharge, and increased body temperature.
  With the onset of infection the immune system is activated, and signs of infection appear.
- With the neutropenic client assess temperature every 4 hours; report a single temperature >38.5°C or three temperatures >38°C in 24 hours.
  The neutropenic client does not produce an adequate inflammatory response; thus fever is usually the first and often the only sign of infection (Wujcik, 1993).
- Note laboratory values (e.g., white blood cell count and differential, serum protein, serum albumin, cultures).
  Laboratory values are correlated with client's history and physical examination to achieve a global view of the client's immune function and nutritional status and to develop an appropriate plan of care for this diagnosis (Lehmann, 1991).
- Encourage intake of a balanced diet, especially proteins, to feed the immune system.
  Immune function is affected by protein (especially arginine intake); the balance between omega-6 and omega-3 fatty acid intake; and adequate amounts of vitamins A, C, and E and the minerals zinc and iron. A deficiency of these nutrients puts the client at an increased risk of infection (Lehmann, 1991).
- Encourage adequate rest to bolster the immune system.
  Chronic disease and physical and emotional stress increase the client's need for rest (Potter, Perry, 1993).
- Wash hands carefully before and after giving care to client and anytime hands become soiled, even if gloves are worn.
  Handwashing is the most important activity in preventing and controlling the spread of infection (McPherson, 1993).

- Follow universal precautions and wear gloves during any contact with body fluids; use goggles and gloves when appropriate.
  Wearing gloves does not obviate the need for scrupulous handwashing; the purpose of wearing gloves is either to protect the hands from becoming contaminated with dirt and microorganisms or to prevent the transfer of organisms that are already present on the hands (Smock, Shiel, 1994).
- Use careful and sterile techniques when using invasive monitoring.
- Use careful sterile techniques wherever there is a loss of skin integrity.
  These important measures prevent infection in at-risk patients (Wujcik, 1993).
- Ensure client's appropriate hygienic care with handwashing, bathing, hair care, nail care, and perineal care, performed by either nurse or client.
  Hygienic care is an important measure to prevent infection in at-risk patients (Wujcik, 1993).

Geriatric

- Recognize that geriatric clients may be seriously infected but have less obvious symptoms.
  Aging and chronic disease may cause depression of the immune system.
- Foot care beyond simple toenail cutting should be performed by a podiatrist.
- Observe client for a low-grade temperature or new onset of confusion.
  The elderly can have infections with low-grade fevers; be suspicious of any temperature rise or sudden confusion—these symptoms may be the only signs of infection.
- Protect the older person from people with obvious infections such as colds and flu.
- Recommend that the geriatric client receive an annual influenza immunization and pneumococcal vaccine.
  These vaccines provide protection against respiratory infection, which is a common cause of infection in the elderly and can result in debilitation or death.
- Recognize that chronically ill geriatric clients have an increased susceptibility to infection; practice meticulous care of all invasive sites.

Client/Family Teaching

- Teach client and family the symptoms of infection that should be promptly reported to a primary medical caregiver (e.g., redness, warmth, swelling, tenderness or pain, new onset of drainage or change in drainage from wound, increased body temperature).
- Assess if client and family know how to read a thermometer; provide instructions if necessary.
- Instruct client and family of the need for good nutrition (especially protein) and proper rest to bolster immune function.
- Teach client and family how to care for site to prevent infection.
- If client has AIDS, discuss the continued need to practice safe sex, avoid unsterile needle use, and maintain a healthy life-style to prevent infection.
- Refer client and family to social services and community resources to obtain support in maintaining a life-style that increases immune function (e.g., adequate nutrition, rest, freedom from excessive stress).

REFERENCES

Lehmann S: Immune function and nutrition: the clinical role of the intravenous nurse, *J Intraven Nurs* 14:406-420, 1991.

McPherson M: Handwashing: why, when and how, *Asepsis' The Infection Prevention Forum* 15:18-21, 1993.

Potter P, Perry A: *Fundamentals of nursing: concepts, process and practice,* St Louis, 1993, Mosby.

Smock M, Shiel M: The role of surgeon and procedure gloves in infection control: A closer look at disposable gloves, *Prof Nurse* 9:324, 326-329, 1994.

Wujcik D: Infection control in oncology patients, *Nurs Clin North Am* 28:639-649, 1993.

Risk for injury

Betty Ackley

Definition The state in which an individual is at risk of injury as a result of the interaction of environmental conditions and the individual's adaptive and defensive resources.
NOTE: There is overlap of this nursing diagnosis and other diagnoses such as **Risk for trauma, Risk for poisoning, Risk for suffocation, Risk for aspiration,** and, if the client is at risk of bleeding, **Altered protection**. Refer to these diagnoses if appropriate.

Defining Characteristics

Presence of risk factors such as evidence of environmental hazards; lack of knowledge regarding environmental hazards; lack of knowledge regarding safety precautions; history of accidents; impaired mobility; sensory deficit; cerebral dysfunction (adapted from Carpenito).

Related Factors (r/t)

Refer to defining characteristics.

Client Outcomes/Goals

- Client is free of injuries.
- Client and family explain ways to prevent injury.

Nursing Interventions and Rationales

- Determine risk of falling by using an evaluation tool.
  An evaluation tool such as the one developed by Spellbring et al can help identify high-risk clients (Kilpack et al, 1991).
- Identify clients likely to fall by placing a "Fall Precautions" sign in the room and by keying the kardex and chart.
  These steps alert the nursing staff of the increased risk of falls (Cohen, Guin, 1991).
- Evaluate client's medications to determine if they increase the risk of falling; consult with physician regarding client's need for medication if appropriate.
- Thoroughly orient client to environment; place call light within reach; show how to call for assistance; answer call light promptly.
- Keep siderails up and maintain bed in low position; ensure that wheels are locked on bed and commode; keep dim light in room at night.
  These safety measures are used as part of a fall-prevention program (Kilpack et al, 1991).
- Assist client with voiding at least every 4 hours; take client to bathroom before bedtime and before administering sedatives.
  Studies have indicated that falls are often linked to the need to eliminate in a hurry (Cohen, Guin, 1991).
- Avoid use of restraints; obtain a physician's order if restraints are necessary.
  Restrained elders often experience an increased number of falls, possibly as a result of muscle deconditioning or loss of coordination (Tinetti, Liu, Ginter, 1992).
- If client is extremely agitated, consider using a special safety bed that surrounds client or, if client has a traumatic brain injury, the Emory cubicle bed.
  Special beds can be an effective alternative to restraints and can help keep the client safe during periods of agitation (Williams, Morton, Patrick, 1990).
- If needed, provide a reality orientation when interacting with client; have family bring in familiar items and clocks and watches from home to maintain orientation.
  Reality orientation can help prevent or decrease the confusion that increases risk of falling.

- Ask family to stay with client to prevent client from accidentally falling or pulling out tubes.
- Remove all possible hazards in the environment such as razors, medications, and matches.
- If client is unsteady on feet, use a walking belt; use two nursing staff members when ambulating client.
- Place an injury-prone client in a room that is near the nurses' station.
  Such placement allows more frequent observation of the client.

Geriatric

- Encourage client to wear glasses and hearing aids and to use walking aids when ambulating.
- Consider use of a "Merri-walker"—an adult walker that surrounds the body if client is mobile but unsafe because of "wobbling."
- Ensure safety in home environment if client has dementia (e.g., ensure that telephone cords are not in walkways, cover slippery tile floors, avoid having stacks of newspapers create obstructions, ensure that chairs have arms for support, cut down on window glare, install handrails in bathrooms and stairways).
  Clients with dementia often do not know where their body is in space, and common obstacles can be particularly hazardous for them in the home (Booth, 1994).
- If client experiences dizziness when getting up due to orthostatic hypotension, teach methods to decrease dizziness such as rising slowly, remaining seated several minutes before arising, flexing feet upward several times while sitting, sitting down immediately if feeling dizzy, and trying to have someone present when rising.
  The elderly cannot compensate for hypotensive stimuli as efficiently as younger people (Carpenito, 1993).

Client/Family Teaching

- Teach how to safely ambulate at home, including using safety measures such as handrails in bathroom.
- Teach caregiver to identify significant places in environment that must be easily located by covering them with bright colors such as yellow or red (e.g., stair edges, stove controls, light switches).

REFERENCES

Booth DE: Many falls among Alzheimer's patients can be avoided, *Advance* 3: pp. 3-4, Winter/Spring 1994.

Carpenito LJ: *Nursing diagnosis: application to clinical practice,* Philadelphia, 1993, JB Lippincott.

Cohen L, Guin P: Implementation of a fall prevention program, *J Neurosci Nurs* 23:315-319, 1991.

Kilpack V et al: Using research-based interventions to decrease patient falls, *Appl Nurs Res* 4:68, 1991.

Spellbring AM et al: Improving safety for hospitalized elderly, *J Gerontol Nurs* 14(2):31-37, 1988.

Tinetti ME, Liu W-L, Ginter SF: Mechanical restraint use and fall-related injuries among residents of skilled nursing facilities, *Ann Intern Med* 116:369-373, 1992.

Williams LM, Morton GA, Patrick CH: The emory cubicle bed: an alternative to restraints for agitated traumatically brain injured clients, *Rehabil Nurs* 15:30-33, 1990.

BIBLIOGRAPHY

Whirret T, Wooldridge P: Home safety and older adults, *Caring* 11:56-58, 1992.

Decreased adaptive capacity: intracranial

Janet Woodruff and Betty Ackley

Definition The clinical state in which intracranial fluid dynamic mechanisms that normally compensate for increases in intracranial volumes are compromised, which results in repeated disproportionate increases in intracranial pressure (ICP) in response to a variety of noxious and non-noxious stimuli.

Defining Characteristics

Major: Repeated increases in ICP of greater than 10 mm Hg for more than 5 minutes following a variety of external stimuli.

Minor: Disproportionate increases in ICP following a single environmental or nursing maneuver stimulus; elevated P2 ICP waveform; volume pressure response test variation (volume-pressure ratio >2, Pressure = volume index <10); baseline ICP equal to or greater than 10 mm Hg; wide amplitude ICP waveform.

Related Factors (r/t)

Brain injuries; sustained increase in ICP ≥10 to 15 mm Hg; decreased cerebral perfusion pressure ≤50 to 60 mm Hg; systemic hypotension with intracranial hypertension.

Client Outcomes/Goals

- Free of undetected, increased intracranial pressure.
- Neurological status remains stable or improves.

Nursing Interventions and Rationales

- Constantly monitor intracranial pressure and vital signs; keep alarm settings on.
  ICP is a dynamic rather than a constant pressure (Hickey, 1992).
- If ICP >20 mm Hg for 5 minutes, evaluate possible causes and take nursing actions to decrease pressure:
  - Evaluate position of client, ensure head of bed at 30 to 45 degrees. Keep client's head in the midline position without neck flexion to prevent kinking of jugular veins.
  - Avoid noxious auditory, visual, or tactile stimuli.
  - Ensure that respiratory status is adequate, and note mixed venous oxygen saturation.
  - Maintain client on fluid restriction and, if possible, slight dehydration to decrease cerebral edema.
  - Have client avoid performing Valsalva's maneuver. If client's movements in bed are causing Valsalva's maneuver, analgesics or paralytics may be needed.
  - Control body temperature; an increased temperature increases cerebral metabolic rate, which increases ICP.

  A sustained ICP above 20 mm Hg can result in brain herniation and death (Vos, 1993).
- Notify physician if nursing interventions do not relieve increased pressure within 20 minutes.
  If ICP remains elevated, a CT scan and various medications (e.g., paralytics, hyperosmolar agents, diuretics) may be needed.
- Compute cerebral perfusion pressure (CPP) and keep it within a range of 50 to 60 mm Hg or greater by regulating ordered vasoactive drips. CPP = MAP (mean arterial pressure) – ICP.
  Cerebral perfusion should be maintained within a prescribed range to ensure adequate perfusion of the brain (American Association of Neuroscience Nurses, 1990).
- Monitor client's level of consciousness, ability to follow commands, and appropriateness of behavior.
  A change in the client's level of consciousness is generally the first sign of neurological deterioration (Mitchell, Ackerman, 1992).

- Check client's pupillary reaction.
In the early stages of increasing ICP, visual changes can occur as a result of hemispheric pressure in the visual pathways of the brain. If client is in a chemical state to decrease ICP, a change in pupil reactions may be the first sign of impending herniation.
- Note any new onset of confusion, dizziness, or syncope.
Confusion occurs as a result of an ICP-related oxygen deficit. The specialized cerebral cortex cells are very sensitive to a decreased oxygen supply (Hickey, 1992).
- Constantly monitor client's vital signs.
Characteristic vital sign changes resulting from increased ICP include increased pulse pressure, slower bounding pulse, decreased respiratory rate, and increased temperature because of pressure damage on vasomotor centers of the brain. These are **later** *signs of increased pressure. Elevated temperature increases the cerebral metabolic rate, which increases ICP (Vos, 1993).*
- Watch client's respiratory patterns for any abnormal patterns such as Cheyne-Stokes respiration; apneustic, cluster, or ataxic breathing patterns; or hyperventilation.
Characteristic respiratory patterns develop depending on the location of the cerebral insult (Mitchell, Ackerman, 1992).
- Monitor motor function by checking grasps, leg strength, and client's ability to move all four extremities. At lower levels of consciousness determine pain response by applying nail bed pressure to all four extremities at least every hour. If paralytics are needed to reduce ICP, consult physician regarding how frequently to let client "up" to check motor function.
- Limit suctioning if possible. If suctioning is necessary, preoxygenate and hyperventilate client, and limit to two suction passes, each no longer than 15 seconds in duration.
Research has shown a strong association between suctioning and increased intracranial pressure (Mitchell, Ackerman, 1992). Careful suctioning can help prevent sustained increases in intracranial pressure (Rudy, Turner, Baun, 1992).
- Recognize the need to keep client on a ventilator and in mild respiratory alkalosis with an increased tidal volume and rate.
Hyperventilation of the ventilatory client is an effective way to reduce ICP. Keeping the P_{CO_2} *around 28 mm Hg provides adequate oxygenation and also assists in vasoconstriction of the cerebral arteries.*
- When positioning client, avoid any flexion of the neck or rotation of the head to the side; keep client's head in a neutral position.
Neck flexion and head rotation decrease venous return, which increases ICP (Williams, Coyne, 1993).
- Position client as ordered, generally in a semi-Fowler's position with a 30-degreee elevation. If turning is necessary, log roll client. Always watch client's response to position changes; if cerebral perfusion pressure decreases when the head of the bed is elevated, consult with physician regarding use of a lower degree of elevation.
Elevated intracranial pressure can be lowered by raising the head of the bed, but elevating the head of the bed may compromise cerebral perfusion pressure (Winkelman, 1994).
- Avoid any knee flexion, and do not raise knee gatch.
Knee flexion traps venous blood in the intra-abdominal space, which increases abdominal and thoracic pressure and reduces venous return from the head (Vos, 1993).

- Sequence nursing care to allow for rest periods between noxious activities such as suctioning and position changing. Allow ICP to return to baseline before initiating any other nursing activities (Mitchell, Ackerman, 1992).
  Rest periods help prevent sustained increases in ICP, which can cause neurological damage.
- Touch client gently and talk quietly while giving care.
  Gentle touching and talking can have a therapeutic effect on clients with increased stability of ICP (Mitchell, Johnson, Haberman-Little, 1985).

REFERENCES

American Association of Neuroscience Nurses, *Core Curriculum for Neuroscience Nursing,* ed 3, Chicago, 1990.

Hickey JV: *Neurological and neurosurgical nursing,* ed 3, Philadelphia, 1992, JB Lippincott.

Mitchell PH, Ackerman LL: Secondary brain injury reduction. In Bulechek GM, McCloskey JC, editors: *Nursing interventions: essential nursing treatments,* ed 2, Philadelphia, 1992, WB Saunders.

Mitchell PH, Johnson FB, Habermann-Little BH: Promoting physiologic stability: touch and ICP, *Commun Nurs Res* 18:93 (Abstr), 1985.

Rudy EB, Turner BS, Baun M: Endotracheal suctioning in adults with head injury, *Heart Lung* 20:667-674, 1992.

Vos HR: Making headway with intracranial hypertension, *Am J Nurs* 93:28-39, 1993.

Williams A, Coyne SM: Effects of neck position on intracranial pressure, *Am J Crit Care* 2:68-71, 1993.

Winkelman C: Advances in managing increased intracranial pressure: a decade of selected research, *AACN Clin Issues* 5:9-14, 1994.

BIBLIOGRAPHY

Rising CJ: The relationship of selected nursing activities to ICP, *J Neurosci Nurs* 25:302-308, 1993.

Knowledge deficit

Suzanne Skowronski

Definition Absence or deficiency of cognitive information related to a specific topic.

Defining Characteristics

Verbalization of the problem; inaccurate follow-through of previous instruction; inaccurate performance of test; inappropriate or exaggerated behaviors (e.g., hysterical, hostile, agitated, apathetic).

Related Factors (r/t)

Lack of exposure; lack of recall; information misinterpretation; cognitive limitation; lack of interest in learning; unfamiliarity with information resources.

Client Outcomes/Goals

- Explains disease state, recognizes need for medications, understands treatments.
- Explains how to incorporate new health regimen into life-style.
- States an ability to deal with health situation and remain in control of life.
- Demonstrates how to perform procedure(s) satisfactorily.
- Lists resources that can be used for more information or support after discharge.

Nursing Interventions and Rationales

- Observe client's ability to learn (e.g., mental acuity, ability to see and hear, no existing pain, emotional readiness, absence of language or cultural barriers).
  Physical and mental readiness are necessary for learning.
- Assess barriers to learning (e.g., perceived change in life-style, financial concerns, cultural patterns, lack of acceptance by peers or coworkers).
  The client's health belief system serves to filter and process new information.
- Determine client's previous knowledge of or skills related to the subject and their influence on their willingness to learn.
  New learning is assimilated into previous assumptions and facts and may involve negotiating, transforming, or stalling.
- When teaching, build on client's existing knowledge base.
  Adults approach new learning experiences in light of a lifetime of accumulated learning; educators must make use of past learning experiences for new content to be relevant (Knowles, 1980).
- Help client write specific learning objectives.
  Objectives focus the content and provide a forum for evaluating outcomes, and the written plan ensures continuity. Client involvement improves compliance with the health regimen and makes teaching and learning a partnership.
- Present material that is most significant to client first, such as how to give injections or change dressings; present additional material once client's most pressing educational needs have been met.
  Adult learners are self-directive in learning, and for them learning is more meaningful and effective when related to what the learner wants to know (Knowles, 1980).
- Give verbal reinforcement for evidence of learning.
  "The learner who receives reinforcement before or after a desired learning behavior will likely repeat that behavior" (Potter, Perry, 1993, p. 204).
- Use visual aids such as programmed learning, charts, and pamphlets; use audiovisual aids such as video and audio tapes.
  Printed material and audiovisual tapes reinforce the spoken word. The client can review and refer to the information when questions arise.

- Provide preadmission self-instruction materials to prepare client for postoperative exercises.
  Providing clients with preadmission information about exercises has been shown to increase positive feelings and the ability to perform prescribed exercises (Rice, Mullin, Jarosz, 1992).
- Explain sensations the client will experience during diagnostic procedures or following surgery.
  Sensory preparation can decrease distress in clients when they experience the actual sensations (Johnson, Lauver, 1989).
- Identify the primary family support person; be aware of that person's ability to learn and incorporate needed changes.
- Assess willingness of family to incorporate new information, immunizations, medical and dental care, and diet modifications as a way to support the client.
  The family as a social unit has its own culture, beliefs, and ways of relating to each other. These are strengths to use when teaching about health care of a family member.
- Provide plenty of time for questions, clarification, and reinforcement when teaching family.
  Each family member has a unique learning style. By getting family support for needed changes in diet, stress management, or life-style, the client will be motivated and successful in implementing new information.
- Help client to identify community resources for continuing information and support.
  Learning occurs through imitation, and persons who are currently involved in life-style changes can help the client anticipate adjustment issues. Community resources can offer financial and educational support.
- Evaluate client's learning through return demonstrations, verbalizations, or the application of skills to new situations.
  The education process is not complete until the learner successfully implements the skill as a tool for health maintenance.

Geriatric

- Adapt the teaching process to meet physical deficits of the aging process (e.g., speak clearly, use a variety of audio-visual-psychomotor methods, use examples, allow time for client to repeat and review).
  Adults are capable of learning at any age. Age modifies but does not inhibit learning (Dellasega et al, 1994).
- Ensure that the client uses necessary reading aids (e.g., glasses, magnifying lenses, large-print texts) or hearing aids.
  Visual and hearing deficits require amplification or clarification of sensory input.
- Use printed material, video tapes, lists, and diagrams that the client can refer to at another time.
  As one ages, short-term memory becomes less effective; these materials reinforce learning.
- Assess client's previous knowledge or resistance or blocks to incorporating new information into the current life-style.
  Long-term memory is strong and affects how well new information is interpreted and used.
- Repeat and reinforce information during several brief sessions.
  Understanding past information is essential to acquiring new knowledge. Brief sessions focus attention on essential information.

- Discuss healthy life-style changes that promote wellness for the older adult.
  It is never too late to stop smoking, lose weight, or modify dietary intake of fats and alcohol. Quality versus quantity of life may be the key issue in teaching self-care health habits.

REFERENCES

Dellasega C et al: Nursing process: teaching elderly clients, *J Gerontol Nurs* 31:20, 1994.

Johnson JE, Lauver DR: Alternative explanations of coping with stressful experiences associated with physical illness, *Adv Nurs Sci* 11(2):39-52, 1989.

Knowles M: *The adult learner: a neglected species,* ed 2, Houston, 1980, Gulf.

Potter P, Perry A: *Fundamentals of nursing: concepts, process, and practice,* St Louis, 1993, Mosby.

Rice VH, Mullin MH, Jarosz P: Preadmission self-instruction effects on postadmission and postoperative indicators in CABG patients: partial replication and extension, *Res Nurs Health* 15:253-259, 1992.

BIBLIOGRAPHY

Pender N: *Health promotion in nursing practice,* ed 2, Norwalk, Conn, 1987, Appleton & Lange.

Redman B: *The process of patient education,* St Louis, 1993, Mosby.

Tarsitano BP: Structured preoperative teaching. In *Nursing interventions: essential nursing treatments,* ed 2, Bulechek G, McCloskey J, editors: Philadelphia, 1992, WB Saunders.

Risk for loneliness

Marty Martin and Jane Curtis

Definition The subjective state in which an individual is at risk of experiencing vague dysphoria.

Defining Characteristics

Presence of risk factors such as affectional deprivation; physical isolation; cathectic deprivation; social isolation.

Related Factors (r/t)

Refer to risk factors.

Client Outcomes/Goals

- Maintains one or more relationships in which he or she is able to self-disclose and demonstrate a balance between emotional dependence and independence.
- Participates in ongoing positive and relevant social activities and interactions that he or she perceives as meaningful.

Nursing Interventions and Rationales

- Assess client's social support system. Use a social support assessment tool if possible.
  Use of social support questionnaire can be helpful to gather relevant information (Norbeck, Lindsey, Carrieri, 1981).
- Evaluate client's desire for social interaction in relation to actual social interaction.
  The concept of loneliness involves a discrepancy between the client's desired and achieved level of social interaction (Christian, Dluhy, O'Neill, 1989).
- Assess the client's interpersonal skills, and intervene according to deficits and behaviors that are blocking communication.
- Encourage involvement in meaningful social relationships that are characteristic of both giving and receiving support.
  It is important to recognize that the positive relevance of social relationship is related to the content and quality of relationships (Gulick, 1994).
- Explore ways to enlarge client's support system and participation in groups and organizations.
  Studies indicate that people with smaller support systems have higher levels of loneliness (Mahon, 1982).
- Encourage client to practice self-disclosure during conversations.
- Encourage client to develop closeness in at least one relationship.
  Dependence and independence should be balanced in healthy relationships. Previous research has indicated that the development of a balanced level of emotional dependence and the ability to self-disclose are important factors in reducing the risk for loneliness (Mahon, 1982; Mahon, Yarcheski, 1992).
- Evaluate the level of character traits, shyness, and self-esteem, particularly for younger and middle adolescent clients.
- For younger and middle adolescent clients, evaluate and encourage close relationships with parents.
- For older adolescents, encourage close relationships with peers and involvement in groups and organizations.
  Research indicates that younger adolescents are at a higher risk for loneliness if they are shy or have low self-esteem. Younger adolescents rely more on parental relationships. An expanded set of relationships becomes increasingly important in alleviating loneliness as adolescents mature (Mahon, Yarcheski, 1992).

Geriatric

- Assess client's adaptive sensory functions or any other health deviations that may limit or decrease his or her ability to interact with others.
- Assess client's potential or actual hearing loss or hearing impairment.
  Research shows that hearing loss is one of the most prevalent chronic health problems of the elderly in the United States (Christian, Dluhy, O'Neill, 1989). Relative to the nature of the sensory deprivation, communication barriers are increased and human intimacy and self-esteem are negatively affected (Chen, 1994). In addition, it is important to note that hearing impairments often go unnoticed and may not evoke public recognition as do more visibly recognized handicaps (Chen, 1994).

REFERENCES

Chen H: Hearing in the elderly, relation of healing loss, loneliness, and self-esteem, *J Gerontol Nurs* 20:22-28, 1994.

Christian E, Dluhy E, O'Neill R: Sounds of silence, *J Gerontol Nurs* 15:4-9, 1989.

Gulick E: Social support among persons with multiple sclerosis, *Res Nurs Health* 17:195-206, 1994.

Mahon NE: The relationship of self disclosure, interpersonal dependency, and life changes to loneliness in young adults, *Nurs Res* 31:343-347, 1982.

Mahon NE, Yarcheski A: Alternate explanations of loneliness in adolescents: a replication and extension study, *Nurs Res* 41:151-156, 1992.

Norbeck J, Lindsey A, Carrieri V: The development of an instrument to measure social support, *Nurs Res* 30:264-269, 1981.

Impaired memory

Betty Ackley

Definition The state in which an individual experiences the inability to remember or recall bits of information or behavioral skills. Impaired memory may be attributed to either temporary or permanent pathophysiological or situational causes.

Defining Characteristics

Major Observed or reported experiences of forgetting; inability to determine if a behavior was performed; inability to learn or retain new skills or information; inability to perform a previously learned skill; inability to recall factual information; inability to recall recent or past events.

Minor Forgets to perform a behavior at a scheduled time.

Related Factors (r/t)

Acute or chronic hypoxia; anemia; decreased cardiac output; fluid and electrolyte imbalance; neurological disturbances; excessive environmental disturbances.

Client Outcomes/Goals

- Demonstrates use of techniques to help with memory loss.
- States has decreased problems with memory loss.

Nursing Interventions and Rationales

- Determine if onset of memory loss is gradual or sudden. If memory loss is sudden, refer client to a physician for evaluation of cause.
  Acute transient memory loss may be associated with neurological disease (Vinson, 1989).
- Determine amount and pattern of alcohol intake.
  Alcohol intake has been associated with "blackouts"—the person may function but not remember actions; long-term alcohol use causes Korsakoff's syndrome with associated memory loss (Vinson, 1989).
- Note client's current medications; some medications such as benzodiazepines have been associated with memory loss.
  Benzodiazepines can produce loss of memory for events that occur after beginning the medication, and information is not stored in long-term memory (Mejo, 1992).
- Note client's current level of stress; determine if there has been a recent traumatic event.
  Post-traumatic stress and stressful and anxiety-inducing general life factors can cause memory problems (Mejo, 1992).
- If signs of depression such as weight loss, insomnia, or sad affect are evident, refer client to psychotherapy.
  Depression is commonly associated with memory loss (Mejo, 1992).
- Encourage client to use a calendar to keep track of appointments, keep reminder lists, place a string around finger or rubber band around wrist to remember needed action, or enlist someone else to remind him or her of important events.
  Using such reminders can help the memory-impaired client just as they help all others to cue needed actions.
- Help client set up a medication box that cues client to take medication at needed times; client will know he or she has taken the medication if the box is empty.
- If safety is an issue (e.g., forgets to turn off stove after use, forgets emergency telephone numbers), suggest alternatives such as using a microwave or whistling teakettle and programming emergency numbers in telephone so that they are readily available.

These measures can be taken to increase client safety (Agostinelli et al, 1994).

- Refer client to a neuropsychologist or occupational therapist who has expertise in working with the memory impaired.
- For memory impairments associated with dementia refer to care plan for **Chronic confusion**.

Geriatric

- Recognize that depression and anxiety are common causes of memory loss in the elderly.
  The elderly often contribute occasional absentmindness to early stages of dementia, which can cause increased anxiety and even depression (Wilson, Moffat, 1992).
- Help family develop a memory aid booklet or wallet that contains pictures and labels from client's life.
  Using memory aids helps clients with dementia make more factual statements and stay on topic and decreases the number of confused, erroneous, and repetitive statements (Bourgeois, 1992).

Client/Family Teaching

- If stress is associated with memory loss, suggest psychotherapy, exercise, or the use of relaxation techniques.
  Nonpharmacological therapy for treatment of stress syndromes is preferable and less likely to aggravate memory loss than commonly used antianxiety medications (Mejo, 1992).
- When teaching client, first determine what the client knows about the topic and build on that knowledge.
  "New material is organized in terms of what already exists, and efficient learning should attempt to take advantage of what is already known in order to graft on new material" (Wilson, Moffat, 1992, p. 21).
- If teaching a skill to client, set up a series of practice attempts. Begin with simple tasks so that they can be positively reinforced and progress to more difficult concepts.
  Distributed practice with correct recall attempts can be a very effective teaching strategy, so that practice is widely distributed over time if possible (Wilson, Moffat, 1992).
- Teach client to use cues to trigger desired behaviors, including alarm watches, electronic organizers, or pocket computers that cue actions at designated times.
  Cuing devices can help remind client of a desired action (Wilson, Moffat, 1992).

REFERENCES

Agostinelli B et al: Targeted interventions, use of the Mini-Mental State Exam, *J Gerontol Nurs* 20:15-23, 1994.

Bourgeois MS: *Conversing with memory impaired individuals using memory aids: a memory aid workbook,* Gaylord, Mich, 1992, Northern Speech Services.

Mejo SL: Anterograde amnesia linked to benzodiazepines, *Nurse Pract* 17:44-50, 1992.

Vinson DC: Acute transient memory loss, *Am Fam Physician* 39:249-253, 1989.

Wilson BA, Moffat N: *Clinical management of memory problems,* San Diego, 1992, Singular.

BIBLIOGRAPHY

Byers PH: Older adults' metamemory: coping, depression, and self-efficacy, *Appl Nurs Res* 6:28-30, 1993.

Paulanka BJ, Griffin LS: Behavioral responses of memory impaired clients to selected nursing interventions, *Phys occup ther geriatr* 12:65-78, 1993.

Impaired physical mobility

Betty Ackley

Definition The state in which an individual experiences a limitation of ability for independent physical movement.

Defining Characteristics

Inability to purposefully move within the physical environment, including bed mobility, transfer, and ambulation; reluctance to attempt movement; limited range of motion; decreased muscle strength, control, or mass; imposed restrictions of movement, including mechanical and medical protocol; impaired coordination.

Related Factors (r/t)

Intolerance to activity; decreased strength and endurance; pain or discomfort; perceptual or cognitive impairment; neuromuscular impairment; musculoskeletal impairment; depression; severe anxiety.

Suggested functional level classification

0, Completely independent
1, Requires use of equipment or device
2, Requires help from another person for assistance, supervision, or teaching
3, Requires help from another person and equipment device
4, Dependent, does not participate in activity

Client Outcomes/Goals

- Participates in required physical activity.
- Meets mutually defined goals of increased mobility.
- Verbalizes feeling of increased strength and an ability to move.
- Demonstrates use of adaptive equipment (e.g., wheelchairs, walkers) to increase mobility.

Nursing Interventions and Rationales

- Observe cause of impaired mobility; determine if cause is physical or psychological.
- Monitor and record client's ability to tolerate activity and to use all four extremities; note pulse rate, blood pressure, dyspnea, and skin color before and after activity. Refer to **Activity intolerance**.
- Observe for pain before activity and if possible treat pain before activity.
  The presence of pain limits mobility; pain is often exacerbated by movement.
- Consult with physical therapy for development of mobility plan.
- Obtain any assistive devices needed before activity such as walking belts, walkers, canes, crutches, or wheelchairs.
  Assistive devices help increase mobility.
- If client is immobile, perform passive range-of-motion exercises at least twice a day unless contraindicated; repeat each maneuver three times.
  Passive range of motion helps to maintain joint mobility, prevent contractures and deformities, increase circulation, and promote a feeling of comfort and well-being (Bolander, 1994; Kottke, Lehman, 1990).
- If client is immobile, consult with physician for a safety evaluation before beginning an exercise program; if program is approved, begin with the following exercises:
  1. Have client perform active range of motion of both upper and lower extremities (e.g., flex and extend at ankles, knees, hips).
  2. Have client perform chin-ups and pull-ups using a trapeze in bed.

3. Have client perform strengthening exercises such as gluteal or quadraceps sitting exercises.
These exercises help prevent weakening and atrophy of muscles.

- Help client to be mobile and walking as soon as possible if not contraindicated because of condition.
The longer a client is immobile, the longer it takes to regain strength, balance, and coordination (Bolander, 1994).
- Use a walking belt when ambulating the client.
With a walking belt the client can walk independently, yet the nurse can rapidly ensure safety if the knees buckle.
- Apply any ordered brace before mobilizing client.
Braces stabilize a body part, which allows increased mobility.
- Increase independence in doing activities of daily living as client gets stronger; discourage helplessness.
Providing unnecessary assistance with transfers and bathing activities may promote dependence and a loss of mobility (Mobily, Kelley, 1991).

Geriatric

- Watch for orthostatic hypotension when mobilizing an elderly client.
Orthostatic hypotension is common in the elderly as a result of cardiovascular system changes, chronic diseases, and medication effects (Mobily, Kelley, 1991).
- Do not routinely assist with transfers or bathing activities unless necessary.
The nursing staff may contribute to impaired mobility by helping too much; encourage independence (Mobily, Kelley, 1991).
- If client is mainly immobile, provide opportunities for socialization and provide sensory stimulation (e.g., television, visits from others).
Recognize that immobility and a lack of social support and sensory input may result in confusion or depression in the elderly (Mobily, Kelly, 1991).

Client/Family Teaching

- Teach client how to get out of bed slowly when transferring from the bed to the chair.
- Teach client relaxation techniques to use during activity.
- Teach client how to use assistive devices such as a cane, a walker, or crutches to increase mobility.
- Develop a mutually agreed on contract with client regarding goals of increased activity; include measurable landmarks of progress, and sign the contract with the client.

REFERENCES

Bolander VB: Meeting mobility needs. In *Sorensen and Luckmann's basic nursing: a psychophysiologic approach,* Philadelphia, 1994, WB Saunders.

Kottke FJ, Lehmann, JF: *Krusen's handbook of physical medicine,* ed 4, Philadelphia, 1990, WB Saunders.

Mobily PR, Kelley LS: Iatrogenesis in the elderly: factors of immobility, *J Gerontol Nurs* 17:5-12, 1991.

BIBLIOGRAPHY

Hummer A: Get your patient moving, *Am J Nurs* 93(6):34-37, 1993.

Kasper CE et al: Alterations in skeletal muscle related to impaired physical mobility: an empirical model, *Res Nurs Health* 16:265-273, 1993.

Ouellet LL, Rush KL: A synthesis of selected literature on mobility: a basis for studying impaired mobility, *Nurs Diag* 3:72-80, 1992.

Noncompliance

Betty Ackley

Definition An individual's informed decision to not adhere to a therapeutic recommendation.

Defining Characteristics

* Behavior indicative of failure to adhere (directly observed or verbalized by patient or significant others); objective tests (e.g., physiological measures, detection of markers); evidence of development of complications; evidence of exacerbation of symptoms; failure to keep appointments; failure to progress. (*Critical)

Related Factors (r/t)

Patient value system; health beliefs; cultural influences; spiritual values; client-provider relationships; lack of financial resources.

Client Outcomes/Goals

- Describes consequence of continued noncompliance with treatment regimen.
- States goals for health and the means by which to obtain them.
- Communicates an understanding of disease and treatment.
- Lists treatment regimens and expectations and agrees to follow through with them.
- Lists alternative ways to meet goals.
- Describes the importance of family participation to help client achieve goals.

Nursing Interventions and Rationales

- Observe for cause of noncompliance with therapeutic protocol; refer to related factors above.
- Determine client's and family's knowledge of illness and treatment. Teach them about the illness and purpose of the treatment regimen if necessary.
  Compliance is increased by knowledge of the therapeutic regimen (Warren, 1992).
- Observe client's cultural influences, values, and beliefs regarding illness, and whether locus of control is internal or external.
  Client may be unable to assume the sick role because of cultural influences, values, or beliefs and may thus reject treatment. Clients with an internal locus of control are more compliant (Warren, 1992).
- Monitor client's ability to follow directions, solve problems, concentrate, and read.
  Clients with cognitive impairments may not be able to follow directions and the prescribed treatment regimen.
- Avoid using threats, pressure, and inappropriate fear arousal to increase compliance.
  These measures are unethical and generally ineffective.
- Determine if client's support system helps or hinders therapy; bring family members and significant others into the educational process as desired by the client.
  A positive social support system is associated with increased compliance (Warren, 1992).
- Develop a therapeutic relationship based on active listening.
  Compliance is increased when the client feels that the health care provider is interested in and genuinely cares how the client is doing (Warren, 1992).
- Listen to client's statements of abilities; encourage client to use these abilities in self-care.
- When dealing with complex health care regimens, start client with small behavioral changes (e.g., have chemotherapy client rinse mouth with a saliva substitute twice daily). When one step has been accomplished, add another step.
  The client is often overwhelmed by what is expected and needs help with managing behavioral changes (Boehm, 1992).

- Make client an active partner in the health care team and allow client to give input on which treatments are acceptable and feasible.
  Recognize that the client has absolute power over whether he or she follows the health care guidelines; health care providers serve to influence behavior.
- Work with client to develop cues that trigger needed health care behaviors (e.g., check blood sugar before putting on makeup each morning).
  Associating cues with a behavior increases the frequency of the desired behavior.
- Work with client to develop an instruction and reminder sheet that fits medications and treatments into the client's life-style.
  The visual reminder helps increase compliance.
- For the chronically ill client, develop a multidisciplinary team to provide care, including a nurse, physician, pharmacist, dietician, and additional therapists as needed. Have team meetings to ensure continuity of care.
  Multidisciplinary team care has been shown to increase compliance (Warren, 1992).
- Develop a mutually agreed on written contract with client regarding needed health care behaviors; give reinforcement as client meets defined goals.
  A client contract that helps the client analyze behavior and choose behavioral strategies can be very effective in changing health care behaviors (Boehm, 1992).
- Consult with primary care practitioner regarding the possibility of simplifying the health care regimen so that it more easily fits into client's life-style (e.g., taking medications one time per day versus four times per day).
  The more complex the regimen, the less likely the client will follow it.

Geriatric

- If client has sensory and coordination deficits, use a medication organizer and have the home-health nurse or family place client's medications in daily compartments.
  A medication organizer can increase the client's ability to take medications as ordered.
- Monitor client for signs of depression associated with noncompliance (e.g., refuses to take medications or eat); refer client for treatment of depression as needed.
  Noncompliance in the elderly may be a form of indirect self-destructive behavior that is associated with depression and leads to suicide (Meisekothen, 1993).
- Use repetition, verbal cues, and memory aids when teaching the health care regimen.
  There may be age-related memory deficits that necessitate an increased use of measures that cue the client to perform needed health care behaviors.

Client/Family Teaching

- Teach medication side effects so that client understands them and feels comfortable discussing their occurrence (e.g., sexual function/dysfunction, mental changes).
  Several medications cause impotence, which can lead to a pattern of noncompliance.

REFERENCES

Boehm S: Patient contracting. In Bulechek GM, McCloskey JC, editors: *Nursing interventions: essential nursing treatments,* Philadelphia, 1992, WB Saunders.

Meisekothen LM: Noncompliance in the elderly: a pathway to suicide, *J Am Acad Nurs Pract* 5:67-71, 1993.

Warren JJ: Ethical concerns about noncompliance in the chronically ill patient, *Prog Cardiovasc Nurs* 7:10-14, 1992.

BIBLIOGRAPHY

Cargill JM: Medication compliance in elderly people: influencing variables and interventions, *J Adv Nurs* 17:422-426, 1992.

Foreman L: Medication: reasons and interventions for noncompliance, *J Psychosoc Nurs Ment Health Serv* 31:23-25, 1993.

Kluckowski JC: Solving medication noncompliance in home care, *Caring* 11:34-41, 1992.

Altered nutrition: less than body requirements

J. Keith Hampton and Gail Ladwig

Definition

The state in which an individual experiences an intake of nutrients insufficient to meet metabolic needs.

Defining Characteristics

Loss of weight with adequate food intake; body weight 20% or more under ideal; reported food intake less than recommended daily allowance; weakness of muscles required for swallowing or mastication; reported or evidence of lack of food; aversion to eating; reported altered taste sensation; satiety immediately after ingesting food; abdominal pain with or without pathology; sore, inflamed buccal cavity; hyperactive bowel sounds; lack of interest in food; perceived inability to ingest food; pale conjunctival and mucous membranes; poor muscle tone; excessive hair loss; lack of information; misinformation; misconceptions.

Related Factors (r/t)

Inability to ingest or digest food or absorb nutrients as a result of biological, psychological, or economic factors.

Client Outcomes/Goals

- Progressively gains weight toward desired goal; weight is within normal range for height and age.
- Describes understanding of any known factors contributing to low weight.
- Verbalizes an understanding of nutritional requirements.
- Able to eat foods high in protein and calories.
- Free of signs of malnutrition.

Nursing Interventions and Rationales

- Observe client's ability to eat (e.g., length of time it takes to eat, ability to: bring food to the mouth, see all the food on the tray, use eating utensils, swallow food, consume foods that vary in texture from liquids to solids).
  Eating is a multifaceted activity; all aspects of the client's eating behavior should be observed (Buelow, Jamieson, 1990).
  NOTE: If client is unable to feed self, refer to nursing interventions and rationales for **Self-care deficit: feeding**. If client has difficulty swallowing, refer to nursing interventions and rationales for **Impaired swallowing**.
- Evaluate laboratory studies (serum albumin, serum total protein, transferrin).
  These values indicate a loss of protein and iron storage and binding capacity (Metheny, 1992).
- Determine ideal body weight for height and age; consult with dietician for measurement of skin fold thickness; observe for muscle atrophy.
  A nutritional assessment is needed to determine the degree of malnutrition.
- Attempt to determine if eating difficulty is physical or psychological.
  It can be difficult to tell if the problem is physical or psychological. Refusing to eat may be the only way the client can express some control, and it may also be a symptom of depression (Evans, 1992).
- Weigh client weekly; have client wear the same clothes and use the same scale at the same time of day.
  Calorie gain is slow, and daily weights can be discouraging. Using the same variables helps monitor the client's response to clinical interventions (Metheny, 1992).

- Monitor food intake; be specific when recording amounts eaten (e.g., 25%, 50%); consult with dietician for an actual calorie count.
- Monitor state of oral cavity (gums, tongue, mucosa, teeth).
- Determine relationship of eating and other events to onset of nausea, vomiting, diarrhea, or abdominal pain.
- Determine the time of day when the client's appetite is the greatest, and plan the highest calorie meal for that time.
- Administer antiemetics as ordered before meals.
  Giving antiemetics before meals reduces the stimulus to vomit and thus potentially increases dietary intake and absorption.
- Work with client to develop a plan for increased activity.
  Immobility leads to negative nitrogen balance, which fosters anorexia.
- Work with the client to determine time of meals, likes and dislikes, food temperature, and eating environment.
  Allowing client input into the dietary plan enhances compliance.
- Provide for and offer good oral hygiene before and after meals.
  Good oral hygiene enhances appetite; the condition of the oral mucosa is critical to the ability to eat (Evans, 1992).
- Use behavior modification. If the problem is anorexia nervosa, offer positive feedback for food eaten.
  Behavior modification is useful in restoring lost weight (Bemis, 1978).
- Observe client's relationship with food and fears about food or eating (e.g., psychotic symptoms, food not tasting good).
- Provide supervision at mealtime to encourage client to eat and drink.
  Eating is ordinarily a time for social interaction (Sanders, 1990).
- Encourage eating by offering small amounts of food at one time; consider six small meals.
  Eating small, frequent meals reduces the sensation of fullness and decreases the stimulus to vomit (Love, Seaton, 1991).
- If client paces or is excessively agitated, offer high carbohydrate foods and fluids that can be carried while pacing. Finger foods such as bananas are helpful.
  If client cannot be still, food can still be consumed if client is in the upright position.
- Ensure that client's environment is pleasant before meals; clear unsightly supplies and avoid invasive procedures before meals.
  A pleasant environment helps maintain the appetite.
- If client lacks endurance, schedule rest periods before meals and open packages and cut up food for client.
  Many clients become quickly fatigued and do not have enough endurance to finish a meal; rest periods before the meal can increase endurance (Evans, 1992).
- If client is lactose intolerant, offer yogurt and ice cream.
  These foods provide the necessary nutrients with less flatulence and cramping.
- Offer foods rich in vitamin C, folic acid, and iron.
  Such foods are necessary if the client is anemic.

Geriatric

- Observe for factors that may be interfering with nutrition (e.g., no transportation, fixed income, high-priced convenience store use).
- Assess fit of dentures (if worn) and insert before meals; provide appropriate food textures for chewing ease.

Poorly fitting dentures deter a client from eating. Refer for a dental consultation if appropriate.

- Encourage increased social contact during meals; consider serving meals in a group setting, or encourage family and friends to visit.
  Social interaction during meals increases food consumption.
- If client has anorexia and dry mouth from medication side-effects, offer fluids shortly before meals to stimulate the appetite and moisten the oral mucosa.
  Small volumes of liquids up to 240 ml stimulate the gastrointestinal tract, which enhances peristalsis and motility (Rogers-Seidel, 1991).
  NOTE: If client is unable to feed self, refer to nursing interventions and rationales for **Self-care deficit: feeding**.

Client/Family Teaching

- Explain the need for consumption of carbohydrates, protein, minerals, fats, and fluids.
  Such explanations help the client identify the impact of a varied diet.
- Teach client to rest before meals.
  Resting reduces systemic energy consumption before meals.
- Provide dietary instructions to client and family.
- Reinforce dietary instructions with written materials.
- Refer client to counseling or family therapy if appropriate.
- Refer to Meals-on-Wheels.
- Teach the client and family home tube feeding or how to manage home parenteral nutrition therapy.

REFERENCES

Bemis K: Current approaches to the etiology and treatment of anorexia nervosa, *Psychol Bull* 85:593-617, 1978.

Buelow JM, Jamieson P: Potential for altered nutritional status in the stroke patient, *Rehabil Nurs* 15:260, 1990.

Evans NJ: *Feeding.* In Bulechek GM, McCloskey JC, editors: *Nursing interventions: essential nursing treatments*, ed 2, Philadelphia, 1992, WB Saunders.

Love CC, Seaton H: Eating disorders: highlights of nursing assessment and therapeutics, *Nurs Clin N Am* 26:677-697, 1991.

Metheny NM: *Fluid and electrolyte balance: nursing considerations*, ed 2, Philadelphia, 1992, Lippincott.

Rogers-Seidel: *Geriatric nursing care plans,* St Louis, 1991, Mosby.

Sanders HN: Feeding dependent eaters among geriatric patients, *J Nutr Elderly* 9:69-74, 1990.

BIBLIOGRAPHY

Norberg A et al: Food refusal amongst nursing home patients as conceptualized by nurses' aides and enrolled nurses: an interview study, *J Adv Nurs* 13:478-483, 1988.

Altered nutrition: more than body requirements

J. Keith Hampton and Gail Ladwig

Definition The state in which an individual experiences an intake of nutrients that exceeds metabolic needs.

Defining Characteristics

*Weight 10% over ideal for height and frame; *weight 20% over ideal for height and frame; *triceps skin fold greater than 15 mm in men or 25 mm in women; sedentary activity level; reported or observed dysfunctional eating pattern; pairing of food with other activities; concentration of food intake at the end of day; eating in response to external cues such as time of day or social situation; eating in response to internal cues other than hunger (e.g., anxiety). (*Critical)

Related Factors (r/t)

Excessive intake in relation to metabolic need.

Client Outcomes/Goals

- States factors that contribute to weight gain.
- Identifies behaviors that remain under client's control.
- Explains current eating patterns.
- Complies with dietary modifications to promote a balanced nutritional intake.
- Accomplishes the desired weight loss over a reasonable length of time (e.g., 1 pound per week).
- States and performs energy-requiring activities into activities of daily living (e.g., exercise 30 minutes daily).

Nursing Interventions and Rationales

- Observe for behaviors that indicate a nutritional intake more than body requirements. *Such observations help gain a clear picture of the client's dietary pattern.*
- Determine client's prehospital eating patterns; ask client what he or she usually ate in a 24-hour period.
- Determine client's knowledge of a nutritional diet.
  Gaining this information helps develop a teaching plan that is based upon the client's level of knowledge.
- Have client keep a "food diary," which states what is eaten and when; identify patterns (e.g., eating when under stress).
  Self-monitoring helps the client assess adherence to self-determined performance criteria and progress toward desired goals. Self-monitoring serves an important role in the maintenance of internal standards of behavior (Fleury, 1991).
- Review client's current exercise level and work to develop an exercise plan that the client is willing to follow.
  If weight loss is to be permanent, an exercise program is essential; the client is more likely to be compliant if he or she has input into the plan (Laguarta, Danish, 1988).
- Consult with dietician to develop a diet that is reasonable and nutritious and can accomplish client's desired weight loss.
  Many clients need assistance in planning meals (Crist, 1992).
- Set attainable goals for weekly weight loss.
  If an unrealistic weight management goal is set, the goal is not attained, and demoralization emerges (Minden, 1993).
- Weigh client twice a week.
  It is important to most clients and their progress to have the tangible reward that the scale shows. Monitoring twice a week keeps the client on the program by not allowing

him or her to eat out of control for a couple of days and then fast to lose weight (Crist, 1992).

- Discuss the importance of an adequate nutritional intake; allow occasional treats.
  Total removal of all treats leads to a negative eating pattern.
- Use the following behavior modification techniques:
  - eat only in a specific location (e.g., dining table)
  - avoid other activities (e.g., television, reading) while eating
  - drink a full glass of liquid before eating
  - use a smaller plate
  - plan eating splurges by saving a portion of calories and having a treat once a week

  Behavior modification focuses on what the client does. Desirable behaviors are rewarded; the reward may be satisfaction in achieving a goal (Barry, 1994).
- Establish a client contract that involves reinforcing and rewarding the attainment of progressive goals and the maintenance of desired weight.
  Contracting provides for mutually agreed on targets, goals, and plans.

Geriatric

- Observe for socioeconomic factors that influence food choices (e.g., carbohydrates are less expensive); plan a menu for a client on a fixed income.
  Food choices in today's food markets are greatly enhanced, even for those on a limited budget (Love, Seaton, 1992).
- Increase client's activity within physiological limits.
  Increased activity stimulates peristalsis and stimulates the appetite (Love, Seaton, 1991).
- Experiment with a variety of flavorings.
  Taste sensation decreases in the elderly, and they crave sweets.
- Involve client in senior citizen groups to occupy time with activities other than eating.
  Generally as people become older they need fewer calories to maintain an adequate body weight (Ringsven, Bond, 1992).

Client/Family Teaching

- Provide the client and family information regarding the nutritional plan.
  Information may make it easier for the client and family to process the therapeutic treatment plan.
- Inform the client of health risks associated with obesity.
  Acknowledgment of risks helps the client to verbalize their overall impact.
- Refer to community resources (e.g., Weight Watchers, Overeaters Anonymous).
- Teach the importance of exercise.
  Exercise increases the metabolic rate so that the body burns more calories, even at rest.
- Teach stress reduction techniques as alternatives to eating.
  Client needs healthy behaviors to substitute for unhealthy behaviors.

REFERENCES

Barry P: *Mental health and mental illness,* ed 5, Philadelphia, 1994, JB Lippincott.

Crist J: *Weight management.* In Bulechek GM, McCloskey JC, editors: *Nursing interventions: essential nursing treatments*, ed 2, Philadelphia, 1992, WB Saunders.

Fleury J: Empowering potential: a theory of wellness motivation, *Nurs Res* 40:288, 1991.

Laguartra I, Danish SJ: A primer for nutritional counseling. In Rankle RT, Yang MU, editors: *Obesity and weight control*, Rockville, Md, 1988, Aspen.

Love C, Seaton H: Eating disorders: highlights of nursing assessment and therapeutics. *Nurs Clin North Am*, 26:677-697, 1991.

Minden S: Weight Management. In National Institute for the Clinical Application of Behavioral Medicine, Fifth International Conference: *The psychology of health, immunity and disease*, vol A, Dec 8-9, 1993, Hilton Head Island, SC.

Ringsven M, Bond D: *Gerontology and leadership skills for nurses,* 1992, Delmar.

Risk for altered nutrition: more than body requirements

J. Keith Hampton and Gail Ladwig

Definition

The state in which an individual is at risk of experiencing an intake of nutrients that exceeds metabolic needs.

Defining Characteristics

Presence of risk factors such as reported or observed obesity in one or both parents; rapid transition across growth percentiles in infants or children; reported use of solid food as major food source before five months of age; observed use of food as reward or comfort measure; reported or observed higher baseline weight at beginning of each pregnancy; dysfunctional eating patterns; pairing of food with other activities; concentration of food intake at end of day; eating in response to external cues such as time of day or social situation; eating in response to internal cues other than hunger (e.g., anxiety).

Related Factors (r/t)

Refer to risk factors.

Client Outcomes/Goals

- Demonstrates an understanding of nutritional concepts for a balanced nutritional intake.
- Explains current eating patterns.
- Complies with dietary modifications to promote a balanced nutritional intake.

Nursing Interventions and Rationales

- Refer to care plan for **Altered nutrition: more than body requirements**.
- Observe for presence of risk factors.
- Increase client's knowledge and awareness of actions that contribute to excessive food intake.
- Observe eating patterns.
- Increase client's activity level to increase calorie use.
- Consult dietician to develop an appropriate diet for the client.
- Alternate rest and moderate activity periods.
- Provide diversional activities.
- Refer client to counseling or to a support group.
- Identify the client's reinforcers for maintaining the reduced weight.
- Encourage client to make decisions regarding changes in eating patterns.
- Encourage client to strive toward realistic goals.

Geriatric

- Plan to decrease calories in the least painful way (e.g., decrease fat in meals rather than eliminating the after-dinner cookie that client has had for years).

Client/Family Teaching

- Educate client about actions that contribute to excess food intake.
  Providing the client with greater knowledge may allow avoidance of excess food intake.
- Teach client behavior modification techniques that decrease calorie intake (e.g., eat slowly, chew food thoroughly, eat only at a specific spot at home, prepare small, one-meal portions, do not eat while doing other activities such as watching television, substitute low-calorie snacks for high-calorie snacks and have them conveniently available, do not keep high-calorie foods in the house).
  Behavior modification techniques can provide alternative stimuli that activate proper eating patterns (Porth, 1992).
- If dietician is not available, educate client about proper nutrition. Clarify misconceptions and discuss the breakdown of protein, fat, and carbohydrates in the diet.
  Accurate information provides the client with a source of reference.

- Instruct client to read nutrition labels; advise clients to overlook cholesterol-free claims and to read the actual label for fat originating from vegetable oil sources; teach client to read "natural food"-product labels for sugar, honey, or concentrated fruit juice content versus sugar free.
  Learning how to read food labels increases the client's knowledge base about food and helps the client identify inappropriate food choices.

REFERENCES Porth CM: Physiology of thirst and drinking: implications for nursing practice, *Heart Lung* 21:273-284, 1992.

Altered oral mucous membranes

Diane Krasner

Definition The state in which an individual experiences disruptions in the tissue layers of the oral cavity.

Defining Characteristics

Oral pain or discomfort; coated tongue; xerostoma (dry mouth); stomatitis; oral lesions or ulcers; lack of or decreased salivation; leukoplakia; edema; hyperemia; oral plaques; desquamation; vesicles; hemorrhagic gingivitis; carious teeth; halitosis.

Related Factors (r/t)

Pathological conditions of oral cavity (irradiation to head or neck); dehydration; trauma (e.g., chemical: acidic foods, drugs, tobacco, noxious agents, alcohol; mechanical: ill-fitting dentures, braces, endotracheal or nasogastric tubes); surgery in oral cavity; NPO for more than 24 hours; ineffective oral hygiene; mouth breathing; malnutrition; infection; lack of or decreased salivation; medication.

Client Outcomes/Goals

- Describes or demonstrates measures to regain or maintain intact oral mucous membranes.
- Reports altered sensation or pain.
- Maintains adequate oral intake.
- Verbalizes a personal plan for maintaining intact oral mucous membranes.

Nursing Interventions and Rationales

- Inspect oral cavity at least once daily and note any discoloration, lesions, edema, bleeding, exudate, or dryness. Refer to a physician or specialist as appropriate.
  Systematic inspection can identify impending problems early.
- Assess for mechanical or chemical agents that could cause or increase trauma to oral mucous membranes.
  Whenever possible, modify plan of care to eliminate causative agents.
- Monitor client's nutritional and fluid status to determine if adequate.
  Dehydration and malnutrition predispose clients to altered oral mucous membranes.
- Determine client's mental status; if client is unable to do self-care, oral hygiene must be provided by the nursing personnel. The nursing diagnosis **Bathing/hygiene self-care deficit** is then also applicable.
- Determine client's usual method of oral care and address any concerns regarding oral hygiene.
  Whenever possible, build on client's existing knowledge base and current practices to develop an individualized plan of care (adult learning theory).
- If client is free from bleeding disorders and able to swallow, encourage client to brush teeth after every meal and floss teeth daily.
- If platelets are decreased or client is unable to swallow, use moistened toothettes to give oral care. Use lemon and glycerine swabs only on intact mucous membranes as a comfort measure for clients who are NPO or are fluid restricted (Wiley, 1969). Avoid using hydrogen peroxide unless needed to remove crusting or debris.
  Hydrogen peroxide can damage oral mucosa and is extremely distasteful to clients (Tombes, Gallucci, 1993).
- Keep inside of mouth moist with frequent sips of water, salt water rinses (1/2 tsp salt in 1 cup warm water), artificial saliva, or prescription medications as ordered by the physician.

Moisture promotes the cleansing effect of saliva and helps avert mucosal drying, which can result in erosions, fissures, or lesions (Shelley, Shelley, 1987).

- Keep lips well lubricated.
- If mouth is severely inflamed, establish a schedule of frequent mouth care every 2 hours while awake. Avoid friction, scrubbing, or the use of harsh chemical agents, which can damage delicate inflamed tissue.
- If mouth is severely inflamed and it is painful to swallow, contact the physician for a topical anesthetic agent or analgesic order. Modification of oral intake (e.g., soft diet, liquid diet) may also be necessary to prevent friction trauma. The nursing diagnosis **Altered nutrition: less than body requirements** may apply.
- If whitish plaques with reddened bases appear in the mouth or on the tongue, suspect a fungal infection and contact the physician for follow-up.
  Oral candidiasis (Monilia) is extremely common secondary to antibiotic therapy and must be treated with oral or systemic antifungal agents (Sauer, 1991; Shelley, Shelley, 1987).
- If client is unable to swallow, keep suction nearby when providing oral care.

Geriatric

- Carefully observe oral cavity and lips for abnormal lesions.
  Malignant lesions are more common in the elderly, especially if there is a history of smoking or alcohol use (Sauer, 1991).
- Ensure that dentures are removed and cleaned, preferably after every meal and before bedtime.
  Dentures left in the mouth at night impede circulation to the palate and predispose the client to skin lesions.

Client/Family Teaching

- Teach how to inspect the oral cavity and how to monitor for signs and symptoms of infection, complications, and healing.
- Teach how to implement a personal plan of oral hygiene, including a schedule of care.

REFERENCES

Shelley WB, Shelley ED: *Advanced dermatologic therapy,* Philadelphia, 1987, WB Saunders.

Sauer, GC: *Manual of skin diseases,* ed 6, Philadelphia, 1991, JB Lippincott.

Tombes MB, Gallucci B: The effects of hydrogen peroxide rinses on the normal oral mucosa, *Nurs Res* 42:332-337, 1993.

Wiley S: Why lemon and glycerol? *Am J Nurs* 69:342-348, 1969.

BIBLIOGRAPHY

Day R: Mouth care in an intensive care unit: a review, *Intensive Crit Care Nurs* 9:246-252, 1993.

Hatton-Smith CK: A last bastion of ritualized practice? A review of nurses' knowledge of oral healthcare, *Professional Nurse* 9:304-308, 1994.

Pain

Christine Pasero and Margo McCaffery

Definition

Pain is whatever the experiencing person says it is, existing whenever he says it does (McCaffery, 1968).

An unpleasant sensory and emotional experience associated with actual or potential tissue damage and described in terms of such damage.

Defining Characteristics

Subjective Pain is always subjective and cannot be proved or disproved. A client's report of pain is the most reliable indicator of pain (Acute Pain Management Guideline Panel, 1992). A client with cognitive ability who can speak or point should use a pain rating scale (e.g., 0 to 10), to identify the current level of pain (self-report) and determine a pain rating goal.

Objective Expressions of pain are extremely variable and cannot be used in lieu of self-report. Neither behavior nor vital signs can substitute for the client's self-report (Acute Pain Management Guideline Panel, 1992); however, the observable responses to pain are helpful in its assessment, especially in clients who cannot or will not use a self-report pain rating scale. Observable responses may be a loss of appetite and an inability to deep breathe, ambulate, sleep, or perform activities of daily living. Clients may exhibit guarded or self-protective behavior, self-focusing or narrowed focus, distraction behavior ranging from crying to laughing, and muscle tension or rigidity. In sudden and severe pain, autonomic responses such as diaphoresis, blood pressure and pulse changes, pupillary dilation, or increases or decreases in respiratory rate and depth may be present.

Related Factors (r/t)

Actual or potential tissue damage (biological, chemical, physical).

Geriatric note: in spite of what many professionals and clients believe, pain is not an expected part of normal aging (Acute Pain Management Guideline Panel, 1992).

Client Outcomes/Goals

- Client with cognitive ability uses pain rating scale to identify current level of pain and determine a pain rating goal.
- Describes how unrelieved pain will be managed.
- Reports that pain management regimen relieves pain to a satisfactory level with minimal or manageable side effects.
- Performs activities of recovery with a reported acceptable level of pain.
- States an ability to obtain sufficient amounts of rest and sleep.
- Describes a nonpharmacological method that can be used to control pain.

Nursing Interventions and Rationales

- Determine if the client is experiencing pain at the time of the initial interview; if so, intervene now to provide pain relief.
  Unrelieved pain causes unnecessary suffering (Jacox et al, 1994).
- Monitor the severity of the pain using a pain rating scale; refer to Appendix D for sample Pain Rating Scales. Note location, quality, and associated manifestations of pain, aggravating factors that increase pain, and factors that alleviate pain.
  The single most reliable indicator of the existence and intensity of pain is the client's self-report (Acute Pain Management Guideline Panel, 1992).
- Ask the client to describe past experiences with pain and the effectiveness of the methods used to manage pain; ask about side effects, typical coping responses, and how client expresses pain.
  A pain history aids in planning and discussing pain control with the client (Acute Pain Management Guideline Panel, 1992).

- Explain the pain management plan, including medication administration, side effects, and complications.
  One of the most important steps toward improved control of pain is for the client to better understand the nature of pain, its treatment, and his or her role in pain control (Jacox, 1994).
- Discuss the client's fears of undertreated pain, overdose, and addiction.
  Because of the many misconceptions regarding pain and its treatment, education about the ability to control pain effectively and correction of myths about the use of opioids should be included as part of the treatment plan (Jacox, 1994). Addiction to opioids is extremely unlikely after using them for acute pain (Acute Pain Management Guideline Panel, 1992).
- Describe the adverse effects of unrelieved pain.
  The physiological and psychological risks associated with untreated pain are great. Pain may lead to shallow breathing and cough suppression followed by retained pulmonary secretions and pneumonia (Acute Pain Management Guideline Panel, 1992).
- Help client use nonpharmacological methods to control pain such as distraction (e.g., music, television, counting to self, reading, stroking, controlled breathing, massage, heat applications, or cold applications as ordered and as therapeutic to client).
  Cognitive and behavioral strategies can restore the client's sense of self-control, personal efficacy, and active participation in care (Jacox, 1994).
- If possible provide ordered pain medication on a schedule that helps prevent onset of pain.
  Pain is easier to manage before it increases in intensity.
- Provide information to decrease anxiety, and allow client to have as much control over pain management as possible.
- Plan care activities around periods of greatest comfort whenever possible.
  Pain diminishes activity (Jacox, 1994).
- Explore the need for both opioid (narcotic) and nonopioid analgesics.
  Some types of pain respond to nonopioid drugs alone; if pain does not respond, add an opioid at increasing doses for increasing severity of pain (American Pain Society, 1992).
- Determine the client's current medication use.
  A medication history aids in planning pain treatment (Acute Pain Management Guideline Panel, 1992).
- Unless contraindicated, obtain a prescription to administer a nonsteroidal anti-inflammatory drug (NSAID) on an around-the-clock schedule.
  The analgesic regimen should include a nonopioid drug, even if pain is severe enough to require the addition of an opioid (American Pain Society, 1992).
- Obtain a prescription to administer opioid analgesic if indicated; administer the analgesic by mouth or intravenously, not by injection. Use a preventive approach to keep pain at or below an acceptable level. Provide a patient-controlled analgesic intravenously or by another route when appropriate and available.
  When pain persists or increases, add an opioid to the NSAID. Use the simplest analgesic dosage schedules and the least invasive pain management modalities first. Avoid the intramuscular route because of unreliable absorption, pain, and inconvenience. Give analgesic around the clock (Jacox, 1994).

- When opioids are administered, assess pain intensity, sedation, and respiratory status on a regular basis.
  Because there is great individual variation in susceptibility to opioid-induced side effects, clinicians should monitor for these potential side effects (Jacox, 1994).
- Review the client's flow sheet and medication records to determine overall degree of pain relief, side effects, and analgesic requirements during the past 24 hours.
  Pain should be assessed at regular intervals to determine the efficacy of the drug interventions, the presence of side effects, or the need for dosage adjustments (Acute Pain Management Guideline Panel, 1992).
- Administer supplemental opioid doses as needed to keep pain ratings at or below an acceptable level.
  A prn order for a supplementary opioid dose between regular doses is an essential backup (American Pain Society, 1992).
- Obtain prescriptions to increase or decrease opioid doses as needed; base these dosage changes on the client's report of pain severity and response to the previous dose in terms of relief, side effects, and ability to perform the activities of recovery.
  Opioid doses should be adjusted in each client to achieve pain relief with an acceptable level of adverse effects (Jacox, 1994).
- As soon as it is feasible to do so, obtain a prescription to change to oral analgesic; use an equianalgesic chart to determine initial dose. Refer to Appendix D for an equianalgesic chart.
  The oral route is preferred because it is the most convenient and cost-effective (Jacox, 1994).
- Ask the client to describe appetite, bowel elimination, and ability to rest and sleep. Administer medications and treatments to improve these functions.
  Because there is great individual variation in the development of opioid-induced side effects, clinicians should monitor for them and prophylactically treat some inevitable ones (Jacox, 1994).

Geriatric

- When assessing pain speak clearly, slowly, and loudly enough for client to hear; repeat information as needed. Be sure client can see well enough to read pain scale and written materials.
- Handle client's body gently; allow client to move at own speed.
- Watch for side effects when using NSAIDs.
  Elders are at increased risk for gastric and renal toxicity from NSAIDs (Acute Pain Management Guideline Panel, 1992). Use NSAIDs with low side-effect profiles such as choline magnesium trisalicylate (Trilisate), diflunisal (Dolobid), and acetaminophen (American Pain Society, 1992; Acute Pain Management Guideline Panel, 1992).
- Use opioids with caution in the elderly client.
  Elders are more sensitive to the analgesic effects of opioid drugs because they experience a higher peak effect and a longer duration of pain relief. Reduce the initial opioid dose by 25% to 50% if the client is frail and debilitated; then increase the dose if safe and necessary (Acute Pain Management Guideline Panel, 1992).

Client/Family Teaching

NOTE: To avoid the negative connotations associated with words "drugs" or "narcotics," use the words "pain medicine" when teaching clients.

- Provide written materials on pain control such as the Agency for Health Care Policy and Research (AHCPR) pamphlet *Pain Control: Patient Guide.*

- Discuss the various discomforts encompassed by the word "pain" and ask client to give examples of pain previously experienced. Explain the pain assessment process and the purpose of the pain rating scale. Teach client to use the pain rating scale to rate the intensity of past or current pain. Ask client to set a pain relief goal by selecting a pain level on the rating scale; instruct client to take action to decrease pain or to notify a member of the health care team if pain increases above this level.
- Demonstrate medication administration and the use of supplies and equipment. If patient-controlled analgesia is ordered, determine client's ability to press the appropriate button.
- Reinforce the importance of taking pain medications to keep the pain under control.
- Reinforce that taking opioids for pain relief is not addiction and that addiction is very unlikely to occur.
- Demonstrate the use of appropriate nonpharmacological approaches for controling pain such as distraction techniques, relaxation breathing, visualization, rocking, stroking, music, and television.

REFERENCES

American Pain Society (APS): *Principles of analgesic use in the treatment of acute pain and cancer pain,* ed 3, Skokie, Ill, 1992, American Pain Society.

Acute Pain Management Guideline Panel: *Acute pain management operative or medical procedures and trauma. Clinical practice guideline,* Rockville, Md, Feb 1992. Agency for Health Care Policy and Research, Public Health Service, US Department of Health and Human Services, Public Health Service, AHCPR Pub. No. 92-0032.

Jacox A et al: *Management of cancer pain.* Rockville, Md, March 1994. Agency for Health Care Policy and Research, US Department of Health and Human Services, Public Health Service, *Clinical practice guideline No 9,* AHCPR Publication No. 94-0592.

McCaffery M: *Nursing practice theories related to cognition, bodily pain and man-environment interactions,* Los Angeles, 1968, University of California at Los Angeles Students' Store.

Chronic pain

Margo McCaffery and Christine Pasero

Definition Pain is whatever the experiencing person says it is, existing whenever he or she says it does (McCaffery, 1968).

The state in which an individual experiences pain that continues for more than 6 months.

NOTE: Some chronic pain syndromes are less than 6 months in duration.

Defining Characteristics

Verbal report of pain experienced for more than 6 months.

Subjective Pain is always subjective and cannot be proved or disproved. The client's report of pain is the most reliable indicator of pain (Acute Pain Management Guideline Panel, 1992). A client with cognitive ability who can speak or point should use a pain rating scale (e.g., 0 to 10) to identify current level of pain (self-report) and determine a pain rating goal.

Objective Expressions of pain are extremely variable and cannot be used in lieu of self-report. Neither behavior nor vital signs can substitute for the client's self-report (Acute Pain Management Guideline Panel, 1992); however, observable responses to pain are helpful in its assessment, especially in the client who cannot or will not use a self-report pain rating scale. Observable responses may be a loss of appetite and an altered ability to ambulate, perform activities of daily living, work, and sleep. The client may show guarded and self-protective behavior, self-focusing or narrowed focus, distraction behavior ranging from crying to laughing, and muscle tension or rigidity. In sudden severe pain, autonomic responses such as diaphoresis, blood pressure and pulse changes, pupillary dilation, and an increase or decrease in respiratory rate and depth may be present; however, these responses are usually not present with relatively stable chronic pain. Clients with chronic pain, cancer or nonmalignant, may experience a threat to their self-image, a perceived lack of options for coping, and worsening helplessness, anxiety, and depression (Jacox, 1994). Chronic pain may affect almost every aspect of the client's daily life, including concentration, work, and relationships.

Related Factors (r/t)

Actual or potential tissue damage; tumor progression and related pathology; diagnostic and therapeutic procedures.

NOTE: The cause of chronic nonmalignant pain may not be known, since pain is a new science and includes diverse types of pain problems.

Geriatric note: In spite of what many professionals and clients believe, pain is not an expected part of normal aging (Acute Pain Management Guideline Panel, 1992).

Client Outcomes/Goals

- Client with cognitive ability uses pain rating scale to identify current level of pain, determines a pain rating goal, and maintains a pain diary.
- Describes the total plan for drug and nondrug pain relief, including how to safely and effectively take medicines and integrate nondrug therapies.
- Demonstrates ability to pace himself or herself and take rest breaks before they are needed.
- Functions at an acceptable level of ability with minimal interference from pain and side effects.

Nursing Interventions and Rationales

- Determine if client is experiencing pain at the time of the initial interview; if so, intervene now to provide pain relief.
  Unrelieved pain causes unnecessary suffering (Jacox, 1994).

- Ask client to describe past and current experiences with pain and the effectiveness of the methods used to manage pain; ask about side effects, typical coping responses, and how client expresses pain.
  A pain history aids in planning and discussing pain control with the client. (Acute Pain Management Guideline Panel, 1992; Jacox, 1994).
- Describe the adverse effects of unrelieved pain.
  Pain prevents productive work, recreation, and enjoyment of the usual role in the family and society (Jacox, 1994).
- Tell the client to report pain location, intensity, and quality when experiencing pain.
  The single most reliable indicator of the existence and intensity of pain is the client's self-report (Acute Pain Management Guideline Panel, 1992).
- Ask client to maintain a diary of pain ratings, times, precipitating events, medications, treatments, and what works best to relieve pain.
  Plans should be made to ensure ongoing assessment of pain and treatment effectiveness in all care settings (Jacox, 1994).
- Explore the need for medications from the three classes of analgesics—opioids (narcotics), nonopioids, and adjuvant medications. For chronic neuropathic pain, consider adjuvants such as anticonvulsants and antidepressants, which are also analgesic.
  Some types of pain respond to nonopioid drugs alone; if not, consider adding an opioid at increasing doses for increasingly severe pain. At any level of pain, analgesic adjuvants may be useful (American Pain Society, 1992).
- Determine the client's current medication use.
  To aid in planning pain treatment, obtain a medication history (Acute Pain Management Guideline Panel, 1992).
- Unless contraindicated, obtain a prescription to administer a nonsteroidal anti-inflammatory drug (NSAID) on an around-the-clock schedule.
  The analgesic regimen should include a nonopioid drug, even if pain is severe enough to require the addition of an opioid (American Pain Society, 1992).
- For persistent cancer pain obtain a prescription to administer opioid analgesics.
  When pain persists or increases, an opioid such as codeine or hydrocodone should be added to the NSAID (Jacox, 1994).
- If the opioid dose is increased, briefly monitor client's sedation and respiratory status.
  A client receiving long-term opioid therapy generally develops a tolerance to the respiratory depressant effects of these agents (Jacox, 1994).
- Explain the prescribed pain management approach, including therapies, medication administration, side effects, and complications.
  One of the most important steps toward improved pain control is for the client to better understand the nature of pain, its treatment, and his or her role in pain control (Jacox, 1994).
- Discuss the client's fears of undertreated pain, addiction, and overdose.
  Because of the many misconceptions regarding pain and its treatment, education about the ability to control pain effectively and the correction of myths about opioid use should be included in the treatment plan. Opioid tolerance and physical dependence are expected with long-term opioid treatment and should not be confused with addiction (Jacox, 1994).

- Review the client's pain diary, flow sheet, and medication records to determine the overall degree of pain relief, side effects, and analgesic requirements over an appropriate time period (e.g., 1 week).
  Pain should be assessed at regular intervals to determine the efficacy of the drug interventions, the presence of side effects, or the need for dosage adjustments (Acute Pain Management Guideline Panel, 1992).
- Administer supplemental opioid doses as needed to keep pain ratings at or below an acceptable level.
  A prn order for a supplementary opioid dose between regular doses is an essential backup (American Pain Society, 1992).
- Obtain prescriptions to increase or decrease analgesic doses, as needed; base these changes on the client's report of pain severity, response to the previous dose in terms of relief and side effects, ability to perform the activities of living, and the prescribed therapeutic regimen.
  Opioid doses should be adjusted in each client to achieve pain relief with an acceptable level of adverse effects (Jacox, 1994).
- If client is on parenteral analgesia, use an equianalgesic chart to convert to an oral or other noninvasive route as smoothly as possible; refer to Appendix D.
  The oral route is the most preferred because it is the most convenient and cost-effective. Avoid the intramuscular route because of unreliable absorption, pain, and inconvenience (Jacox, 1994).
- In addition to the use of analgesics, support the client's use of nonpharmacological methods to control pain such as distraction, imagery, relaxation, massage, and heat and cold application.
  Cognitive-behavioral strategies can restore the client's sense of self-control, personal efficacy, and active participation in his or her own care (Jacox, 1994).
- Plan care activities around periods of greatest comfort whenever possible.
  Pain diminishes activity (Jacox, 1994).
- Ask the client to describe his appetite, bowel habits, and ability to rest and sleep. Administer medications and treatments directed toward improving these functions.
  Because there is great individual variation in the development of opioid-induced side effects, clinicians should monitor for them and prophylactically treat some inevitable ones (Jacox, 1994).
- Explore appropriate resources for long-term pain management (e.g., hospice, pain care center).
  Most clients with cancer or chronic nonmalignant pain are treated for pain in outpatient and home care settings. Plans should be made to ensure ongoing assessment of the pain and the effectiveness of treatments in these settings (Jacox, 1994).
- If the client has progressive cancer pain, help the client and the family to deal with issues related to death and dying.
  Peer support groups and pastoral counseling may increase the client's and family's coping skills and provide needed support (Jacox, 1994).
- If the client has chronic nonmalignant pain, assist the client and family with issues related to minimizing the effect of pain on interpersonal relationships and daily activities (e.g., work, recreation).
  Pain reduces the client's options to exercise control, diminishes psychological well-being, and leads to feelings of helplessness and vulnerability. Therefore clinicians

should support active client involvement in effective and practical methods of pain management (Jacox, 1994).

Geriatric

- Speak clearly, slowly, and loudly enough for client to hear; repeat information as needed. Be sure client can see well enough to read pain scale and written materials.
- When pain cannot be satisfactorily relieved, address own guilt about inability to relieve client's pain so that avoidance of the client or minimization of pain does not occur.
- Teach use of prophylactic medications (e.g., nitroglycerin).

Client/Family Teaching

NOTE: To avoid the negative connotations associated with the words "drugs" or "narcotics," use the words "pain medication" when teaching clients.

- Provide written materials regarding pain control, such as the Agency for Health Care Policy and Research (AHCPR) pamphlet, *Managing Cancer Pain, Patient Guide.*
- Discuss the various discomforts encompassed by the word "pain" and ask the client to give examples of pain previously experienced. Explain the pain assessment process and the purpose of the pain rating scale. Teach the client to use this scale to rate the intensity of past or current pain. Ask client to set a pain relief goal by selecting a pain level on the scale; instruct client to take action to decrease pain or to notify a member of the health care team if pain increases above this level.
- Discuss the total plan for drug and nondrug treatment, including medication administration, maintenance of a pain diary, and the use of supplies and equipment.
- Reinforce the importance of taking pain medications to control pain.
- Reinforce that taking opioids for pain relief is not addiction.
- Explain to the client with chronic neuropathic pain the process of taking tricyclic antidepressants (beginning with a low dose and increasing it gradually). Reinforce that pain relief is delayed and antidepressants must be taken daily. Reassure the client that, although the medicine is an antidepressant, it is being taken for analgesia, not depression. Comparable teaching should occur when an anticonvulsant is prescribed for analgesia.
- Reinforce to the client with chronic nonmalignant pain the importance of participating in a therapeutic regimen, (e.g., physical therapy, group therapy).
- Emphasize to the client the importance of pacing self and taking rest breaks before they are needed.
- Teach client and family distraction-coping techniques for pain management such as relaxation breathing, visualization, hobbies, yoga, meditation, massage, ice applications, exercise, and cutaneous stimulation (touch).
- Discuss the need for exercise to maintain strength, decrease stress, and promote sleep.

REFERENCES

American Pain Society (APS): *Principles of analgesic use in the treatment of acute pain and cancer pain,* ed 3, Skokie, Ill, 1992, American Pain Society.

Acute Pain Management Guideline Panel: *Acute pain management operative or medical procedures and trauma. Clinical practice guideline.* Rockville, Md, March 1992. Agency for Health Care Policy and Research, Public Health Service, US Department of Health and Human Services, Public Health Service, AHCPR Publication No. 92-0032.

Jacox A et al: *Management of cancer pain. Clinical practice guideline No 9.* Rockville, Md, March 1994. Agency for Health Care Policy and Research, US Department of Health and Human Services, Public Health Service, AHCPR Publication No. 94-0592.

McCaffery M: *Nursing practice theories related to cognition, bodily pain and man-environment interactions,* Los Angeles, 1968, University of California at Los Angeles Students' Store.

Risk for altered parent/infant/child attachment

Kathy Wyngarden

Definition Disruption of the interactive process between parent/significant other and infant/child that fosters the development of a protective and nurturing reciprocal relationship.

Defining Characteristics

Presence of risk factors such as inability of parents to meet personal needs; anxiety associated with the parent role; substance abuse; premature infant; ill infant or child who is unable to effectively initiate parental contact because of altered behavioral organization; separation; physical barriers; lack of privacy.

Client Outcomes/Goals

Parent

- Verbalizes feelings about perinatal experience, the infant or child, and the parenting role.
- Identifies unique characteristics of infant or child.
- Initiates interaction and bonding activities with infant or child (e.g., touching, cooing, face-to-face position, caregiving).
- Recognizes infant's or child's approach or withdrawal cues and responds appropriately.
- Identifies strengths and competencies related to parenting.

Infant/child

- Displays approach and interactive behaviors to parent.

Nursing Interventions and Rationales

- Encourage parent to personalize the infant (e.g., call by name, use specific voice or touch cuing, recognize unique characteristics and strengths, bring in clothes, toys, take photographs).
- Encourage parent to see, talk, touch, and hold infant or child, use skin-to-skin contact, and participate in care, as appropriate.
  Parents who participate in bonding activities and skin-to-skin activities are less likely to reject their infant (Hamelin, Ramachandran, 1993; Kemp, 1987; Tomlinson, 1989).
- Explore and validate feelings regarding birth characteristics of infant (e.g., joy, grief, anxiety, guilt).
  Repressed negative feelings can be transmitted to infant through parental behavior and interfere with attachment (Minde, 1980; Ross, 1980; Benfield, Lieb, Reutor, 1976; Boudreaux, 1981).
- Mutually identify responses such as anticipatory grieving and fear regarding poor prognosis and intervene as appropriate (e.g., explore, assess support system, counsel, teach, have parent keep journal).
  Parents often withhold emotional and active involvement until they have a sense that the infant will survive (Kaplan, Mason, 1960; McHaffie, 1990).
- Acknowledge parental identity and facilitate active involvement in support groups and/or extended family.
  There are multiple barriers to the parent seeing self as a parent. If maternal identity is not recognized, input from others is necessary for the mother to see herself as a mother (Zabielski, 1994). Supportive interventions for parents increases visiting and involvement in the parental role (Minde, 1980). Family-centered care is essential since infant and parents are integral members (Lewis et al, 1991; Goodfriend, 1993).
- Develop a mentoring relationship with the parent by encouraging him or her to recognize strengths and competencies as a parent.
  Parental self-esteem and confidence enhance the parent-infant relationship (Lyons-Ruth, Zeanuh, 1993; Lindsay et al, 1993).

- Encourage parent to recognize, interpret, and respond to infant's or child's behaviors in a reciprocal way.
  It is important for parents to know that an infant's inability to respond at times is not a reflection on them. Recognition of the infant as an individual is positively correlated to attachment (Als, 1982; Holaday, 1991; Denehy, 1992).

Client/Family Teaching

- Teach recognition of normal physical and behavioral characteristics of a term or preterm infant.
- Teach how to recognize and support infant's or child's unique self-regulatory and coping strategies.
- Teach developmentally appropriate positioning and handling techniques.
- Teach techniques that modulate the infant or child state.
- Teach the importance of bonding and attachment of infant and child and parent.

REFERENCES

Als H: Toward a synactive theory of development: promise for the assessment and support of infant individuality, *Infant Ment Health J* 2:229-243, 1982.

Benfield D, Lieb S, Reutor J: Grief responses of parents following referral of the critically ill newborn, *N Engl J Med* 194:975-978, 1976.

Boudreaux M. Maternal attachment of high-risk mothers with well newborns: a pilot study, *JOGNN* 10:366-369, 1981.

Denehy J: Interventions related to parent-infant attachment, *Nurs Intervent* 27:425-433, 1992.

Goodfriend MS: Treatment of attachment disorders of infancy in a neonatal intensive care unit, *Pediatrics* 91:139-142, 1993.

Hamelin K, Ramachandran C: Kangaroo care, *Can Nurse* 89:15-17, 1993.

Holaday B: Maternal responses to their chronically ill infants' attachment behavior of crying, *Nurs Res* 30:343-348, 1981.

Kaplan D, Mason E: Maternal reactions to premature birth viewed as an acute emotional disorder, *Am J Orthopsychiatry* 30:539-552, 1960.

Kemp VH: Mothers' perceptions of children's temperament and mother child attachment, *Sch Inquiry Nurs Pract Int J* 1:51-68, 1987.

Lindsay J et al: Creative caring in the NICU parent to parent support, *Neonatal Network* 12:37-44, 1993.

Lewis M et al: Visitation to a neonate intensive care unit, *Pediatrics* 4:795-800, 1991.

Lyons-Ruth K, Zeanuh CH: The family context of infant mental health: affective development in the primary care relationship. In CH Zeanuh, editor: *Handbook of infant mental health,* New York, 1993, Guildford Press.

McHaffie H: Mothers of very low birth weight babies: how do they adjust? *J Adv Nurs* 15:6-11, 1990.

Minde GS: Bonding of parents to premature infants: theory and practice. In PM Taylor, editor: *Parent-infant relationships,* New York, 1980, Grune & Stratton.

Ross GS: Parental responses to infants in intensive care: the separation issue reevaluated, *Clin Perinatol* 7:47-60, 1980.

Tomlinson PS: Verbal behavior associated with indicators of maternal attachment with the neonate, *JOGNN* 18:133-141, 1989.

Zabielski M: Recognition of maternal identity in preterm and fullterm mothers, *Matern Child Nurs J* 22:2-36, 1994.

BIBLIOGRAPHY

Cusson R, Lee A: Parental interventions and the development of the preterm infant, *JOGNN* 23:60-68, 1993.

Klaus MH, Kennell JH: *Parent-infant bonding,* St Louis, Mosby.

Parental role conflict

Catherine Vincent

Definition The state in which a parent experiences role confusion and conflict in response to a crisis.

Defining Characteristics

Major Expresses concerns or feelings of inadequacy regarding the ability to provide for child's physical and emotional needs during hospitalization or at home; demonstrates disruption in caretaking routines; expresses concerns about changes in parental role, family functioning, family communication, or family health.

Minor Expresses concern about perceived loss of control regarding decisions relating to child; reluctant to participate in usual caretaking activities, even with encouragement and support; verbalizes or demonstrates feelings of guilt, anger, fear, anxiety, frustration concerning the effect of the child's illness on family processes.

Related factors (r/t)

Separation from child as a result of chronic illness; intimidation by invasive or restrictive modalities (e.g., isolation, intubation, specialized care center policies); home care of child with special needs (e.g., apnea monitoring, postural drainage, hyperalimentation); change in marital status; interruptions of family life due to home-care regimens (e.g., treatments, caregivers, lack of respite).

Client Outcomes/Goals

- States positive feelings regarding care of child's physical and emotional needs during hospitalization.
- Able to carry out caretaking routines or describe an alternative plan to use during child's hospitalization.
- Participates in care of child.

Nursing Interventions and Rationales

- Assess for any contributing factors or concurrent stressors; refer to defining characteristics and related factors. Consider cultural influences.
- Assess the parent's understanding of family member's illness or crisis and its effect on family functioning.
  A thorough data base is needed to develop nursing interventions and identify strengths and limitations.
- Assess parent's prior coping behaviors.
  Use of prior effective coping behaviors gives the parent a feeling of competence. Identifying ineffective or absent coping behaviors allows development of interventions. Research indicates that a parent who copes successfully is better able to promote the adjustment and recovery of the child (Ladebauche, 1992).
- Identify the parent's needs and concerns and together develop nursing interventions.
  Nursing care is developed in collaboration with the parent. Paying attention to parental observations helps assure the parent that his or her role is important and opinions are valuable (Baker, 1994).
- Encourage and facilitate identification of resources and use of support systems.
  Helping the family to identify resources and support systems facilitates their use, relieves the parent of the burden of child care, and reduces anxiety. Social support lets a person know he or she is loved, cared for, and valued (Austin, 1990; Baker, 1994).
- Plan parental programs geared to the age-appropriate parental concerns: birth to 2 years (transition, sleep, aggression); 3 to 5 years (transition, parent-child relationship, sleep); 6 to 10 years (school, parent-child relationship, divorce); 11 to 18 years (parent-child relationship, divorce, school).

Parents with children of any age seek basic information about a variety of concerns: the nurse can provide ongoing information and support in many areas (Jones, Maestre, McCoy, 1993).

- Determine older mother's support systems and self-expectations of motherhood. Pay particular attention to relationships with spouse or partner, family, and friends.
  Social support has a positive influence to early parenting for primiparas over 35 years of age. Older primiparas with high self-expectations, low satisfaction with parenting, or inadequate social support systems may be at risk (Reece, 1994).
- Be available to discuss concerns; be a good listener.
  The parent is more likely to verbalize concerns when the nurse is not hurried. Open communication is essential for the identification of potential coping problems (Ladebauche, 1992).
- Encourage parent to verbalize feelings and ask questions; help parent recognize normal and healthy responses to stress and conflicts.
  The parent may be reluctant to verbalize feelings that he or she thinks are inappropriate. Helping the parent recognize the normal responses diminishes emotional burdens and allows the nurse to identify feelings that may interfere with learning.
- Structure environment to facilitate parent's comfort.
- Encourage parent to meet own needs of rest, nutrition, and hygiene. Provide facilities so parent may stay with sick child (e.g., cot, reclining chair). Encourage respite from caregiving duties.
  A parent is unable to meet the child's needs when the basic self-needs are unmet.
- Encourage parental involvement in care of child. If possible, arrange unrestricted visiting hours.
- Demonstrate safe places where parent may touch or stroke child. Encourage parent to talk or sing to child. Adjust equipment so that parent is able to hold child; provide a comfortable chair, preferably a rocking chair. Provide opportunities for successful caregiving and offer praise when it is done.
  Involvement in child's care will give the parent a sense of control in the hospital environment.
- Allow parent to bring in familiar items to make the health setting homelike (e.g., favorite toys, pictures, clothing).
- If possible encourage visitation and caregiving by siblings.
- Refer to available telephone counseling services.
  Telephone counseling services can provide confidential advice to families who might otherwise have no access to help in dealing with a child's problems (Jones, Maestri, McCoy, 1993).

Client/Family Teaching

- Provide a clear explanation about the disease, its treatment and prognosis, the child's emotional and physical reaction to illness and hospitalization, and the probable reaction of family members to the crisis. Give a clear explanation of what is expected of the parent. Allow parent to practice skills until comfortable with them. Provide parent with available written materials. Repeat explanations as often as necessary and clarify any misconceptions.
  Providing information to families decreases confusion and anxiety, increases understanding, and allows a feeling of competence and control. Providing information about the disease and treatment process helps build the parent's feelings of confidence (Baker, 1994).

- Refer to home health agencies that specialize in the care needed by the child.
- Refer to social service agencies (e.g., crippled children) for financial support in modifying the home to meet child's health care needs.
- Refer to available counseling and support groups for coping with the chronically ill. *Support groups provide a nonthreatening environment for a parent to express concerns and feelings, and they help diminish the sense of isolation and guilt often felt by the parent of a sick child. Support groups also help the parent cope with the stressors of parenting (Ladebauche, 1992).*
- Refer to nursing interventions and rationales for **Altered parenting**.

REFERENCES

Austin JK: Assessment of coping mechanisms used by parents and children with chronic illness. *MCN* 15:98-102, 1990.

Baker NA: Avoid collisions with challenging families, *MCN* 19:97-101, 1994.

Jones LC, Maestri BO, McCoy K: Why parents use the warm line, *MCN* 18:258-263, 1993.

Ladebauche P: Unit-based family support groups: a reminder, *MCN* 17:18-21, 1992.

Reece SM: Social support and the early maternal experience of primiparas over 35, *Matern Child Nurs J* 21:91-91, 1994.

Altered parenting

Catherine Vincent

Definition The state in which a nurturing figure experiences an inability to create an environment that promotes the optimum growth and development of another human being.

Defining Characteristics

Abandonment; runaway child; inability to control child; incidence of physical and psychological trauma; lack of parental attachment behaviors; inappropriate visual, tactile, and auditory stimulation; negative identification of infant's or child's characteristics; negative attachment of meanings to infant's or child's characteristics; constant verbalization of disappointment about gender or physical characteristics of the infant or child; verbalization of resentment towards the infant or child; verbalization of role inadequacy; *inattentiveness to infant or child needs; verbal disgust at bodily functions of infant or child; noncompliance with health appointments for self, infant, or child; *inappropriate caretaking behavior (e.g., toilet training, sleep, rest, or feeding); inappropriate or inconsistent discipline practices; frequent accidents; frequent illnesses; growth and development lag in the child; *history of child abuse or abandonment by primary caretaker; verbalized desire to have child call parent by first name vs. traditional cultural tendencies; child care given by multiple caretakers without consideration for the needs of the infant or child; compulsive seeking of role approval from others. (*Critical)

Related Factors (r/t)

Lack of available role models; ineffective role models; physical and psychosocial abuse of nurturing figure; lack of support from significant others; unmet social, emotional, and maturational needs of parenting figures; interruption in bonding process (e.g., maternal, paternal); unrealistic expectations of self, infant, or partner; perceived threat to own physical and emotional survival; mental or physical illness; presence of stressors (e.g., finances, legal issues, recent crisis, cultural move); lack of knowledge; limited cognitive functioning; lack of role identity; absent or inappropriate response of child to relationship; multiple pregnancies.

Client Outcomes/Goals

- Initiates bonding process.
- Verbalizes the need to provide a nurturing environment for the child or infant.
- Provides a nurturing environment that promotes the optimum growth and development of the infant or child.

Nursing Interventions and Rationales

- Assess parenting style, interaction with child, and other contributing factors. Refer to defining characteristics and related factors.
  The nurse needs thorough baseline data to develop a plan of care.
- Assess infant's readiness to bond or child's ability to receive parental attention; discuss these abilities with parents.
  Infants give clues to the caregiver that signal needs. An ill or developmentally impaired infant may not emit cues consistent with maternal expectations (Denehy, 1992).
- Assess parent's knowledge of developmental needs.
  If parent does not know what is normal for a child, the parent may have unrealistic expectations for him or her (Denehy, 1992).
- Allow parent to express feelings about infant or child.
- Provide an atmosphere of acceptance; listen attentively.
  It is normal for a parent to have negative feelings about a child, especially a child who has a developmental delay or dysfunction. Underlying feelings must be recognized before learning can be effective.

- Identify and encourage aspects of bonding strength.
  Encouragement strengthens behavior.
- Provide early and repeated parent-infant contact. Identify specific behaviors that can improve bonding.
  Lack of appropriate bonding may be a result of many factors, including a lack of information and contact.
- Orient parent to hospital, unit, and staff.
  Knowledge increases comfort and allows the parent to feel welcome.
- Encourage parent to meet basic self-needs.
  It is exhausting to care for a hospitalized child. A parent who is not meeting his or her own needs of rest, nutrition, and hygiene will be ineffective in caring for the child.
- Encourage parental involvement in care, especially feeding, diapering, and comforting. Assist parent with any interferences (e.g., IVs, monitors).
  Promotion of parenting skills increases confidence and the parent's feelings of control.
- Encourage parent to touch, talk to, hold, and kiss the child.
  Such behaviors are known to promote bonding in infants and comfort in children.
- Provide strategies to reduce separation. Liberalize visiting hours.
  These steps allow maximum contact time with the child.
- Model appropriate behavior for parent.
  Role modeling provides the parent with a visual picture of appropriate behavior.
- Assess parent's resources and availability of support systems, and encourage their use.
  Before adequate interventions can be initiated, the nurse must understand the parent's current support system and concerns (Zacharia, 1994).
- Determine single woman's particular sources of support, especially the availability of her own mother and her partner.
  The mother's own mother and partner are often important sources of support (Zacharia, 1994).
- For mothers with toddlers, assess maternal depression, perceived toddler temperament, and low parental self-efficacy. Self-efficacy is defined as one's judgment of how effectively one can execute a task or manage a situation that may contain novel, unpredictable, and stressful elements.
  A cyclic relationship among depression, perceived difficult temperament, and self-efficacy has been found in mothers or toddlers. Negative feelings about oneself and one's child are likely to negatively influence the parent-child relationship (Gross et al, 1994).
- Determine amount of stress in the family environment, watch for signs of parental substance abuse, and note if the family unit seems isolated from society. Refer to agencies for help with these problems as needed.
  Children are at risk for abuse in families with stress, drug or alcohol abuse, or unrealistic expectations of the child's behavior. A socially isolated parent is more likely to abuse a child (Devlin, Reynolds, 1994). Use of support systems and social services helps allay parental feelings of inadequacy (Baker, 1994).
- Document parent-child interactions.
  Precise documentation is important for communicating with other health care providers and providing legal evidence, if necessary.
- Refer to available telephone counseling services.
  Telephone counseling services can provide confidential advice to families who might otherwise have no access to help in dealing with a child's problems (Jones, Maestri, McCoy, 1993).

Client/Family Teaching

- Provide needed information pertaining to normal growth and developmental behaviors.
  Knowledge of expected behaviors for children reduces unrealistic expectations.
- Teach parenting skills as necessary.
  A parent may feel powerless; helping the parent develop necessary skills or knowledge maintains the integrity of the parental role; and the parent is then less likely to use maladaptive coping styles (Baker, 1994).
- Plan parental programs geared to the following age-appropriate parental concerns: birth to 2 years (transition, sleep, aggression); 3 to 5 years (transition, parent-child relationship, sleep); 6 to 10 years (school, parent-child relationship, divorce); 11 to 18 years (parent-child relationship, divorce, school).
  Parents with children of any age seek basic information about a variety of concerns; the nurse can provide ongoing information and support in many areas (Jones, Maestri, McCoy, 1993).
- Teach stress management.
  Because increased stress is related to child abuse, controling stress may prevent such abuse.
- Refer to support services as needed (e.g., community health nurse, social services, counseling, child protective agencies); refer to support groups.
  The parent needs support to manage angry or inappropriate behaviors. If abuse is suspected, protective services are needed.
- Refer newborns for home-care follow-up.
  As a result of shortened hospital stays, there is inadequate time to assist the parent with new roles (Denehy, 1992).

REFERENCES

Baker NA: Avoid collisions with challenging families, *MCN* 19:97-101, 1994.

Denehy JA: Intervention related to parent-infant attachment, *Nurs Clin North Am* 27:425-433, 1992.

Devlin BK, Reynolds E: Child abuse: how to recognize it, how to intervene, *Am J Nurs* 94:26-31, 1994.

Gross D et al: A longitudinal model of maternal self-efficacy, depression, and difficult temperament during toddlerhood, *Res Nurs Health* 17:207-215, 1994.

Jones LC, Maestri BO, McCoy K: Why parents use the warm line, *MCN* 18:258-263, 1993.

Zachria R: Perceived social support and social network of low-income mothers of infants and preschoolers: pre- and postparenting program, *J Comm Health Nurs* 11:11-20, 1994.

Risk for altered parenting

Definition The state in which a nurturing figure is at risk to experience an inability to create an environment that promotes the optimum growth and development of another human being.

Defining Characteristics

Presence of risk factors such as lack of parental attachment behaviors; inappropriate visual, tactile, or auditory stimulation; negative identification of infant's or child's characteristics; negative attachment of meanings to infant's or child's characteristics; constant verbalization of disappointment about gender or physical characteristics of the infant or child; verbalization of resentment towards the infant or child; verbalization of role inadequacy; *inattentiveness to infant's or child's needs; verbal disgust at bodily functions of infant or child; noncompliance with health appointments for self, infant, or child; *inappropriate caretaking behaviors (e.g., toilet training, sleep, rest, feeding); inappropriate or inconsistent discipline practices; frequent accidents; frequent illnesses; growth and development lag in the child; history of child abuse or abandonment by primary caretaker; verbalized desire to have child call parent by first name vs. traditional cultural tendencies; child care given by multiple caretakers without consideration for the needs of the infant or child; compulsive seeking of role approval from others. (*Critical)

Related Factors (r/t)

Lack of available role models; ineffective role models; physical and psychosocial abuse of nurturing figure; lack of support from significant others; unmet social, emotional, or maturational needs of parenting figures; interruption in bonding process (e.g., maternal, paternal); unrealistic expectations for self, infant, or partner; perceived threat to own physical and emotional survival; mental or physical illness; presence of stressors (e.g., finances, legal issues, recent crisis, cultural move); lack of knowledge; limited cognitive functioning; lack of role identity; absent or inappropriate response of child to relationship; multiple pregnancies.

Client Outcomes/Goals, Nursing Interventions and Rationales, and Client/Family Teaching

Refer to **Altered parenting**.

Risk for perioperative positioning injury

Pamela Emery

Definition The state in which an individual is at risk for injury as a result of the environmental conditions found in the perioperative setting.

Defining Characteristics

Position selected for surgical clients that provides access to the surgical site and to the airway for the administration of anesthetic, and that maintains normal body alignment and function.

Presence of risk factors such as age; weight; nutritional status; preexisting conditions (e.g., diabetes, vascular disease, arthritis, malignancy); effects of anesthetic; duration of procedure. As a result of these factors, there may be a potential for impaired tissue perfusion, impaired skin integrity, or neuromuscular or joint injury related to surgical positioning.

Related Factors (r/t)

Refer to risk factors.

Complications of Surgical Positioning

The systems most frequently affected by surgical positioning are the neurological, musculoskeletal, integumentary, respiratory, and cardiovascular.

Transient physiological reactions to surgical positioning include skin redness, lumbar backache, stiffness in the limbs and neck, and generalized muscle aches that usually resolve within 24 to 48 hours without treatment (Walsh, 1993).

More serious complications of surgical positioning include pressure sores; peripheral nerve injury; deep venous thrombosis; compartment syndrome (impairment of microcirculation in soft tissue); joint injury (Paschal, Strzelecki, 1992; Walsh, 1993).

Client Outcomes/Goals

- Free of injury related to positioning during the surgical procedure.

Nursing Interventions and Rationales

NOTE: Nursing interventions are based on assessing the client for the existence of or potential for injury to any of the above-mentioned systems on the basis of observed or elicited risk factors.

Supine Position (dorsal recumbent)

- Pad all bony prominences (e.g., head, elbows, sacrum, heels) and positioning devices.
  Bony prominences exert pressure on overlying tissue, which predisposes the client to the development of pressure ulcers (Rothrock, 1990). Nerves that pass over or near bony prominences may be injured by compression (Walsh, 1993).
- Support lumbar and popliteal areas.
  Maintaining normal lumbar concavity prevents muscle strain. Support under the knees prevents muscle and ligament strain (Rothrock, 1990).
- Use a firm foam rubber support or padded footboard that extends beyond toes.
  A support or footboard prevents plantar flexion and protects the toes from the weight and pressure of draping materials (Meeker, Rothrock, 1991).
- Use padded foot boards and shoulder braces when Trendelenburg's position or reverse Trendelenburg's position is required.
  Positioning aids help prevent skin injury from shearing forces (opposite parallel force between skin and subcutaneous tissue) (Rothrock, 1990).

NOTE: Either of these two positions (Trendelenburg or reverse Trendelenburg) may have adverse effects on both the circulatory and respiratory systems, which in most circumstances are monitored and controlled by anesthesia personnel. Modifications of both positions may be suggested and implemented by the nurse in collaboration with the surgeon and anesthesiologist.

- Position client's arms with palms up on armboards at less than a 90-degree angle to the body.
  Hyperabduction may damage the brachial plexus and stretch the subclavian and axillary vessels (AORN, 1994; Walsh, 1993).
- Position arms at sides of the body with palms against the body, or pronate and secure arms with a broad lift sheet without flexing the elbow.
  Tucking the arms prevents compression of the fingers if allowed to extend over the edge of the operating table, maintains proper alignment, and prevents compression of the ulnar nerve (Meeker, Rothrock, 1991).
- Protect skin from direct contact with any metal surfaces.
  Faulty or improperly grounded electrosurgical units may seek an alternative pathway through any skin surface in contact with metal and result in an electrical burn (Rothrock, 1990).
- When positioning client, lift rather than pull or slide.
  Sliding and pulling increase the incidence of skin injury from shearing and friction.
- Maintain alignment of head with cervical, thoracic, and lumbar spine.
  Misalignment, flexion, and twisting may cause muscle and nerve damage and airway interference (Meeker, Rothrock, 1991).
- Position client's legs parallel and uncrossed.
  Compression from crossed ankles may injure peroneal and tibial nerves and impede circulation (Walsh, 1993).
- Place leg restraint strap (safety belt) 2 inches above knees.
  Clients may become disoriented and attempt to change position on the narrow operating table.

Prone Position (modifications: kneeling, jackknife, or Kraske position)

- Provide an adequate number of personnel to accomplish "logroll" turning of the anesthetized client.
  Movement and positioning from the supine to the prone position may be safely undertaken by four persons (Meeker, Rothrock, 1991).
- Place chest rolls from clavicles to iliac crests.
  Chest rolls allow for lung expansion and free movement of the diaphragm, and they decrease pressure on female breast tissue (Meeker, Rothrock, 1991; Walsh, 1993).
- Place a bolster or pillow under the pelvis.
  Support of the pelvis decreases abdominal pressure on the inferior vena cava and male genitalia (Meeker, Rothrock, 1991).
- Place a bolster or pillow under client's ankles.
  A cushion prevents plantar flexion and pressure on the toes (Rothrock, 1990).
- Guide client's arms down and forward to rest on armboards that are extended forward from the operating table. Ensure that client's elbows are flexed and padded and hands are placed palm down.
  This movement prevents shoulder dislocation and brachial plexus injury, and padding prevents ulnar and radial nerve compression (Meeker, Rothrock, 1991; Walsh, 1993).
- Place head on foam donut or padded headrest; protect client's ears and eyes.
  Ear cartilage may be damaged if the ear folds or is bent. Corneal abrasions may occur if the eyes are not closed and secured during maneuvering and positioning (Meeker, Rothrock, 1991).

- Avoid severe rotation of client's head to one side.
  Severe head rotation may stretch skeletal muscles and ligaments, causing postoperative pain and limited motion after surgery (Walsh, 1993).

Lateral Position (lateral chest or kidney)

- Provide adequate personnel to properly position the client.
  Lateral positioning requires a four-person team to safely move the client from the supine position (Rothrock, 1990).
- Use a lift sheet to facilitate the turn.
  Lift sheets prevent skin injury resulting from shearing.
- Place a support under the head.
  A pillow or support keeps the head properly aligned with the cervical spine and thoracic vertebrae (Meeker, Rothrock, 1991; Walsh, 1993).
- Flex the bottom leg at the hip and knee.
  Flexing the bottom leg provides a base of support to hold the body in position (Rothrock, 1990).
- Place beanbags, sandbags, or bolsters against the back and abdomen.
  Additional positioning devices provide support and maintain body alignment (Meeker, Rothrock, 1991).
- Pad the lateral aspect of the bottom knee.
  Pressure of the knee against the operating bed may injure the peroneal nerve (Walsh, 1993).
- Place a pillow between the client's legs lengthwise so that the pillow also supports the foot.
  Pressing the bony prominences of one extremity against the other may cause injury to the peroneal and tibial nerves. If the foot extends beyond the pillow it may drop, causing damage to muscles and joints (Meeker, Rothrock, 1991; Walsh, 1993).
- Pad the lower shoulder and bring it forward slightly; the lower arm is extended on a padded armboard.
  All bony prominences should be padded to prevent tissue breakdown. Bringing the shoulder forward relieves pressure on the brachial plexus (Walsh, 1993).
- Place the upper arm on a padded raised armboard or padded Mayo stand.
  Raising the upper arm elevates the scapula and widens the intercostal spaces, which provides access to the upper thoracic cavity (Rothrock, 1990).
- Place an axillary roll at the apex of the scapula in the axillary space of the dependent arm.
  A soft roll relieves pressure on the arm and facilitates chest expansion (Meeker, Rothrock, 1991; AORN, 1994).

NOTE: Some surgeons prefer the use of wide adhesive tape to secure the hips, arms, and legs. This practice would be contraindicated in clients with tape allergies or in the frail elderly with fragile skin.

Lithotomy Position

- Loosely secure client's arms across the abdomen or extend on padded armboards.
  Arms must not be placed at the client's sides since the table will be "broken" for the procedure, and fingers may extend beyond the break (Meeker, Rothrock, 1991; Rothrock, 1990).
- Pad the sacral area and provide a small lumbar roll.
  Bony prominences must be padded to prevent soft tissue damage. A lumbar roll helps maintain normal lumbar concavity (AORN, 1994; Meeker, Rothrock, 1991).

- Place client's legs in the stirrups simultaneously.
  Raising the legs together requires two persons and helps prevent stress on hip joints (Walsh, 1993).
- Lower client's legs simultaneously and slowly.
  Blood pools result from this position, and lowering the legs slowly helps decrease the hypotension experienced (Paschal, Strzelecki, 1992).
- Avoid acute flexion of the thigh. Acute flexion of the thigh increases intra-abdominal pressure against the diaphragm, thus decreasing tidal volume, which is a more pronounced problem in the obese client (Meeker, Rothrock, 1991).
  Severe flexion may also strain the lumbar spine, damage the prosthetic hip joint, and cause nerve damage (Walsh, 1993).
- Pad all bony prominences and surfaces that may contact the leg support system.
  Pressure on the lateral aspect of the knee may damage the peroneal nerve (Paschal, Strzelecki, 1992).
  Contact with metal at any point during use of the electrosurgical unit may result in an electrical burn (Rothrock, 1990).
  Compression of soft tissue may predispose client to venous thrombosis; prolonged compression may result in compartment syndrome (Paschal, Strzelecki, 1992).

NOTE: If assessment reveals conditions that place the client at increased risk for injury in this position, positioning complications may be prevented by attempting this position while the client is awake and able to report any discomfort.

REFERENCES

Association of Operating Room Nurses: *AORN standards and recommended practices for perioperative nursing,* Denver, 1994, The Association of Operating Room Nurses.

Meeker M, Rothrock J: *Alexander's care of the patient in surgery,* ed 9, St Louis, 1991, Mosby.

Paschal C, Strzelecki L: Lithotomy positioning devices, factors that contribute to patient injury, *AORN J* 55:1011, 1992.

Rothrock J: *Perioperative nursing care planning,* St Louis, 1990, Mosby.

Walsh J: Postoperative effects of O.R. positioning, *RN* 56:50, 1993.

Risk for peripheral neurovascular dysfunction

Betty Ackley

Definition The state in which an individual is at risk of experiencing a disruption in circulation, sensation, or motion.

Related Factors (r/t)

Fractures; mechanical compression (e.g., tourniquet, cast, brace, dressing, restraints); orthopedic surgery; trauma; immobilization; burns; vascular obstruction.

Client Outcomes/Goals

- Circulation, sensation, and movement of an extremity within client's normal limits.
- Explains signs of neurovascular compromise and ways to prevent venous stasis.

Nursing Interventions and Rationales

- Perform neurovascular assessment q___h or minutes. Use the five Ps of assessment:

  Pain—Assess severity (on scale of 1 to 10), quality, radiation, and relief by medications.
  Pain that is unrelieved by medication can be an early symptom of compartment syndrome or may indicate that client needs more effective pain medication (Dykes, 1993).

  Pulses—Check the pulses distal to the injury. Check uninjured side first to establish a baseline for a bilateral comparison.
  An intact pulse generally indicates a good blood supply to the extremity (Dykes, 1993).

  Pallor—Check color and temperature changes below the fracture site. Check capillary refill.
  A cold, pale, or bluish extremity indicates arterial insufficiency or arterial damage. Normal capillary refill is 3 seconds (Dykes, 1993).

  Parasthesia (change in sensation)—Check by lightly touching the skin proximal and distal to the injury. Refer to the following chart for guidelines on how to best assess sensation. Ask if client has any unusual sensations such as hypersensitivity, tingling, prickling, decreased feelings, or numbness accompanied by a lack of sensation.
  Changes in sensation are indicative of nerve compression and damage and can also indicate compartment syndrome (Dykes, 1993).

  Paralysis—Ask client to do appropriate range of motion in the unaffected and then the affected extremity. Refer to the following chart.

How to Check for Nerve Damage with Common Fractures

Fracture	Nerve Damaged	Sensation	Motion
Humerus	Radial	Check over dorsum of index finger	Ask to hyperextend thumb
Radial	Radial	See above	See above
	Medial	Check over palmar surface of fingers	Ask to touch thumb to tip of little finger
Ulnar	Ulnar	Check little finger to ring finger	Ask to spread fingers
Femoral	Peroneal	Check over top foot between 1st and 2nd toes	Ask to point toes toward head
Fibular	Peroneal	See above	See above
Tibial	Tibial	Ask if medial side of sole of foot feels warm	Ask to point toes downward

(Dykes, 1993).

- Monitor client for symptoms of compartment syndrome evidenced by decreased sensation, weakness, loss of movement, pain with passive movement, pain greater than expected, pulselessness, and tenseness of the skin that surrounds the muscle compartment.
  Compartment syndrome is characterized by increased pressure within the compartment, which compromises circulation, viability, and function of tissues (Slye, 1991; Andrews, 1993).
- Monitor appropriate application and function of corrective device (e.g., cast, splint, traction) q____h.
- Position extremity in correct alignment with each position change; check q____h to ensure appropriate alignment.
- Monitor for signs of deep vein thrombosis evidenced by pain, deep tenderness, swelling, and redness in the involved extremity, usually the calf. If there is no sensation in the area, take serial leg measurements of the thigh and leg circumferences. Do not rely on Homan's sign.
  Thrombosis with clot formation is usually first detected as swelling of the involved leg and then as pain. Leg measurement discrepancies greater than 2 cm warrant further investigation. Homan's sign is not reliable (Slye, 1991; Herzog, 1992).
- Monitor for any signs of infection (e.g., edema, warmth, elevated temperature or white blood cell count).
- Help client perform prescribed exercises q____h.
- Provide a nutritious diet and adequate fluid replacement.
  Good nutrition and sufficient fluids are needed to promote healing and prevent complications.

Geriatric

- Use heat and cold therapies cautiously.
  Elderly clients often have decreased sensation and circulation.

Client/Family Teaching

- Teach client and family to recognize signs of neurovascular dysfunction and to report signs immediately to the appropriate person.
- Emphasize proper nutrition to promote healing.
- If necessary, refer to rehabilitation facility for proper use of assistive devices and measures to improve mobility without compromising neurovascular function.

REFERENCES

Andrews HA: Common musculoskeletal interventions. In *Luckmann and Sorensen's Medical-surgical nursing: a psychophysiologic approach,* Philadelphia, 1993, WB Saunders.

Dykes PC: Minding the five *p*'s of neurovascular assessment, *Am J Nurs* 93(6):38-39, 1993.

Herzog JA: Deep vein thrombosis in the rehabilitation client, *Rehabil Nurs* 17:196-197, 1992.

Slye DA: Orthopedic complications: compartment syndrome, fat embolism syndrome, and venous thromboembolism, *Nurs Clin North Am* 26:113-128, 1991.

BIBLIOGRAPHY

Donnor C: Critical difference: detecting venous thrombosis, *Am J Nurs* 93:48, 1993.

Personal identity disturbance

Gail Ladwig

Definition The inability to distinguish between self and nonself.

Defining Characteristics

Withdrawal from social contact; change in ability to determine relationship of body to environment; inappropriate or grandiose behavior (adapted from Carpenito).

Related Factors (r/t)

Situational crisis; psychological impairment; chronic illness; pain.

Client Outcomes/Goals

- Shows interest in surroundings.
- Responds to stimuli with appropriate affect.
- Performs self-care and self-control activities appropriate for age.
- Acknowledges personal strengths.
- Engages in interpersonal relationships.
- Verbalizes willingness to change life-style and use appropriate community resources.

Nursing Interventions and Rationales

- Address client by name; let client know who is approaching and orient him or her to surroundings.
  These interventions help a client with a loss of ego boundaries to identify the boundaries between himself or herself and the environment (Haber et al, 1992).
- Have client describe his or her perceptions of the environment as concretely as possible.
  These descriptions provide feedback that confirms the client's existence.
- Use touch only after a thorough assessment.
  Some clients may touch people to identify separateness from others; other clients experience fusion with others when they touch (Haber et al, 1992).
- Have all team members approach client in a consistent manner.
  Consistency promotes trust, which is necessary in establishing a therapeutic relationship that helps the client develop interpersonal relationships.
- Provide time for one-to-one interactions to establish a therapeutic relationship.
  The one-to-one relationship provides the basis for a therapeutic relationship and includes the use of "self."
- Encourage client to verbalize feelings about self and body image; have client make a list of positive strengths.
  These verbalizations help the client recognize "self"; listing strengths aids the client in self-exploration.
- Hold client responsible for age-appropriate behavior; involve client in planning of self-care.
  Involving client in care gives him or her a sense of control and helps the client gain "ego strength" (Preston, 1994).
- Give positive feedback when appropriate self-control is used.
  Positive reinforcement encourages repetition of behavior.
- Encourage participation in group therapy to receive feedback from others regarding behavior and to build skills for relationships.
  Group feedback enhances changes in behavior (Bulechek, McCloskey, 1992).
- Use a daily diary to set achievable and realistic goals and monitor successes.
  Small successes reinforce visible and achievable change.

Geriatric

- Monitor for signs of depression, grief, and withdrawal.
  The personal identity disturbance may mask underlying depression.
- Address the client by his or her full name preceded by the proper title (Mr., Mrs., Ms., Miss); use nickname or first name only if suggested by the client; do not use terms of endearment (e.g., "honey").
  Addressing the client in this way helps the client identify ego boundaries and shows respect.
- Practice reality orientation principles; ask specifically how the client feels about events that are happening.
  These steps help define ego boundaries.
- Ask client about important past experiences.
  Reconsideration of past experiences, missed opportunities, and mistakes allows the aged to reach ego integrity (Bulechek, McCloskey, 1992).

Client/Family Teaching

- Teach stress reduction and relaxation techniques.
  These techniques can be used when the client becomes anxious about the loss of self.
- Refer to community resources or other self-help groups appropriate to client's underlying problem (e.g., Adult Children of Alcoholics, parent effectiveness group).
  Peer groups can support positive change and help reduce regression to previous behaviors.

REFERENCES

Bulechek G, McCloskey J: *Nursing interventions: essential nursing treatments,* ed 2, Philadelphia, 1992, WB Saunders.

Carpenito JL: *Nursing diagnosis: application to clinical practice,* ed 5, Philadelphia, 1993, JB Lippincott.

Haber J et al: *Psychiatric nursing,* ed 4, St Louis, 1992, Mosby.

Preston K: Rehabilitation nursing: a client-centered philosophy, *Am J Nurs* 94:66-70, 1994.

Risk for poisoning

Catherine Vincent

Definition Accentuated risk of accidental exposure to or ingestion of drugs or dangerous products in doses sufficient to cause poisoning.

Defining Characteristics

Presence of risk factors such as

Internal (individual)

Reduced vision; verbalization of an occupational setting that lacks adequate safeguards; lack of safety or drug education; lack of proper precautions; cognitive or emotional difficulties; insufficient finances.

External (environmental)

Large supplies of drugs in house; medicines or dangerous products placed or stored within the reach of confused persons; availability of illicit drugs potentially contaminated by poisonous additives; chemical contamination of food and water; unprotected or unventilated areas; presence of poisonous vegetation; presence of atmospheric pollutants.

Related factors (r/t)

Refer to risk factors.

Client Outcomes/Goals

- States and uses safety measures to prevent accidental exposure to or ingestion of drugs or dangerous products.
- Shows no evidence of accidental poisoning.
- Locks drugs and harmful substances out of reach of children and others with cognitive or emotional difficulties.
- Labels all poisonous substances.

Nursing Interventions and Rationales

- Provide labels with large print for the visually impaired.
- Have caregiver be in charge of medications for clients with emotional or cognitive difficulties.
- Provide "Mr. Yuk" labels for families with children.
  Collaborate with community agencies to develop, implement, and evaluate poison prevention programs (Jones, 1993).
- If poisoning occurs, place victim with head turned to the side.
  If victim vomits, this position prevents aspiration.
- Monitor respiratory, circulatory, and mental status of client.
  Some toxic substances may alter vital signs and level of consciousness (Morelli, 1993).
- Attempt to identify the type and amount of substance ingested.
  The correct treatment is correlated with the type of substance ingested.
- Before performing any other interventions, call the posion control center.
  Rapid initiation of treatment reduces mortality and morbidity and lowers emergency room visits and hospital admissions (Jones, 1993).
- If an acidic substance has been ingested, the caregiver may be instructed to give milk; if the substance was an alkaline, lemon juice or vinegar may be recommended.
- Follow poison control center's directions (e.g., induce vomiting, save vomitus, bring person to the emergency room).

Geriatric

- Instruct not to store medications with similar appearances near each other (e.g., nitroglycerin ointment tube near toothpaste tube).

Client/Family Teaching

- Teach family to always call medicine by name when giving it to children and not to refer to it as candy.
- Caution persons to keep purses containing medication out of reach of infants and children.
  Frequently purses contain medications without childproof caps.
- Remove ointments, creams, and talcum from infants' reach.
  Even in small quantities, many common over-the-counter remedies can be fatal to children (Liebelt, Shannon, 1993; Morelli, 1993).
- Teach family to keep potentially dangerous substances out of reach of children and confused persons; a high cupboard for an infant or a locked cupboard for a toddler, preschooler, or confused person may be required.
  Once they learn to crawl, infants can explore and are persistent. Once children begin to walk and climb and develop the concept of object permanence, they can reach most heights and open cupboards and unscrew lids. Many toxic substances are not protected with safety caps (Liebelt, Shannon, 1993).
- Teach family to always store potentially harmful substances in their original containers.
  Poisonous substances are required by law to have antidotes on the label.
- Teach family never to store medication or poisonous substances in food containers.
- Teach family to keep poisonous houseplants out of the reach of children; keep infants away from plants.
  Many plants are toxic to infants. Infants have a high level of hand-to-mouth behavior and will eat anything.
- Teach children to avoid eating out of containers with the "Mr. Yuk" label.
- Teach client and family to only take medicine prescribed specifically for them.
- Teach family to read and follow labels on all products before using them and to adjust doses for age.
- Instruct family with young children to keep syrup of ipecac on hand at all times—two doses for each child.
  Ipecac induces vomiting.
- Give family the phone number of the local poison control center; instruct family to place the number near phone for all caregivers and to always call Poison Control before performing any other interventions.
  Always call Poison Control before treating a child who has had a possible ingestion. Rapid initiation of treatment reduces mortality and morbidity and lowers emergency room visits and hospital admissions (Jones, 1993).
- Teach family to follow poison control center's directions. If an acidic substance has been ingested, the caregiver may be instructed to give milk; if the substance was an alkaline, lemon juice or vinegar may be recommended.
- Refer clients with substance abuse problems to appropriate community agencies.
  Clients with substance abuse problems are at risk for overdosing on potentially toxic substances.

REFERENCES

Jones NE: Childhood residential injuries, *MCN* 18:1168-1172, 1993.

Liebelt E, Shannon MW: Small doses, big problems: a selected review of highly toxic common medications, *Pediatr Emerg Care* 9:292-297, 1993.

Morelli J: Pediatric poisoning: the 10 most toxic prescription drugs, *Am J Nurs* 93:26-29, 1993.

Whaley L, Wong D: *Nursing care of infants and children,* ed 4, St Louis, 1991, Mosby.

Post-trauma response

Judith Rizzo

Definition The state in which an individual experiences a sustained painful response to an overwhelming traumatic event. This response can occur immediately following an event, years later, or anytime in between.

Defining Characteristics

Major: Intrusive responses; reexperience of the traumatic event, which may be identified in cognitive, affective, behavioral, or sensory motor activities (e.g., flashbacks, intrusive thoughts, repetitive dreams or nightmares); excessive verbalization of the traumatic event; verbalization of survival guilt or guilt about behavior required for survival.

Minor: Avoidance responses; psychic or emotional numbness (e.g., impaired interpretation of reality, confusion, dissociation, amnesia, vagueness about traumatic event, constricted affect); altered life-style (self-destructive behaviors such as substance abuse, suicide attempt, or other acting-out behaviors); difficulty with interpersonal relationships; development of phobia regarding trauma; poor impulse control; irritability; explosiveness; obsessive-compulsive behaviors; panic. The most common symptoms are sleeplessness, nightmares of the event, and anxiety, especially immediately following the event.

Related Factors (r/t)

Natural or manmade disasters; wars; epidemics; rape; assault; torture; catastrophic illnesses or accidents.

Client Outcomes/Goals

- Returns to baseline level of functioning as quickly as possible.
- Acknowledges the traumatic event and begins to work with the trauma by talking about the experience and expressing feelings of fear, anger, and guilt.
- Directs anger at event instead of at a significant other.
- Acknowledges that feelings are personal, real, and individual.
- Identifies and connects with support persons and resources.
- Assimilates the experience into a meaningful whole and goes on to set goals and pursue them.

Nursing Interventions and Rationales

- Observe client's response, its severity, and its effect on current functioning.
- Provide a safe and therapeutic environment in which client can regain control.
  A common symptom is fearfulness that the event may recur or a feeling of profound vulnerability to future occurrences.
- Stay with client and offer support during episodes of high anxiety.
  Client may initially be in shock and may appear dazed or confused.
- Use touch with client's permission (e.g., hand on shoulder, holding of hand).
  In Ricci's study of personal space invasion in the nurse-client relationship, anxiety scores of the experimental group showed a definite downward trend, indicating that the intrusion of a nurse into a client's space had a calming rather than a stimulating effect (Ricci, 1981).
- Provide a safe and structured environment for client to describe the traumatic experience and express feelings.
- Help client ventilate feelings verbally or through other channels; spend one-to-one time with client.
  These steps promote trust and open expression of feelings.
- Explore available support systems.

Support systems decrease isolation, encourage communication, and provide diversional activity.

- Provide or arrange for follow-up treatment.
- Restore sleep.
  Disrupted sleep is the most prevalent symptom following a traumatic event.
- Help client use positive cognitive restructuring to reestablish feelings of self-worth.
  After a traumatic event, thinking often becomes negative, and the client feels devalued.
- Normalize symptoms; help client to understand that these feelings and thoughts are a result of the trauma and do not indicate mental illness.
  Many symptoms of a trauma response are mistaken for mental illness, when actually they are normal responses to an abnormal event.

Geriatric

- Observe client for concurrent losses that may affect coping skills.
  As the elderly age, the number of losses are multiplied and compounded.
- Allow client more time to establish trust and to express anger, guilt, and shame about the trauma.
- Review past coping skills and give client positive reinforcement for successfully dealing with other life crises.
  Those who have had positive adjustments in life and to aging and who can put events into proper perspective may be more positive in adjusting to loss.
- Monitor client for clinical signs of depression and anxiety; refer to physician for medication if appropriate.
  Depression in the elderly is underestimated in this country.

Client/Family Teaching

- Explain to client and family what to expect the first few days after the traumatic event and in the long term.
  Knowing what to expect can minimize much of the anxiety that accompanies a traumatic response.
- Teach positive coping skills and avoidance of negative coping skills such as alcohol use. Teach relaxation skills to decrease anxiety when flashbacks or intrusive thoughts occur.
  Following a traumatic event, it is tempting for clients to maladaptively cope with their overwhelming emotions, which can set unhealthy patterns for the future.
- Refer to peer support groups.
  Support groups decrease the sense of social isolation.

REFERENCES

Ricci, MS: An experiment with personal space invasion in the nurse-patient relationship and its effect on anxiety, *Issues Ment Health Nurs* 3:203-218, 1981.

BIBLIOGRAPHY

Bille D: Post-traumatic stress disorder: the hidden victim, *J Psychosoc Nurs* 31:19-28, 1993.

Cox H et al: *Clinical applications of nursing diagnosis: adult, child, women's, psychiatric, gerontic and home health considerations,* ed 2, Philadelphia, 1993, FA Davis.

Mitchell J: Stress: development and functions of a critical incident stress debriefing team, *J Emerg Med Serv* 13:43-46, 1988.

National Organization for Victim Assistance Training Manual. (N.O.V.A.) "Coordinating a Community Crisis Response," 1988.

Schwartz J, Kettley J, Rizzo J: Predictors of vulnerability after trauma, unpublished manuscript, 1992.

Powerlessness

Gail Ladwig

Definition Perception that one's own action will not significantly affect an outcome; a perceived lack of control over a current situation or immediate happening.

Defining Characteristics

Severe — Verbalized inability to control or influence situation; verbalized inability to control self-care; depression regarding physical deterioration that occurs despite client compliance with regimens; apathy.

Moderate — Nonparticipation in care or decision-making when opportunities are provided; verbalized dissatisfaction regarding inability to perform previous tasks or activities; does not monitor progress; verbalized doubt regarding role performance; reluctance to express true feelings; fear of alienation from caregivers; passivity; inability to seek information regarding care; dependence on others that may result in irritability, resentment, anger, and guilt; no defense of self-care practices when challenged.

Related Factors (r/t)

Health care environment; interpersonal interactions; life-style of helplessness; illness-related regimen.

Client Outcomes/Goals

- States feelings of powerlessness and other feelings related to powerlessness (e.g., anger, sadness, hopelessness).
- Identifies things that he or she can control.
- Participates in planning care; makes decisions regarding care and treatment when possible.
- Asks questions about care and treatment.
- Verbalizes a hopeful future.

Nursing Interventions and Rationales

- Observe for factors contributing to powerlessness (e.g., immobility; hospitalization; unfavorable prognosis; no support system; misinformation about situation; inflexible routine).
  Correctly identifying the actual or perceived problem is essential to providing the correct support measures.
- Establish therapeutic relationship with client by spending time one-to-one, assigning the same caregiver, and keeping commitments (e.g., "I will be back to answer your questions in the next hour").
  The trust and consistency fostered by a therapeutic relationship provides the client with a secure environment in which to deal with problems and develop adaptation skills (Johnson, 1993).
- Allow client to express hope, which may range from "I hope my coffee will be hot" to "I hope I will die with my significant other here." Listen to client's priorities.
  Hope is a way of coping with a stressful situation and motivates the client to continue. Motivation is necessary in the change process.
- Allow time for questions (15 to 20 minutes each shift); have client write down questions.
  Allowing for questions encourages the client to take some control of the situation (Roberts, White, 1990).
- Have client assist in planning of care if possible (e.g., what time to bathe, pain medication before uncomfortable procedures, food and fluid preferences); document specifics in care plan.

Assisting in care planning encourages the client to take some control of the situation (Roberts, White, 1990).

- Keep items client uses and needs within reach such as urinal, tissues, phone, television controls.
  Client is able to participate in own care if care devices are accessible. Participation in care enhances a sense of control.
- Work with client to set achievable short-term goals such as walking to window to wave to children by the end of the week.
  Setting goals that a client can achieve helps increase hope that things can change and that there are things he or she can still accomplish.
- Have client write goals and plans to achieve them (e.g., dangle legs at bedside 10 minutes for 2 days, and then sit in chair 10 minutes for 2 days, and then walk to window).
  Active participation enhances a feeling of power.
- Give praise for accomplishments.
  Positive reinforcement encourages repetition of behavior.
- Help client identify those things he or she can control.
  Identifying items within client's control encourages the client to take some control of the situation.
- Keep interactions with client focused on client, not on family or physician; actively listen to client.
  Such a focus helps the client to maintain a sense of "self." The client can use a lot of energy by holding in unacceptable or frightening feelings; by listening to the client and allowing these feelings to be expressed, that energy is released and can be used in different ways (Clark, 1993).
- Acknowledge subjective concerns or fears.
  All feelings are personal and have meaning for the client.
- Allow client to take control of as many activities of daily living as possible; keep client informed of all care that will be given.
  Clients are more amenable to therapy if they know what to expect and can perform some tasks independently.
- Help client to develop realistic goals within the limitations of illness; do not emphasize limitations.
  Setting goals that the client can achieve helps increase the hope that things can change and that there are things he or she can still accomplish.
- Develop contract with client that states client's and nurse's responsibilities and privileges.
  A contract helps give the situation structure and clarifies what may or may not happen and who has responsibility for the client's care.

Client/Family Teaching

- Explain all procedures, treatments, and expected outcomes.
  Clients are more amenable to therapy if they know what to expect.
- Provide written instructions for treatments and procedures for which the client will be responsible.
  A written record provides a concrete reference so that the client and family can clarify any verbal information that was given. People tend to forget half of what they hear within a few minutes; thus it is important for nurses to supplement oral instructions with written material (Wong, 1992).

- Help client practice assertive communication techniques; use role-playing (e.g., "Tell me what you are going to ask your doctor").
  Role-playing is the most commonly used technique in assertiveness training and deconditions the anxiety that arises from interpersonal encounters.
- Refer to support groups, pastoral care, or social services.
  These services help decrease levels of stress and increase levels of self-esteem and also help the client to know that he or she is "not alone."

REFERENCES

Clark, S: Challenges in critical care nursing: helping patients and families cope, *Crit Care Nurse* (suppl) 2:3-24, Aug 1993.

Johnson BS: *Adaptation and growth: psychiatric-mental health nursing,* Philadelphia, 1993, JB Lippincott.

Roberts S, White BS: Powerlessness and personal control model applied to the myocardial infarction patient, *Prog Cardiovasc Nurs* 5:84-94, 1990.

Wong M: Self-care instructions: do patients understand educational materials? *Focus Criti Care* 19:47, 1992.

BIBLIOGRAPHY

Burnard P: *Counseling: a guide to practice in nursing,* Oxford, 1992, Butterworth-Heinemann.

Clemons S, Cummings S: Helplessness and powerlessness: caring for clients in pain, *Holistic Nurs Pract* 6:76-85, 1991.

Drew B: Differentiation of hopeless, helplessness, and powerlessness using Erik Erikson's "Roots of Virtue," *Arch Psychiatr Nurs* 4:332-337, 1990.

Townsend M: *Psychiatric mental health nursing concepts of care,* Philadelphia, 1992, FA Davis.

Altered protection

Betty Ackley

Definition The state in which an individual experiences a decrease in the ability to guard the self from internal or external threats such as illness or injury.

Defining Characteristics

Major Deficient immunity; impaired healing; altered clotting; maladaptive stress response; neurosensory alteration.

Minor Chilling; perspiring; dyspnea; cough; itching; restlessness; insomnia; fatigue; anorexia; weakness; immobility; disorientation; pressure sores.

Related Factors (r/t)

Extremes of age; inadequate nutrition; alcohol abuse; abnormal blood profiles (e.g., leukopenia, thrombocytopenia, anemia, coagulation); drug therapies (e.g., antineoplastic, corticosteroid, immune, anticoagulant, thrombolytic); treatments (e.g., surgery, radiation); diseases (e.g., cancer, immune disorders).

Client Outcomes/Goals

- Free of infection.
- Free of any evidence of bleeding.
- Explains precautions to take to prevent infection.
- Explains precautions to take to prevent bleeding.

Nursing Interventions and Rationales

- Take temperature, pulse, and blood pressure q_____h.
- Observe nutritional status (e.g., weight, serum protein and albumin, muscle mass size, usual food intake). Refer to dietician if not well nourished.
  Good nutrition is needed to maintain immune function and to support formation of clotting elements.
- Observe sleep pattern; if altered, refer to nursing interventions and rationales for **Sleep pattern disturbance**.
- Observe for stress in client's life.

Prevention of Infection

- Monitor for signs of infection (e.g., fever, chills, flushed skin, edema, redness).
  With the onset of infection, the immune system is stimulated, resulting in classic signs of infection.
- If immune system is depressed, notify physician of elevated temperature, even in the absence of other symptoms of infection.
  Clients with depressed immune function are unable to mount the usual immune responses to the onset of infection; fever may be the only sign of infection present (Wujcik, 1993).
- If white blood cell count is severely decreased (absolute neutrophil count less than 1000 per mm^3), initiate the following precautions:
  - Take vital signs q4h.
  - Complete a head-to-toe assessment twice daily, including inspection of oral mucosa, invasive sites, wounds, urine, and stool; monitor for onset of new complaints of pain.
  - Avoid using urinary catheters, injections, or rectal or vaginal manipulations.
  - Maintain meticulous care of all invasive sites.
  - Have client wear a mask when leaving room.
  - Limit and screen visitors to minimize exposure to contagion.
  - Help client bathe daily and complete oral hygiene frequently.

- Serve client only cooked fruits and vegetables.
- Help client to cough and deep breathe regularly; maintain appropriate activity level.
- Obtain a private room for client.

A client with an absolute neutrophil count less than 1000 per mm^3 is severely neutropenic, has an impaired immune function, and is very prone to infection. Precautions are taken to limit exposure to pathogens (Wujcik, 1993).

- Refer to care plan for **Risk for infection** for more interventions regarding prevention of infection.

Prevention of Bleeding

- Monitor client's risk for bleeding; evaluate clotting studies and platelet counts.
  Laboratory studies give a good indication of the seriousness of the bleeding disorder.
- Watch for hematuria, melena, hematemesis, epistaxis, bleeding from mucosa, blood from suctioning, increased petechia, increased areas of ecchymosis.
  These areas of bleeding can be detected in a bleeding disorder (Paschall, 1993).
- Apply pressure for a longer time than usual to invasive sites such as venipuncture or injection sites.
  With a bleeding disorder, additional pressure is needed to stop bleeding of invasive sites.
- Take vital signs frequently; watch for changes associated with fluid-volume loss.
  Excessive bleeding causes a decreased blood pressure and an increased pulse and respiratory rate.
- Monitor menstrual flow if relevant; have client use pads instead of tampons.
  Menstruation can be excessive with bleeding disorders; tampons can increase trauma to the vagina.
- Initiate the following bleeding precautions:
  - Have client use a moistened toothette instead of a toothbrush; have client avoid flossing.
  - Ask client either not to shave or to only use an electric razor.
  - Avoid giving injections or rectal or vaginal suppositories if possible; consult with physician to give medications orally or intravenously.

  Such steps help prevent any unnecessary trauma that could result in bleeding.
- To decrease risk of bleeding, avoid administering salicylates or nonsteroidal anti-inflammatory medications.

Client/Family Teaching

Depressed Immune Function

- Teach precautions to take to decrease the chance of infection (e.g., avoid uncooked fruits or vegetables, observe appropriate self-care, ensure a safe environment for immunodeficient client).
- Teach client and family how to take a temperature, and encourage family to take client's temperature between 3 PM and 7 PM at least once daily.
  The client's temperature is more likely to be elevated in the evening hours because the circadian rhythm peaks during this time (Samples, 1985).
- Teach client and family to notify physician of elevated temperature, even in the absence of other symptoms of infection.
  Clients with depressed immune function are unable to mount the usual immune response to the onset of infection; fever may be the only sign present of infection (Wujcik, 1993).

- Teach client to avoid crowds and contact with persons who have infections.
- Teach the need for good nutrition, avoidance of stress, and adequate rest to maintain immune system function.
  Client education to increase nutrition, manage stress, and perform self-care can reduce the risk of neutropenic infection (Carter, 1993).

Bleeding Disorder

- Teach client to wear Medic-Alert bracelet and notify all health care personnel of the bleeding disorder.
- Teach client and family the signs of bleeding and precautions to take to prevent bleeding.
- Caution client to avoid taking over-the-counter medications without permission of physician.
  Medications containing salicylates or nonsteroidal anti-inflammatory medications can increase bleeding.

REFERENCES

Carter LW: Influences of nutrition and stress on people at risk for neutropenia: nursing implications, *Oncol Nurs Forum* 20:1241-1249, 1993.

Samples JF et al: Circadian rhythms: basis for screening for fever, *Nurs Res* 34:377-379, 1985.

Paschall FE: Thrombotic thrombocytopenic purpura: the challenges of a complex disease process, *AACN Clin Issues* 4:655-663, 1993.

Wujcik D: Infection control in oncology patients, *Nurs Clin North Am* 28:639-649, 1993.

BIBLIOGRAPHY

Pavel J, Plunkett A, Sink B: Nursing care of clients with hematologic disorders. In Black J, Matassarin-Jacobs E, editors: *Luckmann and Sorensen's medical-surgical nursing: a psychophysiologic approach,* Philadelphia, 1993, WB Saunders.

Rape trauma syndrome

Nancee Bender Radtke

Definition The trauma syndrome that develops after actual or attempted forced violent sexual penetration against the victim's will and consent. The syndrome includes an acute phase of disorganization of the victim's life-style and a long-term process of reorganization of life-style.

NOTE: Recent research challenges the two-phase theory of trauma processing that is part of the NANDA diagnosis of **Rape trauma syndrome**. Kilpatrick, Veronen, and Best (1985) found that a victim's level of distress resulting from tension, depression, anger, fatigue, and confusion between 6 and 21 days following trauma was highly predictive of the distress level at 3 months following the trauma; this distress level remained relatively stable up to 4 years. This syndrome may include two other components: rape trauma, compound reaction, and rape trauma, silent reaction. There are additional nursing careplans for each of these diagnoses.

Defining Characteristics

Acute phase Emotional reactions (e.g., anger, embarrassment, fear of physical violence and death, humiliation, revenge, self-blame); multiple physical symptoms (e.g., gastrointestinal irritability, genitourinary discomfort, muscle tension, sleep pattern disturbance); anxiety; fear; shame; pale complexion; weak pulse; shallow breathing; subdued feelings; numbness; disbelief; slow and inaudible speech; crying.

Long-term phase

Changes in life-style (e.g., changing residence, dealing with repetitive nightmares and phobias, seeking family support, seeking social network support). Rape victims experience emotional, physical, and cognitive reactions to the trauma of rape. During adjustment, clients resume activities, deal with practical matters, deny feelings about rape, experience daydreams and flashbacks, and are less interested in talking about the rape. During integration clients may suddenly become depressed and unable to stop thinking about the rape. Experiences trigger memories and nightmares, and clients may experience difficulty working through feelings. The trial of the rapist may also cause problems. As clients recover, they return to their level of functioning before the assault. Unfortunately, persistent depressive symptoms and suicide ideations and attempts are frequent (Tyra, 1993).

Client Outcomes/Goals

- Shares feelings, concerns, and fears.
- Recognizes that the rape or the attempt was not own fault.
- States that no matter what the situation, no one has the right to assault another.
- Identifies behaviors and situations within own control to prevent or reduce risk of recurrence.
- Describes treatment procedures and reasons for treatment.
- Reports absence of physical complications or pain.
- Identifies support systems and is able to ask them for help in dealing with this trauma.
- Functions at same level as before crisis, including sexual functioning.
- Recognizes that it is normal for full recovery to take a year.

Nursing Interventions and Rationales

- Observe client's responses, including anger, fear, self-blame, sleep pattern disturbances, and phobias.
- Monitor client's verbal and nonverbal psychological state (e.g., crying, wringing hands, avoiding interactions or eye contact with staff).

The most depressed victims are those most concerned with being stigmatized and blamed for the crime (Frable, Blackstone, Sherbaum, 1990).

- Stay with client initially or have a trusted person stay with client; if a law enforcement interview is permitted, provide support by staying with client.
  Early crisis intervention involves helping client decide who to tell about the rape and regain the control lost during the assault.
- Explain each part of treatment. Discuss importance of pelvic examination; if this is first examination, explain instruments and let client know when and where you will touch.
  Do not wait for the client to ask questions; explain everything you are doing and why it must be done; explain when and where you will touch. Eye contact is very important because it helps the client feel worthy and alive (Ruckman, 1992).
- Observe for signs of physical injury. Ask questions such as, "Did he push you?" "Did he hit you?" " Did he choke you?" and "Do you feel sore anywhere?" Instruct the client to return for additional photos if bruises become more pronounced in a few days.
  It is important to carefully document that force was used and that sexual contact was not consensual. Sore areas are not visible in photos.
- Encourage client to verbalize feelings.
  Being listened to helps the client gain self-control by feeling acceptance from others (Ruckman, 1992).
- Provide privacy for client to express feelings. Limit the number of nurses, escort to treatment room as soon as possible, do not question in triage area, close curtains and door, avoid other interruptions during contact with client (e.g., telephone calls, leaving the room, outside stimuli such as radios).
- Document a one- or two-sentence capsule of what happened; getting the details of the sequence of events is the police officer's job.
  If some details are not mentioned in the nurse notes but were told to police, the defense attorney may attempt in court to make this look like a discrepancy to cause reasonable doubt and thus obtain an acquittal (Ledry, 1992).
- Enlist the help of supportive counselors who are experienced with rape trauma; refer to a rape crisis counselor, mental health clinic, or psychotherapist.
  After physical needs are attended to, the client should be placed in the care of a counselor who can maintain a relationship long after discharge from the Emergency Department (Ruckman, 1992).
- Instead of saying, "Do you want me to call?", describe the community rape crisis center person and how that person will be available after the client goes home.
  The client wants control but may have difficulty making decisions during the initial time in the Emergency Department.
- Explain collection of specimens for evidence; provide for self-care needs after examination (e.g., cleansing the vaginal and rectal area).
  A card with the victim's name and date is held next to the injury in each picture for identification; direct quotes rather than summaries or paraphrases should be used. Most states provide Sexual Assault Evidence Collection kits, which prevent any inconsistencies in the collection of evidence that will be used in court.
- Explain that client's undergarments may need to be kept for evidence; instruct client to put other clothing in a paper bag once at home and to not wash it until it is known if it will be needed for evidence.
  Do not place clothes in plastic because moisture may accumulate and cause deterioration.

- Discuss the possibility of pregnancy and sexually transmitted diseases (STDs) and the treatments available.
  Administering a urine pregnancy test is routine before giving medications to prevent pregnancy or treat STDs. Most clients prefer to prevent pregnancy rather than face the possibility of terminating it in the future. The risk of human immunodeficiency virus (HIV) exposure is a special concern to rape victims; the nurse should bring the issue up and inform the client of locations and schedules for HIV testing.
- Explain that it is the client's choice whether or not to report rape.
  The first step in evidence collection is obtaining a signed consent from the client to do an examination and release collected evidence to police.
- Encourage client to report rape.
  It is important for rape victims to recognize that they are victims of a crime that is not their fault (Ledry, 1992). Reporting is an issue separate from prosecution; even if victims report, they will not be forced to appear as a witness.
- Discuss client's support system; involve support system if appropriate and if client grants permission. Nonsupport and victim-blaming attitudes by significant others are common responses.
  Research indicates that significant others are coping with their own responses to trauma and may be incapable of supporting the victim (Mackey et al, 1992).
- Obtain blood alcohol level if indicated.

Geriatric

- Build a trusting relationship.
  Recognize the attitudes and values of an older generation; stigmatization may cause a self-view of disgust and shame (DeLorey, Wolf, 1993).
- Explain reporting and encourage client to report.
  Embarrassment may prevent reporting; respect client's choice. Older rape victims have reported having a greater fear of people finding out about their rape than younger women (Tyra, 1993).
- Observe for psychosocial distress (e.g., memory impairment, sleep disturbances, regression, changes in bodily functions).
  Exacerbation of a chronic illness may be a major consequence of sexual assault.
- Identify new injuries related to the assault and their immediate effects on the client's existing health problems (e.g., cardiovascular disease, arthritis, respiratory disease).
  A review of the client's current medications may add to the nurse's understanding of relevant health problems.
- Modify the rape protocol to promote comfort of the geriatric client and to accommodate changes of age; consider positioning the female client with pillows rather than with stirrups, and consider appropriate speculum size.
  Effects of aging result in decreased muscle tone and thinning of the vaginal wall.
- Assess for mobility limitations and cognitive impairment.
  Elicit information from family or caregivers to verify level of functioning before sexual assault.
- Respect client's need for privacy.
  Older clients may be reluctant to have their children or younger family members present during examination and treatment; give clients a choice.
- Consider arrangements for temporary housing.
  Most sexual assaults of older clients occur in the home.

NOTE: Older age makes a client more powerless, especially if isolated as a result of living alone. Physical frailty or physical injury can have a much greater effect on an older victim, and the victim may experience a compound reaction because she is older. Sexual violence against an older female is a reflection of antiage and antiwoman attitudes. Sixty percent of sexually assaulted older females are severely injured—10% are murdered, 7% are stabbed, and 43% are beaten (Delorey, Wolf, 1993).

Male Rape Reactions to male rape are either disbelief or an assumption that males who are raped are gay.

Most females are aware of the possibility that they may be raped, males are not. The care required is very similar to the care of females who have been raped (Laurent, 1993).

Client/Family Teaching

- Discharge instructions should be written.
  Anxiety can hamper comprehension and retention of information; repeat instructions and provide written instructions.
- Provide instructions to significant others.
  Significant others need many of the same supportive and caring interventions as the client; suggest that they, too, might benefit from counseling.
- Explain purpose of "morning after pill."
  Norgestrel (Ovral) prevents pregnancy and is only used in emergencies. It must be taken within 72 hours (3 days) of sexual contact for it to work; it will not cause a miscarriage if client is already pregnant, but it could harm the baby.
- Explain potential for common side effects related to treatment with "morning after pill," (norgestrel) such as breast swelling or nausea and vomiting (call the Emergency Department if client vomits within 1 hour of taking pill, because pill may need to be repeated); period may take 3 to 30 days to start; if period has not started in 30 days, contact physician.
- Explain potential for severe side effects related to treatment with "morning after pill" (norgestrel) such as severe leg or chest pain; breathing trouble; coughing up of blood; severe headache or dizziness; trouble seeing or talking.
- Advise client to call or return if new problems develop.
  Physical injuries may not be recognized as a result of client's "numbness" during the initial examination, or client may have forgotten or not understood some of the instructions.
- Teach relaxation techniques.
- Discuss practical life-style changes within client's control to reduce the risk of future attacks. Financial limitations can limit some alternatives such as moving to another home. Provide other alternatives such as keeping doors locked, checking car before getting in, not walking alone at night, keeping someone informed of whereabouts, asking someone to check if client has not arrived within reasonable amount of time, keeping lights on in entryway, having keys in hand when approaching car or house, having a remote key–entry car or garage.
- Teach client to use self-defense techniques to surprise attacker and then run for help. Refer client to self-defense school.
- Teach client appropriate outlets for anger.
- Encourage significant other to direct anger at event and attacker, not at the client.
- Emphasize vulnerability of client and ensure that reactions are appropriate for the victim of sexual assault.
  Females are at higher risk for depression than males, and the risk is significantly higher between the ages of 18 and 44 (Mackey et al, 1992).

NOTE: Post traumatic stress disorder (PTSD) has a high probability of being a psychological sequelae to rape. Research by Foa, Steketee, and Roghbaum (1991) demonstrated two effective treatments for improvement of PTSD in rape victims—prolonged exposure and stress inoculation training. Prolonged exposure involves reliving the rape scene by imagining it as vividly as possible, describing it aloud in the present tense, taping this description, and listening to the tape at least once daily. Stress inoculation training involves breathing exercises to diminish anxiety and instruction in coping skills, thought stopping, cognitive restructuring, self-dialogue, modeling, and role-playing. Research suggests that a combination of both treatments may provide the optimal effect.

REFERENCES

Delorey C, Wolf, KA: Sexual violence and older women, *AWHONNS Clin Iss Perinatal Women's Health Nurs* 4:173-179, 1993.

Foa EB, Skeketee G, Roghbaum BD: Behavioral/cognitive conceptualization of posttraumatic stress disorder, *Behav Ther* 20:155-176, 1989.

Frable D, Blackstone T, Sherbaum C: Marginal and mindful: deviants in social interaction, *J Pers Soc Psychol* 59:140-149, 1990.

Kilpatrick DG, Vereonen LJ, Best CL: *Factors predicting psychological distress among rape victims.* In Figley GR, editor: *Trauma and its wake: the study and treatment of post-traumatic stress disorder,* New York, 1985, Brunner/Mazel.

Laurent C: Male rape, *Nurs Time*, 89(10), 1993.

Ledry L: The sexual assault nurse clinician: a fifteen-year experience in Minneapolis, *JEN* 18:217-229, 1992.

Mackey T et al: Factors associated with long-term depressive symptoms of sexual assault victims, *Arch Psychiatr Nurs* 6:10-25, 1992.

Ruckman LM: Rape: how to begin the healing, *Am J Nurs* 92:48-52, 1992.

Tyra PA: Older women: victims of rape, *J Gerontol Nurs* pp. 7-12, 1993.

BIBLIOGRAPHY

Burgess AW, Holstrom, LL: *Rape victims of crisis,* Bowie, Md, 1974, Robert J Brady.

Rape trauma syndrome: compound reaction

Nancee Bender Radtke

Definition Refer to **Rape trauma syndrome**.

Defining Characteristics

Refer to **Rape trauma syndrome**. Additional characteristics include reactivated symptoms of previous conditions (e.g., physical illness, psychiatric illness, reliance on alcohol or drugs).

Related Factors (r/t)

Rape.

Client Outcomes/Goals

Refer to **Rape trauma syndrome**.

Nursing Interventions and Rationales

Refer to **Rape trauma syndrome; Powerlessness; Ineffective individual coping; Dysfunctional grieving; Anxiety; Fear; Violence: self-directed; Sexual dysfunction**.

Geriatric (risk for compound reaction)

- Refer to **Rape trauma syndrome**.

Client/Family Teaching

- Teach client what reactions to expect during the acute and long-term phase; acute phase: anger, fear, self-blame, embarrassment, vengeful feelings, physical symptoms, muscle tension, sleeplessness, stomach upset, genitourinary discomfort; long-term phase: changes in life-style or residence, nightmares, phobias, seeking of family and social network support.
  Of assessed rape victims, 16.5% were diagnosed with posttraumatic stress disorder an average of 17 years after the assault (Mackey et al, 1992).
- Encourage psychiatric consultation if client is suicidal, violent, or unable to continue activities of daily living.
  Rape victims are four times more likely to attempt suicide, which is 8.7% higher than nonvictims (Mackey et al, 1992).
- Discuss any of the client's current stress-relieving medications that may result in substance abuse.
  The initial response to trauma is for the noradrenergic system to maintain the arousal state, increase vigilance, and be "protective" to prevent subsequent trauma. Following massive traumatization, neurotransmitters are depleted at the synapse level, which is associated with long-term depression and numbing; this depletion also leaves the client with a different threshold, increasing vulnerability to subsequent stress (Mackey et al, 1992).

REFERENCES

Mackey et al: Factors associated with long-term depressive symptoms of sexual assault victims, *Arch Psychiatr Nurs* 6:10-25, 1992.

Refer to **Rape trauma syndrome**.

Rape trauma syndrome: silent reaction

Nancee Bender Radtke

Definition Refer to **Rape trauma syndrome**.

Defining Characteristics

Abrupt changes in relationships with males; increased nightmares; increased anxiety during interview (e.g., blocking of associations, long periods of silence, minor stuttering, physical distress); pronounced changes in sexual behavior; no verbalization of the rape; sudden onset of phobic reactions.

Related Factors (r/t)

Rape.

Client Outcomes/Goals

Refer to **Rape-trauma syndrome**.

- Resumes previous level of relationships with significant others.
- States improvement in sleep without nightmares.
- Able to express feelings about and discuss the rape.
  Nondisclosure about a sexual assault may arise out of self-protection, but this defensive coping style acts as a pressure cooker and is associated with more intense depressive symptoms (Mackey et al, 1992).
- Returns to usual pattern of sexual behavior.
  Women who are sexually active after the assault report lower levels of depression (Mackey et al, 1992). However, being sexually active cannot be construed to mean that the client has adjusted to or resolved the sexual trauma.
- Free of phobic reactions.

Nursing Interventions and Rationales

Refer to nursing diagnoses for **Rape trauma syndrome; Powerlessness; Ineffective individual coping; Dysfunctional grieving; Anxiety; Fear; Violence: self-directed; Sexual dysfunction;** or **Impaired communication**.

- Observe disruptions in relationships with significant others.
  Poorly adjusted clients may elicit unsupportive behavior from others or perceive actions of others in a negative way.
- Monitor for signs of increased anxiety (e.g., silence, stuttering, physical distress, irritability, unexplained crying spells).
  Focus on coping strengths of the client.
- Observe for changes in sexual behavior.
  More than 80% of sexually active victims reported some sexual dysfunction as a result of the assault (Mackey et al, 1992). Some victims engage in sexual intimacy to prove to themselves and their partners that they are normal or unaffected by the assault.
- Identify phobic reactions to objects in environment (e.g., strangers, doorbells, being with groups of people, knives).
- Provide support by listening when client is ready to talk.
  Controlled clients may not be believed because they do not fit the stereotypical picture of rape victims.
- Be nonjudgmental when feelings are expressed; explain that anger is normal and needs to be verbalized. Reassure client with phrases such as, "I'm sorry this happened to you."
- Remain with client while anxious even if client is silent. Be gentle in speech and actions; move slowly.
- Evaluate somatic complaints.
  Women are at higher risk for depression than men (Mackey et al, 1992).

Geriatric Refer to **Rape trauma syndrome**.

Client/Family Teaching

Refer to **Rape trauma syndrome**.

- Reassure that client is not "bad" and is not at fault. Avoid questions beginning with "Why."
  "Why" questions may sound judgmental and feed into self-blame.
- Refer to sexual assault counselor.
  Long-term counseling may need to be recommended.
- Offer information about pregnancy, Hepatitis B, and sexually transmitted disease testing, treatment, and procedures. Do not wait for victim to request information.

REFERENCES Mackey et al: Factors associated with long-term depressive symptoms of sexual assault victims, *Arch Psychiatr Nurs* 6:10-25, 1992.

Refer to **Rape trauma syndrome**.

Relocation stress syndrome

Betty Ackley

Definition Physiological or psychosocial disturbances that result from a transfer from one environment to another.

Defining Characteristics

Major Anxiety; apprehension; increased confusion (elderly); depression; loneliness.

Minor Verbalization of unwillingness to relocate; sleep disturbances; change in eating habits; dependency; gastrointestinal disturbances; increased verbalization of needs; insecurity; lack of trust; restlessness; sad affect; unfavorable comparison of posttransfer and pretransfer staff; verbalization of concern or unhappiness about transfer; vigilance; weight change; withdrawal.

Related Factors (r/t)

Past, concurrent, and recent losses; losses involved with the decision to move; feeling of powerlessness; lack of adequate support system; little or no preparation for the impending move; moderate-to-high degree of environmental change; history and types of previous transfers; impaired psychosocial health status; decreased physical health status.

Client Outcomes/Goals

- States anxiety is decreased.
- Oriented to person, place, and time.
- Able to share feelings of sadness or loneliness.
- Seeks out staff or one identified person for 30 minutes daily.
- States benefits of new living situation.
- Able to carry out activities of daily living in usual manner.
- Maintains previous health status (e.g., elimination, nutrition, sleep, social interaction).

Nursing Interventions and Rationales

- Obtain a nursing history, including reason for the move, how client has handled previous transfers, history of losses, and family support for the client.
  A history helps determine the amount of support needed and appropriate interventions to decrease relocation stress.
- Observe the following procedures if client is being transferred to a nursing home or adult foster care:
  - Allow client to have a choice of placement and preadmission visits if possible.
    Having some control over the event elicits problem-solving coping strategies (Oleson, Shadick, 1993).
  - If client cannot choose placement, arrange for a visit or phone call by a member of the staff to welcome client, or at least provide pictures of the new care facility.
  - Have a familiar person accompany client to the new facility.
- After the transfer, determine client's mental status; document status and observe for any new onset of confusion.
- Use reality orientation if needed (e.g., today is _____, the date is _____, you are at _____ facility); repeat information as needed; provide clock or calendar.
- Establish how the client would like to be addressed (Mr., Mrs., Miss, by first name, by nickname).
- Give a thorough orientation to the new environment and routines; repeat directions prn.
  The stress of the move may interfere with client's ability to remember directions (Harkulich, 1992).

- Spend one-to-one time with client; allow client to express feelings and convey acceptance of them; emphasize that the client's feelings are real and individual and that it is acceptable to be sad or angry about moving.
  Expressing feelings helps the client adjust to the situation.
- Assign the same staff to client; maintain consistency in routines of care.
  Consistency hastens adjustment (Harkulich, 1992).
- Have client state one positive aspect of the new living situation each day.
  Helping the client to focus on the positive aspects of the move can help change attitudes.
- Monitor client's health status and provide appropriate interventions for problems with social interaction, nutrition, sleep, or elimination.
  Stress from the transfer can cause physiological and psychological disturbances (Barnhouse, Brugler, Harkulich, 1992).
- If client is being transferred within a facility, have staff from new unit visit client before the transfer.
- Once client is transferred, have previous staff make occasional visits until client is comfortable in new surroundings.
- Watch for coping problems (e.g., withdrawn, regressive, or angry behavior) and intervene immediately.
  Failure to cope in a timely manner may cause a permanent pattern of impaired adjustment (Oleson, Shadick, 1993).
- Allow client to grieve for old situation; explain that it is normal to feel sadness over change and loss.
- Allow client to participate in care as much as possible and to make decisions when possible (e.g., location of bed, choice of roommate, bathing routines); make an effort to accommodate the client.

Geriatric

- Monitor need for transfer, and transfer only when necessary.
  Some clients adapt poorly to transfer and can lose areas of functioning.
- Protect client from injuries such as falls.
  Falls and increased accidents are common with relocation.

Client/Family Teaching

- Teach about the grief process associated with change and loss and about normal and abnormal responses to a transfer.
- Help significant others learn how to support client with the move by setting up a schedule of visits, dealing with holidays, bringing familiar items from home, and establishing a system for contact when client needs support.

REFERENCES

Barnhouse AH, Brugler CJ, Harkulich JT: Relocation stress syndrome, *Nurs Diag* 3:166-167, 1992.

Harkulich JT: *Relocation stress.* In Gettrust K, Brabeck PD, editors: *Nursing diagnosis in clinical practice: guides for care planning,* Albany, NY 1992, Delmar.

Oleson M, Shadick KM: Application of Moos and Schaefer's model to nursing care of elderly persons relocating to a nursing home, *J Adv Nurs,* 18:479-485, 1993.

BIBLIOGRAPHY

Aroin KJ: A model of psychological adaptation to migration and resettlement, *Nurs Res* 39:5-9, 1990.

Rantz M, Egan K: Reducing death from translocation syndrome, *Am J Nurs* 87(10):1351-1352, 1987.

Thomasma M, Yeaworth RC, McCabe BW: Moving day: relocation and anxiety in institutionalized elderly, *J Gerontol Nurs* 16:18-25, 1990.

Altered role performance

Gail Ladwig

Definition Disruption in the way one perceives one's role performance.

Defining Characteristics

Change in self-perception of role; change in others' perception of role; conflict in roles; change in physical capacity to resume role; lack of knowledge regarding role; change in usual patterns of responsibility.

Related Factors (r/t)

To be developed.

Client Outcomes/Goals

- Identifies realistic perception of role.
- States personal strengths.
- Acknowledges problems contributing to inability to carry out usual role.
- Accepts physical limitations regarding role responsibility and considers ways to change life-style to accomplish goals associated with role performance.
- Demonstrates knowledge of appropriate behaviors associated with new or changed role.
- States knowledge of change in responsibility and new behaviors associated with new responsibility.
- Verbalizes acceptance of new responsibility.

Nursing Interventions and Rationales

- Observe client's knowledge of behaviors associated with role.
  Ability to perform perceived roles is easily hampered by illness; it is important to note whether or not the client feels capable of functioning in the usual role.
- Allow client to express feelings regarding the role change.
  The client may experience disappointment and feelings of grief because of a role change; it is therapeutic for the client to express these feelings.
- Ask client direct questions regarding the new role and how the health care system can help him or her continue in this role.
  To maintain self-esteem, it is important to accurately assess the client's needs and ways to meet them; direct questions help elicit factual information.
- Have client make a list of strengths that are needed for the new role; acknowledge which strengths client has and which strengths need to be developed; work with client to set goals for desired role.
  In setting valued goals, people adapt their world to self-generated needs and projects rather than adapting themselves to a given world (Nuttin, 1992). Focusing on strengths helps the client to enhance behaviors associated with role performance in a positive way.
- Have client list problems associated with the new role and look at ways of overcoming them (e.g., if pain is worse late in day have client complete necessary role tasks early in day).
  There are many ways to accomplish tasks; it is helpful to help the client recognize this and make the appropriate accommodations.
- Look at ways to compensate for a physical disability (e.g., have a ramp built to provide access to house, put household objects within client's reach from wheelchair).
  Helping the client to help himself or herself by modifying the environment enhances self-esteem and fosters a sense of power by remaining able to function in his or her role.

Geriatric

- Explore community needs after assessing client's strengths; suggest functional activities (e.g., being a foster grandparent or a mentor for small businesses).
  If physical strength is declining, activities that require less physical prowess and more mental expertise are sometimes appropriate (Ringsven, Bond, 1991).
- Refer to family counseling as needed for adjustment to role changes.
  The family needs to be helped as a system because a change in one person's role affects the entire family.

Client/Family Teaching

- Help client identify resources for assistance in caring for a disabled or aging parent (e.g., adult day care).
  There are varying levels of assistance for the aging, and the client and family needs assistance in identifying these levels.
- Refer to appropriate community agencies to learn skills for functioning in the new or changed role (e.g., vocational rehabilitation, parenting classes, hospice, respite care).
  As one person changes, the other family members need to alter their patterns of communication and behavior to maintain balance in the family. Family members also need assistance to develop these new skills (Barry, 1994).

REFERENCES

Barry P: *Mental health and mental illness,* ed 5, Philadelphia, 1994, JB Lippincott.

Nuttin, JR: *Motivation, intention and voliton.* In Fleury J, editor: The application of motivational theory to cardiovascular risk reduction, *Image: J Nurs Schol* 24:229-239, 1992.

Ringsven M, Bond D: Gerontology and leadership skills for nurses, Albany, NY, 1991, Delmar.

Self-care deficit, bathing/hygiene

Linda Williams

Definition

The state in which an individual experiences an impaired ability to perform or complete bathing and hygiene activities.

Defining Characteristics

*Inability to wash body or body parts; inability to obtain or get to water source; inability to regulate temperature or flow. (*Critical)

Impaired physical mobility—Functional level classification

- 0—Completely independent
- 1—Requires use of equipment or device
- 2—Requires help from another person for assistance, supervision, or teaching
- 3—Requires help from another person and equipment device
- 4—Dependent, does not participate in activity

Related Factors (r/t)

Intolerance to activity; decreased strength and endurance; pain; discomfort; perceptual or cognitive impairment; neuromuscular impairment; musculoskeletal impairment; depression; severe anxiety.

Client Outcomes/Goals

- Free of body odor; skin intact.
- States satisfaction with ability to use adaptive devices to bathe.
- Bathes with assistance of caregiver as needed without anxiety.
- Explains and uses methods to bathe safely and with minimal difficulty.

Nursing Interventions and Rationales

- Observe for cause of inability to bathe; refer to related factors.
  Self-care requires multisystem competence, and restorative program planning is specific to problems that interfere with self-care.
- Assess client's ability to bathe self, noting specific deficits.
  Functional assessment provides activities of daily living task analysis data for goal and intervention planning.
- Ask client for input on bathing methods and timing of bath.
  Providing the client with opportunities for guiding own care increases control and prevents learned helplessness (LeSage et al, 1989).
- Request referrals for occupational and physical therapy.
  Collaboration and correlation of activities with interdisciplinary team members increases the client's mastery of self-care tasks.
- Plan activities to prevent fatigue during bathing.
  Energy conservation increases activity tolerance and promotes self-care.
- Medicate for pain 45 minutes before bathing, if needed.
  Pain relief promotes participation in self-care.
- Place all bathing equipment within easy reach.
  Environmental modifications promote safety and conserve energy.
- Use any necessary adaptive bathing equipment (e.g., long-handled brushes, soap-on-a-rope, washcloth mitt, wall bars, tub bench, shower chair, commode chair without pan in shower).
  Adaptive devices extend the client's reach, increase speed and safety, and decrease exertion.
- Provide privacy; give towel bath if appropriate, and use bath blanket if body-size towel is unavailable.
  Towel bathing increases privacy, which conveys respect during bathing (Wright, 1990).

- Allow client to participate as able in bathing, and provide praise for accomplishments; increase tasks as able.
  The client's expenditure of energy provides the caregiver the opportunity to convey respect for a well-done task, which increases the client's self-esteem.
- Inspect skin condition during bathing.
  Observation of skin allows detection of skin problems.
- Use or encourage caregiver to use an unhurried and caring touch.
  The basic human need of touch offers reassurance and comfort.
- If client is bathing alone, place assistance call light within client's reach.
  A readily available signaling device promotes safety and provides reassurance for the client.
- Monitor for fatigue, frustration, or inability to complete bathing tasks, and assist client as needed.
  The activity of bathing can produce atypical responses in acutely ill patients (Robichaud-Ekstrand, 1991).

Geriatric

- Assess for grieving resulting from loss of function.
  Grief resulting from loss of function can inhibit relearning of self-care.
- Allow client or caregiver adequate time to complete the bathing activity.
  Aging increases the time required to complete a task; thus elderly individuals with a self-care deficit require more time to complete a task.
- Use only a mild soap on genital and axillary areas; rinse well.
  Soap can alter skin pH and may increase the skin dryness that results from decreased oil production and perspiration in the elderly.
- Limit bathing to once or twice a week; provide a partial bath at other times.
  Frequent bathing promotes skin dryness.
- Use tepid water; test water temperature before use.
  Hot water promotes skin dryness and may burn a client who has decreased sensation.
- Use a gentle touch when bathing; avoid vigorous scrubbing motions.
  Aging skin is thinner, more fragile, and less able to withstand mechanical friction.
- Apply an emollient to wet skin after bathing.
  Applying an emollient to wet skin decreases skin dryness by preventing the loss of moisture that occurs during bathing (Fenske, Grayson, Newcomer, 1989).

Client/Family Teaching

- Teach how to use adaptive devices for bathing.
  Adaptive devices can provide independence, safety, and speed.
- Teach bathing techniques that promote safety (e.g., getting into tub before filling it with water, emptying water before getting out, antislip mat, wall-grab bars, tub bench).
  Safety devices decrease fear of injury and increase independence.
- Teach client and family an individualized bathing routine that includes a schedule, privacy, skin inspection, soap or lubricant, chill prevention.
  Understanding the client's needs and teaching the methods to meet these needs increases the client's satisfaction with the bathing experience.

REFERENCES

Fenske N, Grayson L, Newcomer V: Common problems of aging skin, *Patient Care* 23:225, 1989.

LeSage J et al: Learned helplessness, *J Gerontol Nurs* 15:9, 1989.

Robichaud-Ekstrand S: Shower versus sink bath: evaluation of heart rate, blood pressure and subjective response of the patient with myocardial infarction, *Heart Lung* 20:375, 1991.

Wright L: Bathing by towel, *Nurs Time* 86:36, 1990.

Self-care deficit, dressing/grooming

Linda Williams

Definition The state in which an individual experiences an impaired ability to perform or complete dressing and grooming activities.

Defining Characteristics

*Impaired ability to put on or take off necessary items of clothing; impaired ability to obtain or replace articles of clothing; impaired ability to fasten clothing; inability to maintain appearance at a satisfactory level. (*Critical)

Related Factors (r/t)

Intolerance to activity; decreased strength and endurance; pain; discomfort; perceptual or cognitive impairment; neuromuscular impairment; musculoskeletal impairment; depression; severe anxiety.

Client Outcomes/Goals

- Dresses and grooms self to optimal potential.
- Able to use adaptive devices to dress and groom.
- Explains and uses methods to enhance strengths during dressing and grooming.
- Dresses and grooms with assistance of caregiver as needed.

Nursing Interventions and Rationales

- Observe for cause of inability to dress and groom self; refer to related factors.
  Self-care requires multisystem competence, and restorative program planning is specific to problems that interfere with self-care.
- Assess client's ability to dress and groom self; note specific deficits.
  Functional assessment provides activities of daily living task analysis data for goal and intervention planning.
- Identify and include client's strengths in dressing and grooming.
  Incorporating the client's strengths into a dressing and grooming program increases self-care independence.
- Ask client for input on clothing choices and how to increase the ease of dressing self.
  Providing the client with opportunities for guiding own care increases control and prevents learned helplessness (LeSage et al, 1989).
- Request referrals for occupational and physical therapy.
  Collaboration and correlation of activities with interdisciplinary team members increases the client's mastery of self-care tasks.
- Medicate for pain 45 minutes before dressing and grooming, if needed.
  Pain relief promotes participation in self-care.
- Plan activities to prevent fatigue while dressing and grooming.
  Energy conservation increases activity tolerance and promotes self-care.
- Help client store clothing and grooming devices within easy reach; closet rods or drawers between eye and hip level and turntables are helpful.
  Environmental modifications minimize bending and conserve energy (Lorig, Fries, 1990).
- Select larger-sized clothing and clothing with elastic waistbands, Velcro fasteners, or wide sleeves and pant legs.
  Simplified dressing promotes independence.
- Use adaptive dressing and grooming equipment as needed (e.g., long-handled brushes, grasping devices, Velcro closures, zipper pulls, button hooks, elastic shoelaces, large buttons, soap-on-a-rope, suction holders).
  Adaptive devices increase speed and safety and decrease exertion.

- Lay clothing out in the order that it will be put on by the client.
  Simplified dressing tasks increase self-care ability.
- Encourage client to dress appropriately for time of day.
- Perform dressing and grooming activities in a consistent sequence each day.
  An established routine of awakening and dressing provides a sense of normalcy and increases motivation to perform self-care. Prolonged repetition promotes increased relearning of self-care tasks (Giles, Shore, 1989).
- Encourage participation; guide client's hand through task if necessary.
  Experiencing the normal process of a task through guided practice facilitates optimal relearning.

Geriatric

- Assess for grieving resulting from loss of function.
  Grief resulting from loss of function can inhibit relearning of self-care.
- Frequently assess client's pain; provide pain relief as needed before dressing and grooming activities.
  Elderly people have twice the incidence of pain; they often have more than one pain source, which commonly includes arthritis (Acute Pain Management Guideline Panel, 1992).
- Allow client or caregiver adequate time to complete dressing (e.g., do not insist that client is dressed at an early hour).
  Aging increases the time required to complete a task; the elderly client with a self-care deficit requires more time to complete a task.

Client/Family Teaching

- Teach client to dress the affected side first, then the unaffected side.
  Dressing the affected side first allows for easier manipulation of clothing.
- Teach the simplest step in a task until mastered, and then proceed to more complicated steps.
  Simplified dressing and grooming tasks that consist of many small steps promotes mastery.
- Teach how to use adaptive devices for dressing and grooming.
  Assistive devices can provide independence, safety, and speed.
- Teach client and family to select clothes appropriate for the season, temperature, and weather.
  Clients with altered sensation need to understand the factors that influence body temperature and the environment.

REFERENCES

Acute Pain Management Guideline Panel. *Acute pain management: operative or medical procedures and trauma.* Clinical Practice Guideline, Rockville, Md, 1992, Agency for Health Care Policy and Research, Public Health Service, US Department of Health and Human Services (ACHPR Publication No 92-0032).

Giles G, Shore M: A rapid method for teaching severely brain injured adults how to wash and dress, *Arch Phys Med Rehabil* 70:156, 1989.

LeSage J et al: Learned helplessness, *J Gerontol Nurs* 15:9, 1989.

Lorig K, Fries J: *The arthritis helpbook*, ed 3, Reading, Mass, 1990, Addison-Wesley.

BIBLIOGRAPHY

Carnevali D, Patrick M: *Nursing management of the elderly*, ed 3, Philadelphia, 1993, JB Lippincott.

Dittmar S: *Rehabilitation nursing*, St Louis, 1989, Mosby.

Hopkins H, Smith H: *Willard and Spackman's occupational therapy*, ed 7, Philadelphia, 1988, JB Lippincott.

Self-care deficit, feeding

Linda Williams

Definition The state in which an individual experiences an impaired ability to perform or complete feeding activities for oneself.

Defining Characteristics

Inability to bring food from a receptacle to the mouth.

Related Factors (r/t)

Intolerance to activity; decreased strength and endurance; pain; discomfort; perceptual or cognitive impairment; neuromuscular impairment; musculoskeletal impairment; depression; severe anxiety.

Client Outcomes/Goals

- Feeds self.
- States satisfaction with ability to use adaptive devices for feeding.
- Caregiver provides assistance with feeding when necessary.

Nursing Interventions and Rationales

- Observe for cause of inability to feed self independently; refer to related factors.
  Self-care requires multisystem competence, and restorative program planning is specific to problems that interfere with self-care.
- Assess client's ability to feed self; bilaterally test gag reflex; note specific deficits.
  Functional assessment provides activities of daily living task analysis data for goal and intervention planning.
- Ask client for input on methods to facilitate eating and feeding (e.g., cultural foods, food and fluid preferences).
  Providing the client with opportunities for guiding one's care increases control and prevents learned helplessness (LeSage et al, 1989).
- Request referral for occupational and physical therapy; request a dietician.
  Collaboration and correlation of activities with interdisciplinary team members increases the client's mastery of self-care tasks.
- Use any necessary adaptive feeding equipment (e.g., rocker knives, plate guards, suction mats, built-up handles on utensils, scoop dishes, large-handled cups).
  Adaptive devices increase independence.
- Ensure that client has dentures, hearing aids, and glasses in place.
  Adaptive devices increase self-care.
- Help client into sitting position; ensure that client's head is flexed slightly forward and shoulders are supported while eating and for 1 hour after a meal.
  Gravity assists with swallowing, and aspiration is decreased when sitting upright.
- Prepare meal items before client begins eating.
  Preparing items for the client conserves energy for hand-to-mouth activities.
- Allow client to participate in feeding as able, and provide praise for all feeding attempts; increase tasks as able.
  Client's expenditure of energy provides caregiver the opportunity to convey respect for a well-done task, which increases self-esteem.
- When assisting with meal, caregiver should sit beside client on the unaffected side.
  Sitting beside the client makes the caregiver more comfortable and less likely to hurry and it encourages the client to eat more (Kolodny, Malek, 1991).
- Encourage participation; guide client's hand through task if needed.
  Experiencing the normal process of a task through guided practice facilitates optimal relearning.

- Plan activities to prevent fatigue before meals.
  Energy conservation increases activity tolerance and promotes self-care.
- Medicate for pain before meals, if needed.
  Pain relief promotes participation in self-care.
- Provide client with a pleasant meal environment; keep the environment free of toileting devices and odors, avoid painful procedures before meals, remove lids from tray, provide clean utensils for separate courses, and maintain a social environment.
  Attention to the aesthetics of feeding increases feeding success.
- Encourage client to keep food on the unaffected side or in the center of mouth while chewing.
  Keeping food away from the affected side of the mouth prevents pocketing of food.
- Provide oral hygiene after eating and check for pocketing of food.
  Aspiration can occur from food left in the mouth.

Geriatric

- Allow client with dentures adequate time to chew.
  Chewing with dentures takes four times longer to reach a certain level of mastication than chewing with natural teeth.
- Be prepared to intervene if choking occurs; have suction equipment readily available, and know the Heimlich maneuver.
  Frail and elderly clients are at an increased risk of choking.
- Choose soft foods rather than liquids, or use dietary thickeners.
  Choking occurs more easily on clear liquids than on solid or soft foods (Hogstel, Robinson, 1989).
- Provide finger foods.
  Finger foods can be nutritious and they allow independence and the choice of what and when to eat.

Client/Family Teaching

- Teach client how to use adaptive devices.
  Adaptive devices increase independence.
- Teach client with hemianopsia to scan the plate by turning head so that plate is in line of vision.
  Compensation for hemianopsia is done by turning head to place items in line of vision (Needham, 1993).
- Teach the visually impaired client to locate foods according to numbers on a clock.
  For visually impaired clients, food is placed on the plate using the clock method.
- Teach caregiver feeding techniques that prevent choking (e.g., sit beside client on the unaffected side, feed client slowly, check food temperature, provide fluid between bites, establish a method to communicate readiness for next bite, limit conversation while chewing).
  Sitting beside the client makes the caregiver more comfortable and less likely to hurry (Kolodny, Malek, 1991).

REFERENCES

Hogstel M, Robinson N: Feeding the frail elderly, *J Gerontol Nurs* 15:16, 1989.
Kolodny V, Malek A: Improving feeding skills, *J Gerontol Nurs* 17:20, 1991.
LeSage J et al: Learned helplessness, *J Gerontol Nurs* 15:9, 1989.
Needham J: *Gerontological nursing: a restorative approach*, Albany, NY, 1993, Delmar.

BIBLIOGRAPHY

Carnevali D, Patrick M: *Nursing management of the elderly*, ed 3, Philadelphia, 1993, JB Lippincott.
Dittmar S: *Rehabilitation nursing*, St Louis, 1989, Mosby.
Hopkins H, Smith H: *Willard and Spackman's occupational therapy*, ed 7, Philadelphia, 1988, JB Lippincott.

Self-care deficit, toileting

Linda Williams

Definition The state in which an individual experiences an impaired ability to perform or complete toileting activities for oneself.

Defining Characteristics

*Inability to get to toilet or commode; *inability to sit on or rise from toilet or commode; *inability to manipulate clothing for toileting; *inability to carry out proper toileting hygiene; inability to flush toilet or commode. (*Critical)

Related Factors (r/t)

Impaired transfer ability; impaired mobility status; intolerance to activity; decreased strength and endurance; pain; discomfort; perceptual or cognitive impairment; neuromuscular impairment; musculoskeletal impairment; depression; severe anxiety.

Client Outcomes/Goals

- Free of incontinence and impaction with no urine or stool on skin.
- States satisfaction with ability to use adaptive devices for toileting.
- Explains and uses methods to be safe and independent in toileting.

Nursing Interventions and Rationales

- Observe cause of inability to toilet independently; refer to related factors.
  Self-care requires multisystem competence, and restorative program planning is specific to problems that interfere with self-care.
- Assess ability to toilet; note specific deficits.
  Functional assessment provides activities of daily living task analysis data for goal and intervention planning.
- Ask client for input on toileting methods and timing and how to better provide toileting activities.
  Providing the client with opportunities for guiding own care increases control and prevents learned helplessness (LeSage et al, 1989).
- Assess client's usual bowel and bladder toileting patterns and the terminology used for toileting.
  Individuals develop a unique pattern of toileting over time for faster, normal elimination.
- Request referral for occupational and physical therapy for help in working with client to transfer from bed to commode.
  Collaboration and correlation of activities with interdisciplinary team members increases the client's mastery of self-care tasks.
- Use any necessary assistive toileting equipment (e.g., toilet risers, raised toilet seat, suction mats, spill-proof urinals, support rails next to toilet, toilet safety frames, Sanifems [allow a woman to void standing], fracture bedpans).
  Adaptive devices promote independence and safety.
- Provide privacy.
  Privacy can prevent suppression of elimination resulting from embarrassment about noise and odor.
- Schedule toileting to occur when defecation urge is strongest or voiding is likely (e.g., in the morning, every 2 hours, after meals, at bedtime). Assist client until self-care ability increases.
  The defecation urge is strongest in morning or within 1 hour after meals or warm beverages. Approximately 50 to 75 ml of urine are produced hourly, and the urge to void occurs at 200 ml; thus a 2-hour schedule can reduce incontinence.
- Allow client to participate as able in toileting, and provide praise for accomplishments; increase tasks as able; work with client to aim toward independence in toileting.

Client's expenditure of energy provides caregiver the opportunity to convey respect for a well-done task, which increases self-esteem.

- Obtain a bedside commode if necessary; avoid bedpans if possible. If client is acutely ill, provide bedpan at appropriate intervals.
  A sitting position uses gravity and is more conducive to normal elimination.
- Make assistance call light readily available to client, and answer light promptly; remove environmental barriers to toilet.
  To decrease incontinence, the client needs rapid access to toileting facilities; navigational barriers can increase incontinence episodes (Noelker, 1987).
- Keep toilet paper and handwashing items within easy reach of client.
- Inspect skin condition.
  Observation of skin allows detection of skin problems.
- Provide prompt skin care and linen changes after incontinence episodes.
  The presence of urine or stool on the skin leads to skin breakdown.

Geriatric

- Assess client's mobility status and speed of movement.
  Elderly women with slower mobility experience more incontinent episodes (Wyman, Eiswick, 1993).
- Reassure client that call light will be answered promptly.
  The elderly cannot respond quickly to the urge to void as a result of limited functional ability and environmental barriers; they are also unable to delay voiding as a result of decreased muscle tone and neurological changes.
- Provide a small footstool in front of toilet or commode.
  Intra-abdominal pressure is increased by elevating knees above the hips, which facilitates elimination in the elderly person with weak abdominal muscles.
- Assess client's functional ability to manipulate clothing for toileting; modify clothing with Velcro fasteners and elastic waistbands.
  Delays resulting from manipulating zippers and buttons may cause functional incontinence (Wold, 1993).
- Avoid use of indwelling or condom catheters, if possible.
  An indwelling urinary catheter is a source of infection and keeps the bladder empty, which reduces bladder capacity and decreases the opportunity for independence.
- Help client develop a regular toileting schedule; use verbal prompting to impart awareness of need.

Client/Family Teaching

- Teach client and family how to toilet client with adaptive and safety devices.
  Adaptive devices can provide independence, safety, and speed.
- Prepare client for toileting needs by teaching the action of medications such as diuretics.
  Medications that promote elimination require prompt responses to toileting needs.
- Teach family how to help client toilet, including the use of a bedpan, commode, and appropriate toileting schedule.

REFERENCES

LeSage J et al: Learned helplessness, *J Gerontol Nurs* 15:9, 1989.

Noelker L: Incontinence in elderly cared for by the family, *Gerontologist* 27:194, 1987.

Wold G: *Basic geriatric nursing,* St Louis, 1993, Mosby.

Wyman J, Eiswick R: Influence of functional, urological and environmental characteristics on urinary incontinence in community-dwelling older women, *Nurs Res* 42:270, 1993.

BIBLIOGRAPHY

Hamilton LW, Creason NS: Mental status and functional abilities: change in institutionalized elderly women, *Nurs Diag* 3:81-86, 1992.

Chronic low self-esteem

Helen Kelley

Definition Long-standing negative self-evaluations and negative feelings about self or capabilities.

Defining Characteristics

Major — Self-negating verbalizations; expressions of shame or guilt; evaluation of self as unable to deal with events; rationalization or rejection of positive feedback about self; exaggeration of negative feedback about self; hesitancy about new things or situations.

Minor — Frequent lack of success in work or other life events; excessive adherence to or dependency on others' opinions; lack of eye contact; nonassertive or passive nature; indecisiveness; excessive searches for reassurance.

Related Factors (r/t)

Childhood abuse or neglect (physical, sexual, or emotional); abusive adult relationships; elder abuse; mental illness (especially depression); drug or alcohol use or dependence; eating disorders.

Client Outcomes/Goals

- Demonstrates improved ability to interact with others (e.g., maintains eye contact, expresses feelings).
- Verbalizes increased self-acceptance through use of positive self-statements.
- Identifies personal strengths.
- Able to set small, achievable goals.
- Attempts independent decision making.

Nursing Interventions and Rationales

- Actively listen to and respect the client.
  Attentive attitude conveys acceptance (Norris, 1992).
- Assess existing strengths and coping abilities, and provide opportunities for their expression and recognition.
  Self-esteem is enhanced by the ability to perform competently (Coopersmith, 1981).
- Identify and limit client's expressions of negative self-assessment.
  These limitations disrupt the pattern of negative distortion.
- Encourage realistic and achievable goal setting; recognize the value of attempts and accomplishments.
  Reframe "failures" as opportunities to learn and change tactics.
- Demonstrate and promote effective communication techniques.
  Effective communication increases the opportunity to receive positive validation from others.
- Encourage independent decision making by reviewing options and their possible consequences with client.
  Autonomy enhances self-esteem (Crouch, 1983).

Geriatric

- Support client in identifying and adapting to functional changes.
  Accurate evaluation allows the client to establish realistic expectations of self.
- Use reminiscence to identify patterns of strength and accomplishment.
  Identifying strengths and accomplishments counteracts pervasive negativity.
- Encourage participation in peer group activities.
  Withdrawal and social isolation are detrimental to feelings of self-worth.

Client/Family Teaching

- Refer to community agencies for psychotherapeutic counseling.
- Refer to psychoeducational groups on stress reduction and coping skills.

REFERENCES

Coopersmith S: The antecedents of self-esteem, Palo Alto, Calif, 1981, *Consulting Psychologist Press.*

Crouch MA, Straub V: Enhancement of self-esteem in adults, *Fam Community Health* 6:65-72, 1983.

Norris J: Nursing interventions for self-esteem disturbance, *Nurs Diag* 3:48-53, 1992.

BIBLIOGRAPHY

Stanwyck DJ: Self-esteem through the life span, *Fam Community Health* 8:11-23, 1983.

Wesorick B: Disturbances in self-concept. In *Standards of nursing care: a model for nursing practice*, Philadelphia, 1990, JB Lippincott.

Self-esteem disturbance

Helen Kelley

Definition Negative self-evaluation and negative feelings about self or capabilities, which may be directly or indirectly expressed.

Defining Characteristics

Self-negating verbalization; expressions of shame or guilt; evaluation of self as unable to deal with events; rationalization or rejection of positive feedback about self; exaggeration of negative feedback about self; rationalization of personal failures; hesitancy about new things or situations; denial of problems obvious to others; projection of blame or responsibility for problems; hypersensitivity to slight criticism; grandiosity.

Client Outcomes/Goals

- Able to accurately assess own strengths and weaknesses.
- Able to admit own error without excessive guilt or defensiveness.
- Able to accept compliments.
- Willing to take risks and try new things or situations.
- Accepts responsibility for own actions.
- Accepts criticism and attempts to correct problems.

Nursing Interventions and Rationales

- Ask client to list one positive attribute for each negative attribute that he or she generates.
  Such a list promotes a realistic and balanced perspective of self.
- Treat client in a nonjudgmental way; acknowledge client's right to have personal values and beliefs.
  Such treatment encourages honesty and appreciation of unique qualities (Norris, 1992).
- Help client identify origins of self-esteem.
  Self-esteem is learned behavior and can be changed.
- Have client participate in a daily grooming routine.
  Positive feelings are generated when a person is well groomed.
- Reframe mistakes and errors (own and others') as natural and human experiences.
  Modeling acceptance of self and others lessens the need for defensive responses when errors are made.
- Have client practice making positive statements about self and responding in a positive way when compliments are given; role-play may be used.
- Encourage a problem-solving approach rather than an expression of doubt or defensiveness.
  A problem-solving approach promotes constructive action.
- Encourage client to ask for feedback rather than dread criticism.
  Feedback promotes self-control.
- Give recognition to appropriate risk-taking attempts and encourage the practice of new behaviors.
  Change requires a willingness to tolerate the discomfort of unfamiliar behavior and responses for a period of time (Wilson, Kneisel, 1992).

Geriatric

- Promote a positive self-image; compliment client on appearance; help client look his or her best.
- Do not appear rushed; encourage verbalization of client's fears about the illness or dysfunction.

The elderly client's response time may be slower; multiple losses lead to fear about the illness or dysfunction.

- Help client to review life and identify successes; encourage participation in support-reminiscence groups.
  Reminiscence is very therapeutic for the elderly client.
- Assist in planning a schedule for regular visits by family and significant others.

Client/Family Teaching

- Teach that self-esteem is a learned behavior and that any learned behavior can be changed.
- Refer to community agencies, self-help groups, or counseling as needed.

REFERENCES Norris J: Nursing intervention for self-esteem disturbance, *Nurs Diag* 3:48-53, 1992.
Wilson HS, Kneisel CR: *Psychiatric nursing*, Menlo Park, Calif, 1992, Addison-Wesley.

Situational low self-esteem

Helen Kelley

Definition Negative self-evaluation or feelings about self that develop in response to a loss or change in an individual who previously had a positive self-evaluation.

Defining Characteristics

Major: Episodic occurrence of negative self-appraisal in response to life events in a client with a previously positive self-appraisal.

Minor: Self-evaluation; verbalization of negative feelings about the self (e.g., helplessness, uselessness).

Self-negating verbalizations; expressions of shame or guilt; evaluation of self as unable to handle situations or events; difficulty making decisions.

Related Factors (r/t)

Situational crisis; significant losses; persons; roles; stressful changes; work; family; body image and appearance; health problems; disability.

Client Outcomes/Goals

- States effect of life events on feelings about self.
- States positive personal strengths.
- Acknowledges presence of guilt and does not blame self if action was related to another person's appraisal.
- Seeks help for situations when necessary.

Nursing Interventions and Rationales

- Actively listen to and demonstrate respect for and acceptance of client.
  Clarification of thoughts and feelings promotes self-acceptance (LeMone, 1991).
- Help client recognize that he or she is the only person he or she can control; say to the client "No one can make you feel guilty without your consent."
- Mutually identify strengths, resources, and previously effective coping strategies.
  Acknowledgment of competence enhances self-esteem (Miller, 1983).
- Have client list strengths.
- Accept client's own pace in working through grief or crisis situations.
  Pressuring the client to prematurely resolve feelings increases the client's sense of inadequacy (Kus, 1985).
- Assess client for symptoms of depression and potential for suicide or violence; immediately notify appropriate personnel of symptoms. Refer to **Risk for violence**.
  Safety measures and psychiatric interventions are essential when a risk is present.
- Refer to **Self-esteem disturbance** and **Chronic low self-esteem**.

Client/Family Teaching

- Educate client and family regarding the grief process.
  Understanding this process normalizes responses of sadness, anger, guilt, and helplessness.
- Teach client and family that the crisis is temporary.
  Knowing that the crisis is temporary provides a sense of hope for future resolution.
- Refer to appropriate community resources or crisis intervention centers.

REFERENCES

Kus RJ: *Crisis intervention.* In Bulechek GM, McCloskey JC, editors: *Nursing interventions: treatments for nursing diagnoses*, Philadelphia, 1985, WB Saunders.

LeMone P: Analysis of a human phenomenon: self-concept, *Nurs Diag* 2:126, 1991.

Miller JF: *Coping with chronic illness: overcoming powerlessness*, Philadelphia, 1983, FA Davis.

Risk for self-mutilation

Gail Ladwig

Definition The state in which an individual is at high risk to perform a deliberate act on the self with the intent not to kill but to injure, which produces immediate tissue damage to the body.

Risk Factors (r/t)

Groups at risk Clients with borderline personality disorders (especially females 16 to 25 years of age); clients in a psychotic state (frequently males in young adulthood); emotionally disturbed or battered children; mentally retarded and autistic children; clients with a history of self-injury.

Risk factors Inability to properly cope with increased psychological or physiological tension; feelings of depression, rejection, self-hatred, separation anxiety, guilt, and depersonalization; fluctuating emotions; command hallucinations; need for sensory stimuli; parental emotional deprivation; dysfunctional family.

Client Outcomes/Goals

- States appropriate ways to cope with increased psychological or physiological tension.
- Able to express feelings.
- Seeks help when hallucinations are present.
- Uses appropriate community agencies when caregivers are unable to attend to emotional needs.

Nursing Interventions and Rationales

- Assess for family history of substance abuse.
  Self-mutilation and heavy use of mental health services have been correlated with having an alcoholic parent (Rose et al, 1991).
- Monitor the client's behavior; do 15-minute checks at irregular times so client does not notice a pattern.
  When there is lack of control, safety of the client is an important issue and close observation is essential. Not following a pattern prevents the client from being self-abusive when he or she knows the caregiver will not be present.
- Secure a written or verbal contract from client to notify staff when experiencing feelings of self-mutilation.
  Discussing feelings of self-harm with a trusted person provides relief for the client. A contract gets the subject out in the open and places some of the responsibility for safety with the client.
- Monitor for presence of hallucinations; ask specifically, "Do you hear voices that other people do not hear?"
  Brief, reversible psychotic episodes tend to occur as a response to stress. (First et al, 1994). An accurate assessment of the client's contact with reality is important in planning care; acknowledging that the client may hear something that others do not may open up communication and help to establish trust.
- Assure client that he or she will not be alone and will be safe during the hallucinations; provide referrals for medication.
  Hallucinations can be very frightening, and the client needs reassurance that he or she will not be left alone.
- If self-mutilation does occur, care for the wounds in a matter-of-fact way.
  This approach does not support inappropriate attention-getting behavior and may decrease repetition of the behavior.
- When client is experiencing extreme anxiety, provide for one-to-one staffing.
  The presence of a trusted individual may calm fears about personal safety.

- Reinforce alternative ways of dealing with anxiety such as exercise, engaging in unit activities, or talking about feelings.
  With practice, clients can substitute other behaviors when feeling anxious. If inappropriate ways of handling life situations can be learned, appropriate ways can also be learned.
- Keep environment safe; remove all harmful objects from the area.
  Client safety is a nursing priority.
- If client is unable to control behavior, time out in a quiet room may be necessary; ensure safety by providing staff observation.
  Because of extreme fear of abandonment, leaving a client alone may cause extreme anxiety; however, the client may need to be away from other external stimuli when very agitated.
- Give positive reinforcement when client makes appropriate behavioral choices; confront inappropriate behavior.
  It is important to reinforce appropriate behavior to encourage repetition.
- Involve client in planning of care and emphasize that client can make choices.
  Involving the client in planning of care places some of the responsibility for improvement with the client.
- Emphasize that client must comply with the rules of the unit; give positive reinforcement for compliance and minimize attention to disruptive behavior.
  It is important to reinforce appropriate behavior to encourage repetition.
- Concentrate on client's strengths; have client list strengths and carry the list on a 3×5 card to refer to when negative thoughts occur.
  Positive reinforcement enhances self-esteem and encourages repetition of behavior; listing strengths encourages the client to get reinforcement from within instead of from external sources.
- Refer to protective services if there is evidence of abuse.
  It is the nurse's legal responsibility to report abuse.

Client/Family Teaching

- Teach stress reduction techniques such as imagery and controlled breathing (breathing in on "re" and breathing out on "lax"); teach client to sustain the breathing-out phase.
  Anxiety lessens when relaxation is used, and the use of imagery enhances the experience.
- Provide client and family with phone numbers of appropriate community agencies for therapy and counseling.
  Continuous follow-up care may be necessary, and the method to access this care must be given to the client.
- Give client positive things on which to focus by referring to appropriate agencies for job-training skills or education.
  Alternative coping skills and the means to access them are essential for continued good mental health.

REFERENCES

First MB et al: Changes in mood, anxiety, and personality disorders *Psychiatr Nurs*, 1(1), 1994.

Rose SM, Peabody CG, Strategies B: Undetected abuse among intensive case management clients, *Hosp Community Psychiatry*, 42:5, 1991.

BIBLIOGRAPHY

Bulechek G, McCloskey J: *Nursing interventions: essential nursing treatments,* ed 2, Philadelphia, 1992, WB Saunders.

Johnson, BS: *Adaptation and growth psychiatric-mental health nursing* Philadelphia, 1993, JB Lippincott.

Townsend, M: *Psychiatric mental health nursing: concepts of care,* 1993, FA Davis.

Sensory/perceptual alterations (specify): visual, auditory, kinesthetic, gustatory, tactile, olfactory

Betty Ackley

Definition The state in which an individual experiences a change in the amount or patterning of oncoming stimuli accompanied by a diminished, exaggerated, distorted, or impaired response to such stimuli.

Defining Characteristics

Major Disorientation regarding time, place, or persons; altered abstraction; altered conceptualization; change in problem-solving abilities; reported or measured change in sensory acuity; change in behavior pattern; anxiety; apathy; change in usual response to stimuli; indication of body image alteration; restlessness; irritability; altered communication patterns.

Minor Complaints of fatigue; alterations in posture; changes in muscular tension; inappropriate responses; hallucinations.

Related Factors (r/t)

Altered, excessive, or insufficient environmental stimuli; altered sensory reception, transmission, or integration; endogenous chemical alterations (e.g., electrolytes), exogenous chemical alterations (e.g., drugs); psychological stress.

Client Outcomes/Goals

- Demonstrates understanding by a verbal, written, or signed response.
- Demonstrates relaxed body movements and facial expressions.
- Explains plan to modify life-style to accommodate visual or hearing impairment.
- Remains free of physical harm resulting from decreased balance or a loss of vision, hearing, or tactile sensation.
- Has contact with appropriate community resources.

Nursing Interventions and Rationales

Sensory Deprivation/Overload

- Observe for factors that can cause sensory/perceptual alterations (e.g., insufficient sleep, sensory deprivation, sensory overload with excessive noise and stimuli, substance abuse, medications, electrolyte imbalance, normal aging process).
  Sensory/perceptual alterations are common in critical care, surgical care (especially cardiac surgery), and in hospitalized elderly clients (Wilson, 1993).
- Assess orientation, attention, concentration, memory, ability to think, overall appearance, body movements, speech, use of appropriate language, mood, and affect.
  A complete bedside assessment is necessary to determine the presence of sensory/perceptual alteration (Inaba-Roland, Maricle, 1992).
- Orient to time, place, and person; inform of current weather, news items, family visits, or telephone calls.
  Reality orientation can help prevent an onset of confusion or sensory/perceptual alteration.
- Converse with client when entering the room, touch the client as appropriate and within client's cultural norms, and explain all procedures. Do not discuss client's situation with physician or fellow staff without including client in the conversation.
  Meaningful human contact within the framework of the client's culture may help decrease the incidence of confusion (Kloosterman, 1991).
- Provide radio, television, clocks, or calendars to encourage orientation.

- Encourage visits from significant others; encourage client to keep pictures of family and friends at bedside.
  Hospitalized clients who have less contact with significant others have an increase in sensory/perceptual alterations (Foreman, 1986).
- Decrease noise pollution as much as possible (e.g., place pulse oximeter away from client's head, turn off suction when not in use, hang IVs before the alarm sounds).
  Constant noxious noise can lead to sensory overload (Halm, Alpen, 1993).
- Cluster activities to provide rest periods; morning naps are especially helpful. Ensure *at least* 2 hours of uninterrupted sleep at night. Refer to nursing interventions for **Sleep pattern disturbance**.

Auditory

- Observe emotional needs and encourage expression of feelings.
  Hearing impairments may cause frustration, anger, fear, and self-imposed isolation (Taylor, 1993).
- Keep background noise to a minimum; turn off television and radio when communicating with client.
  Background noise significantly interferes with hearing in the hearing-impaired client.
- Stand or sit directly in front of client if possible; make sure adequate light is on nurse's face, establish eye contact, and use nonverbal gestures.
  These measures make it easier to read lips and watch nonverbal communication, which is a large component of all communication.
- Speak distinctly in lower voice tones if possible.
  In many kinds of hearing loss, clients lose the ability to hear higher-pitched tones but can still hear lower-pitched tones.
- If necessary, provide a communication board or personnel who know sign language.
  These alternative forms of communication help decrease social isolation.
- Refer to appropriate resources such as a speech and hearing clinic, audiologist, or ear, nose, and throat physician.
- Assist client with placement of hearing aid if necessary.

Visual

- Observe client's emotional needs; encourage expression of feelings; expect grieving behavior.
  Blind people grieve the loss of vision and experience a loss of identity and control over their lives (Vader, 1992).
- Identify name and purpose when entering client's room.
  Identifying self when entering the room helps the client feel secure and lessens social isolation.
- Orient to time, place, person, and surroundings; provide a radio or talking books.
- If client has decreased vision, keep environment well lit but reduce glare (e.g., waxed floors, blinding sunlight in room).
  Glare "wipes out" vision, and the client sees only a blurred image.
- Keep doors completely open or closed; keep furniture out of path to bathroom; do not rearrange furniture.
  These actions maintain a safe environment for the client.
- Feed client at mealtimes if blindness is temporary.
- Keep siderails up for client's safety; explain this precaution to client.

- Converse with and touch client frequently during care if frequent touch is within client's cultural norm.
  Appropriate touch can decrease social isolation.
- Walk client by having client grasp nurse's elbow and walk partly behind nurse.
- Walk a frightened or confused client by having client put both hands on nurse's shoulders; back up in desired direction while holding client around the waist.
  This method helps the client feel secure and ensures safety.
- Keep call light within client's reach; check location of call light before leaving the room.
- Ensure access to any necessary eyeglasses or magnifying glasses.
- Refer to optometrist or ophthalmologist for vision care if needed.
  NOTE: For **Sensory perceptual alteration: kinesthetic and tactile**, refer to **Potential for injury**. For **Sensory perceptual alteration: olfactory and gustatory** refer to **Altered nutrition: less than body requirements**.

Geriatric

- Keep environment quiet, soothing, and familiar.
  Recognize that the elderly client may become more agitated and wander in the late afternoon and evening.
- Avoid using extremely hot or cold foods or bathwater.
- If client has a sensory deprivation, encourage family to give sensory stimulation by providing music, voices, photographs, touch, and familiar smells.
- If client has a hearing or vision loss, work with client to ensure contact with others and to strengthen the social network.
  Severe loneliness can accompany hearing or vision loss in the elderly as a result of self-imposed isolation (Christian, Dluhy, O'Neill, 1989; Foxall et al, 1992).

Client/Family Teaching

- Teach family how to provide appropriate stimuli in the home environment to prevent sensory/perceptual alterations.
- Teach blind client how to feed self; identify food placement as the hours on a clock.
- Teach client and family ways to deal with the vision or hearing loss.
- Refer to community agencies for help in dealing with sensory/perceptual losses.

REFERENCES

Christian E, Dluhy N, O'Neill R: Sounds of silence: coping with hearing loss and loneliness, *J Gerontol Nurse* 15:4-9, 1989.

Foreman M: Acute confusional states in hospitalized elderly: a research dilemma, *Nurs Res* 35:34, 1986.

Foxall MJ et al: Predictors of loneliness in low vision adults, *West J Nurs Res* 14:86-99, 1992.

Halm MA, Alpen MA: The impact of technology on patients and families, *Adv Clin Nurs Research* 28:443-457, 1993.

Inaba-Roland K, Maricle R: Assessing delirium in the acute care setting, *Heart Lung* 21:48, 1992.

Kloosterman ND: Cultural care: the missing link in severe sensory alteration, *Nurs Sci Q,* 4:119-121, 1991.

Taylor KS: Geriatric hearing loss: management strategies for nurses, *Geriatr Nurs* 14:74-76, 1993.

Vader LA: Vision and vision loss, *Nurs Clin North Am* 27:705-714, 1992.

Wilson LD: Sensory perceptual alteration: diagnosis, prediction and intervention in the hospitalized adult, *Nurs Clin North Am* 28:747-765, 1993.

BIBLIOGRAPHY

Alberti PW et al: New reasons for hope in hearing loss, *Patient Care* 26:75-78, 1992.

Sexual dysfunction

Gail Ladwig

Definition The state in which an individual experiences a change in sexual function that is unsatisfying, unrewarding, and inadequate.

Defining Characteristics

Verbalization of problem; alteration in achieving perceived sex role; actual or perceived limitation imposed by disease or therapy; value conflict; alteration in achieving sexual satisfaction; inability to achieve desired satisfaction; seeking of confirmation of desirability; alteration in relationship with significant other; change of interest in self and others.

Related Factors (r/t)

Biopsychosocial alteration of sexuality; ineffectual or absent role models; physical abuse; psychosocial abuse (e.g., harmful relationships); vulnerability; value conflict; lack of privacy; lack of significant other; altered body structure or function (e.g., pregnancy, recent childbirth, drugs, surgery, anomalies, disease process, trauma, irradiation); misinformation; knowledge deficit.

Client Outcomes/Goals

- Identifies individual cause of sexual dysfunction.
- Identifies stresses that contribute to dysfunction.
- Discusses alternative, satisfying, and acceptable sexual practices for self and partner.
- Able to discuss with partner concerns about body image and sex role.

Nursing Interventions and Rationales

- Gather client's sexual history, noting normal patterns of functioning and client's vocabulary.
  This history begins the process of helping the client with actual or perceived needs.
- Determine client's and partner's current knowledge.
  One of the most frequent nursing interventions is education.
- Observe for stress, anxiety, and depression as a possible cause of dysfunction.
  Sexual dysfunction can be attributed to many psychological factors.
- Observe for grief related to loss (e.g., amputation, mastectomy, ostomy).
  A change in body image often precedes sexual dysfunction.
- Explore physical causes such as diabetes, arteriosclerotic heart disease, drug or medication side effects, or smoking in males.
  Sexual dysfunction may be related to a physical illness.
- Provide privacy and be verbally and nonverbally nonjudgmental.
  Privacy is important in ensuring confidentiality. To facilitate communication it is also vital that the nurse clarify personal values and remain nonjudgmental.
- Provide privacy to allow sexual expression between client and partner (e.g., private room, Do Not Disturb sign for a specified length of time).
  The hospital setting has little opportunity for privacy, so the nurse must ensure that it is available.
- Explain need for client to share concerns with partner.
  Regardless of the experience of sexual function, maintaining the relationship is important for meeting intimacy needs (Lemone, 1991).
- Validate normalcy of client's feelings and correct misinformation.
  A sensitive nurse who has an understanding of sexual health, functioning, and interferences can direct those who need help toward treatment (Lewis, 1992).

Geriatric

- Discuss with client and partner their present role adjustments.
  This discussion assists client and partner with coping.
- Assess the possibility of erectile dysfunction.
  Erectile dysfunction occurs in men of any age but is more common in older men. Sexual function can almost always be restored, but many men never seek help (Lewis, 1992).
- Explore with client and partner various sexual gratification alternatives (e.g., caressing, sharing feelings).
  There are many satisfying alternatives for expressing sexual feelings. The many losses associated with aging leave the elderly with special needs for love and affection.
- Discuss the difference between sexual function and sexuality.
  All individuals possess sexuality from birth to death, regardless of the changes that occur over the life span.
- If prescribed, teach how to use nitroglycerin before sexual activity.
  Pain inhibits satisfying sexual activity.

Client/Family Teaching

- Teach the importance of resting before sexual activity; for some clients, mornings are the best time for sexual activity.
  A more satisfying experience may occur if the client is not tired.
- Teach that usual or previous types of activity may be resumed when client can climb two flights of stairs without symptoms (e.g., change in breathing pattern or heart rate, pain).
  This parameter is accepted and used by most health care providers.
- Teach client to take prescribed pain medications before sexual activity.
  Pain inhibits satisfying sexual activity.
- Teach possible need for modifying positions (e.g., side-to-side, limited resting on arms, heavier person on bottom).
  Changes in position can enhance satisfaction and comfort.
- Refer to appropriate literature on sexuality and sexual function.
  Inappropriate knowledge contributes to dissatisfaction.
- Refer to appropriate community resources such as a clinical specialist, family counselor, or sexual counselor; if appropriate, include both partners in the discussion.
  A high percentage of women report a need for more information after a cancer surgery that affected sexual response. They also express a need for partners to be included in the discussions (Corney, 1992).
- Teach how drug therapy affects sexual response; teach the possible side effects and the need to report them.
  Some medications have side effects that may affect sexual function.

REFERENCES

Corney R et al: The care of patients undergoing surgery for gynecological cancer: the need for information, emotional support and counseling, *J Adv Nurs*, 17:667-671, 1992.

Lemone, P: Transforming: patterns of sexual function in adults with insulin-dependent diabetes mellitus, Birmingham, 1991, University of Alabama.

Lewis JH: Treatment options for men with sexual dysfunction, *J ET Nurs*, 19:131-142, 1992.

BIBLIOGRAPHY

Bulechek G, McCloskey J: *Nursing interventions: essential nursing treatments*, ed 2, Philadelphia, 1992, WB Saunders.

Johnson BS: *Adaptation and growth: psychiatric-mental health nursing,* Philadelphia, 1993, JB Lippincott.

Altered sexuality pattern

Gail Ladwig

Definition The state in which an individual expresses concern regarding his or her sexuality.

Defining Characteristics

Reported difficulties, limitations, or changes in sexual behaviors or activities.

Related Factors (r/t)

Knowledge or skill deficit regarding alternative responses to health-related transitions; altered body functioning or structure; illness or medical cause; lack of privacy; lack of significant other; ineffective or absent role models; conflicts with sexual orientation; variant preferences; fear of pregnancy or of acquiring a sexually transmitted disease; impaired relationship with significant other.

Client Outcomes/Goals

- States knowledge of difficulties, limitations, or changes in sexual behaviors or activities.
- States knowledge of sexual anatomy and functioning.
- States acceptance of altered body structure or functioning.
- Describes acceptable alternative sexual practices.
- Identifies importance of discussing sexual issues with significant other.
- Describes practice of "safe sex" in regard to pregnancy and avoidance of sexually transmitted diseases.

Nursing Interventions and Rationales

- After establishing rapport or a therapeutic relationship, give client permission to discuss issues dealing with sexuality; ask client specifically, "Have you been or are you concerned about functioning sexually because of your health status?"
  This information helps identify any sexual problems or concerns. It is necessary information in formulating the plan of care.
- Observe client's perception of normal functioning and what client thinks is the cause of difficulties, limitations, or changes.
  The nurse needs to know if the client has accurate information.
- Teach normal anatomy and sexual functioning if needed.
  Many people have beliefs about sex that originate from family, friends, or culture; often these ideas are not true and not based on scientific data.
- Discuss alternative sexual expressions for altered body functioning or structure; closeness and touching are other forms of expression, and some clients choose masturbation for sexual release.
  Nursing intervention is important in helping the client discover possible alternatives for sexual expression.
- If mutual masturbation is a choice of expression, provide latex gloves.
  Latex gloves prevent possible exposure to infection through cuts on hands (Tucker et al, 1992).
- Discuss modifying positions to accommodate the altered physical state; instruct in the use of pillows for comfort.
  Modified positions can enable and enhance sexual satisfaction otherwise impeded by physical disability.
- Encourage client to discuss concerns with significant other.
  Open communication enhances appropriate expression of needs.

- Provide the client privacy for sexual expressions (e.g., close the door when significant other visits and put a "Do Not Disturb" sign on the door).
  The hospital environment needs to allow for sexual expression between partners.

Geriatric

- Discuss the difference between sexual functioning and sexuality.
  All humans have needs related to sexuality, not just sexual performance; these differences need to be recognized and addressed.
- Allow client to verbalize feelings regarding loss of sexual partner or significant other.
  The elderly experience many losses and need to be able to express grief over these losses.

Client/Family Teaching

- Refer to appropriate community agencies (e.g., certified sex counselor, Reach to Recovery, Ostomy Association).
  There may be needs that either are beyond the nurse's skill and ability to address or are related to a particular situation (e.g., presence of an ostomy that requires intervention from specialized sources) (Lewis, 1992).
- Discuss contraceptive choices, refer to appropriate health professional (e.g., gynecologist, nurse practitioner).
  Specialists may be needed for complex situations.
- Teach "safe sex," which includes using latex condoms, applying spermicide nonoxynol 9 inside and outside of the condom (*this appears to give added protection if the condom breaks*), washing with soap immediately after sexual contact, not ingesting semen, avoiding oral-genital contact, not exchanging saliva, avoiding multiple partners, abstaining from sexual activity when ill, and avoiding recreational drugs and alcohol when engaging in sexual activity.
  Accurate information regarding "safe sex" is essential for sexually active clients (Tucker, 1992).

REFERENCES

Lewis JH: Treatment options for men with sexual dysfunction, *J ET Nurs*, 19:131-42, 1992.

Tucker M et al: *Patient care standards: nursing process, diagnosis, and outcome,* St Louis, 1992, Mosby.

BIBLIOGRAPHY

Bulechek G, McCloskey J: *Nursing interventions: essential nursing treatments,* ed 2, Philadelphia, 1992, WB Saunders.

Johnson BS: *Adaptation and growth: psychiatric-mental health nursing,* Philadelphia, 1993, JB Lippincott.

Impaired skin integrity

Diane Krasner

Definition The state in which an individual's skin is adversely altered.

Defining Characteristics

Disruption of skin surface; destruction of skin layers.

Related Factors (r/t)

External (environmental)

Hyperthermia; hypothermia; chemical substance; mechanical factors (e.g., shearing forces, pressure, restraint); irradiation; physical immobilization; humidity.

Internal (somatic)

Medication; altered nutritional state (e.g., obesity, emaciation); altered metabolic state; altered circulation; altered sensation; altered pigmentation; skeletal prominence; developmental factors; immunological deficit; altered skin turgor (change in elasticity).

Client Outcomes/Goals

- Regains integrity of skin surface.
- Reports any altered sensation or pain at site of skin impairment.
- Demonstrates understanding of plan to heal skin and prevent reinjury.
- Describes measures to protect and heal the skin and to care for any skin lesion.

Nursing Interventions and Rationales

- Assess site of skin impairment and determine etiology (e.g., acute or chronic wound, burn, dermatological lesion, pressure ulcer, skin tear).
  Prior assessment of wound etiology is critical for proper identification of nursing interventions (Krasner, 1990).
- Determine that the skin impairment involves skin damage only (e.g., a partial-thickness wound, a stage-I or stage-II pressure ulcer). Classify superficial pressure ulcers in the following manner:
  - **Stage I:** Nonblanchable erythema of intact skin; the heralding lesion of skin ulceration
  - **Stage II:** Partial-thickness skin loss involving epidermis or dermis. This ulcer is superficial and appears as an abrasion, blister, or shallow crater (Adapted from the National Pressure Ulcer Advisory Panel Consensus Development Conference Statement, 1989).
- For deeper wounds into subcutaneous tissue, muscle, or bone (stage III or stage IV), refer to the nursing diagnosis **Impaired tissue integrity**.
- Monitor site of skin impairment at least once a day for color changes, redness, swelling, warmth, pain, or other signs of infection. Determine if client is experiencing changes in sensation or pain.
  Systematic inspection can identify impending problems early (Bryant, 1993).
- Monitor client's skin care practices, noting type of soap or other cleansing agents used, temperature of water, and frequency of skin cleansing.
  Individualize plan according to client's skin condition, needs, and preferences. Avoid harsh cleansing agents, hot water, extreme friction or force, or too-frequent cleansing (Panel for the Prediction and Prevention of Pressure Ulcers in Adults, 1992).
- Monitor client's continence status and minimize exposure of the site of skin impairment and other areas to moisture from incontinence, perspiration, or wound drainage.

If client is incontinent, implement an incontinence management plan to prevent exposure to chemicals in urine and stool that can strip or erode the skin; refer to a physician (e.g., urologist, gastroenterologist) for an incontinence work-up (Doughty, 1991; Urinary Incontinence Guideline Panel, 1992; Wound, Ostomy, and Continence Nurses Society, 1992, 1994).

- For clients with limited mobility, use a risk-assessment tool to systematically assess immobility-related risk factors.
  A validated risk-assessment tool such as the Norton Scale or the Braden Scale should be used to identify clients at risk for immobility-related skin breakdown (Panel for the Prediction and Prevention of Pressure Ulcers in Adults, 1992).
- Implement a written treatment plan for topical treatment of the site of skin impairment.
  A written plan assures consistency in care and documentation (Maklebust, Sieggreen, 1991). Topical treatments must be matched to the client, to the wound, and to the setting (Krasner, 1990).
- Select a topical treatment that will maintain a moist wound-healing environment that is balanced with the need to absorb exudate.
  Caution should always be taken not to dry out the wound (Bergstrom et al, 1994).
- Position the client off the site of skin impairment. If consistent with overall client management goals, turn and position client at least every 2 hours; transfer client with care to protect against the adverse effects of external mechanical forces such as pressure, friction, and shear.
  If the goal of care is to keep the client comfortable (e.g., a terminally ill client), turning and repositioning may not be appropriate. Maintain the head of the bed at the lowest possible degree of elevation to reduce shear and friction, and use lift devices, pillows, foam wedges, and pressure-reducing devices in the bed (Panel for the Prediction and Prevention of Pressure Ulcers in Adults, 1992).
- Avoid massaging around the site of skin impairment and over bony prominences.
  Research suggests that massage may lead to deep-tissue trauma (Panel for the Prediction and Prevention of Pressure Ulcers in Adults, 1992).
- Assess client's nutritional status; refer for a nutritional consult and/or institute dietary supplements.
  Inadequate nutritional intake places individuals at risk for skin breakdown and compromises healing (Krasner, 1990).

Client/Family Teaching

- Teach skin and wound assessment and ways to monitor for signs and symptoms of infection, complications, and healing.
  Early assessment and intervention helps prevent serious problems from developing.
- Teach use of a topical treatment that is matched to the client, the wound, and the setting.
  The topical treatment must be adjusted as the status of the wound changes.
- If consistent with overall client management goals, teach how to turn and reposition at least every 2 hours.
  If the goal of care is to keep the client comfortable (e.g., terminally ill client), turning and repositioning may not be appropriate (Panel for the Prediction and Prevention of Pressure Ulcers in Adults, 1992).
- Teach the use of pillows, foam wedges, and pressure-reducing devices to prevent pressure injury.

REFERENCES

Bergstrom N et al: *Treatment of Pressure Ulcers.* Clinical Practice Guideline, No 15. Rockville, Md, Dec 1994, Public Health Service, Agency for Health Care Policy and Research, US Department of Health and Human Services (AHCPR Publication No 95-0652).

Bryant R: Acute and chronic wounds, St Louis, 1993, Mosby.

Consensus Development Conference Statement. Buffalo, NY, 1989, National Pressure Ulcer Advisory Panel.

Doughty D: *Urinary and fecal incontinence: nursing management,* St Louis, 1991, Mosby.

Krasner D: *Chronic wound care: a clinical source book for healthcare professionals,* King of Prussia, Pa, 1990, Health Management Publications.

Maklebust J, Sieggreen M: *Pressure ulcers: guidelines for prevention and nursing management,* West Dundee, Ill, 1991, S-N.

Panel for the Prediction and Prevention of Pressure Ulcers in Adults: *Pressure ulcers in adults: prediction and prevention.* Clinical Practice Guideline, No 3. Rockville, Md, May 1992; Agency for Health Care Policy and Research, Public Health Service, US Department of Health and Human Services (AHCPR Publication No. 92-0047).

Urinary Incontinence Guideline Panel. *Urinary Incontinence in Adults:* Clinical Practice Guideline. Rockville, Md, March 1992, Agency for Health Care Policy Research, Public Health Service, US Department of Health and Human Services (AHCPR Publication No. 92-0038).

Risk for impaired skin integrity

Diane Krasner

Definition The state in which an individual's skin is at risk of being adversely altered.

Defining Characteristics

Presence of risk factors such as

External (environmental)

Hypothermia; hyperthermia; chemical substance; mechanical factors (e.g., shearing forces, pressure, restraint); irradiation; physical immobilization; humidity.

Internal (somatic)

Medication; altered nutritional state (e.g., obesity, emaciation); altered metabolic state; altered circulation; altered sensation; altered pigmentation; skeletal prominence; developmental factors; immunological deficit; altered skin turgor (change in elasticity) psychogenic factors; immunological deficit.

Related Factors (r/t)

Refer to risk factors.

Client Outcomes/Goals

- Reports altered sensation or pain at risk areas.
- Demonstrates understanding of personal risk factors for impaired skin integrity.
- Verbalizes a personal plan for preventing impaired skin integrity.

Nursing Interventions and Rationales

- Monitor skin condition at least once a day for color or texture changes, dermatological conditions, or lesions. Determine if client is experiencing loss of sensation or pain.
  Systematic inspection can identify impending problems early (Bryant, 1993).
- Identify clients at risk for impaired skin integrity as a result of compromised perfusion, immunocompromise, or chronic medical conditions such as diabetes mellitus or renal failure.
  These patient populations are known to be at high risk for impaired skin integrity (Krasner, 1990).
- Monitor client's skin care practices, noting type of soap or other cleansing agents used, temperature of water, and frequency of skin cleansing.
  Individualize plan according to client's skin condition, needs, and preferences. Avoid harsh cleansing agents, hot water, extreme friction or force, or too-frequent cleansing (Panel for the Prediction and Prevention of Pressure Ulcers in Adults, 1992).
- Monitor client's continence status and minimize exposure of the site of skin impairment and other areas to moisture from incontinence, perspiration, or wound drainage.
  If client is incontinent, implement an incontinence management plan to prevent exposure to chemicals in urine and stool that can strip or erode the skin; refer to a physician (e.g., urologist, gastroenterologist) for an incontinence work-up (Doughty, 1991; Urinary Incontinence Guideline Panel, 1992; Wound, Ostomy and Continence Nurses Society, 1992, 1994).
- For clients with limited mobility, monitor condition of skin over bony prominences.
  Pressure ulcers usually occur over bony prominences such as the sacrum, coccyx, trochanter, and heels as a result of unrelieved pressure between the prominence and the support surface (Krasner, 1990).
- Use a risk-assessment tool to systematically assess immobility-related risk factors.
  A validated risk-assessment tool such as the Norton Scale or the Braden Scale should be used to identify clients at risk for immobility-related skin breakdown (Panel for the Prediction and Prevention of Pressure Ulcers in Adults, 1992).

- Implement a written prevention plan.
  A written plan ensures consistency in care and documentation (Maklebust, Sieggreen, 1991).
- If consistent with overall client management goals, turn and position client at least every 2 hours; transfer client with care to protect against the adverse effects of external mechanical forces (e.g., pressure, friction, shear).
  If the goal of care is to keep the client comfortable (e.g., a terminally ill client), turning and repositioning may not be appropriate. Maintain the head of the bed at the lowest possible degree of elevation to reduce shear and friction and use lift devices, pillows, foam wedges, and pressure-reducing devices in the bed (Panel for the Prediction and Prevention of Pressure Ulcers in Adults, 1992).
- Avoid massaging over bony prominences.
  Research suggests that massage may lead to deep-tissue trauma (Panel for the Prediction and Prevention of Pressure Ulcers in Adults, 1992).
- Assess client's nutritional status; refer for a nutritional consult and/or institute dietary supplements.
  Inadequate nutritional intake places individuals at risk for skin breakdown and compromises healing (Krasner, 1990).

Geriatric

- Limit number of complete baths to 2 or 3 per week, and alternate them with partial baths. Use a tepid water temperature (between 90°F and 105°F) for bathing.
  Excessive bathing, especially in hot water, depletes the aging skin of moisture and increases dryness.
- Use superfatted soaps such as Dove, Tone, or Caress.
  Superfatted soaps help retain moisture in dry, aging skin (Hardy, 1992).
- Increase fluid intake within cardiac and renal limits to a minimum of 1500 ml/day.
  Dry skin is caused by loss of fluid in the skin; increasing fluid intake hydrates the skin.
- Increase humidity in the environment, especially during the winter, by using a humidifier or placing a container of water on a warm environment.
  Increasing the moisture in the air helps keep moisture in the skin (Fenske, Grayson, Newcomer, 1989).

Client/Family Teaching

- Teach skin assessment and ways to monitor for impending skin breakdown.
  Early assessment and intervention helps prevent the development of serious problems.
- If consistent with overall client management goals, teach how to turn and reposition client at least every two hours.
  If the goal of care is to keep the client comfortable (e.g., a terminally ill client), turning and repositioning may not be appropriate (Panel for the Prediction and Prevention of Pressure Ulcers in Adults, 1992).
- Teach the use of pillows, foam wedges, and pressure-reducing devices to prevent pressure injury.

REFERENCES

Bryant R: *Acute and chronic wounds,* St Louis, 1993, Mosby.

Doughty D: *Urinary and fecal incontinence: nursing management,* St Louis, 1991, Mosby.

Fenske NA, Grayson LD, Newcomer VD: Common problems of aging skin, *Patient Care* 23:225, 1989.

Hardy MA: *Dry skin care.* In Bulechek GM, McCloskey JC, editors: *Nursing interventions: essential nursing treatments,* ed 2, Philadelphia, 1992, WB Saunders.

Krasner D: *Chronic wound care: a clinical source book for healthcare professionals,* King of Prussia, Pa, 1990, Health Management Publications.

Maklebust J, Sieggreen M: *Pressure ulcers: guidelines for prevention and nursing management,* West Dundee, Ill, 1991, S-N.

Panel for the Prediction and Prevention of Pressure Ulcers in Adults: *Pressure ulcers in adults: prediction and prevention.* Clinical Practice Guideline, No 3. Rockville, Md, May 1992, Agency for Health Care Policy and Research, Public Health Service, US Department of Health and Human Services (AHCPR Publication No. 92-0047).

Urinary Incontinence Guideline Panel. *Urinary Incontinence in Adults:* Clinical Practice Guideline. Rockville, Md, March 1992, Agency for Health Care Policy and Research, Public Health Service, US Department of Health and Human Services (AHCPR Publication No. 92-0038).

Wound, Ostomy, and Continence Nurses Society: *Standards of care: dermal wounds: pressure ulcers,* Costa Mesa, CA, 1992, WOCN.

Wound, Ostomy, and Continence Nurses Society: *Standards of care: patient with fecal incontinence,* Cosa Mesa, CA, 1994, WOCN.

Wound, Ostomy, and Continence Nurses Society: *Standards of care: patient with urinary incontinence,* Costa Mesa, CA, 1992, WOCN.

Sleep pattern disturbance

Gwethalyn Edwards and Betty Ackley

Definition Disruption of sleep time that causes discomfort or interferes with desired life-style.

Defining Characteristics

*Verbal complaints of difficulty falling asleep; *awakening earlier or later than desired; *interrupted sleep; *verbal complaints of not feeling well-rested; changes in behavior and performance (e.g., increasing irritability, restlessness, disorientation, lethargy, listlessness); physical signs (e.g., mild or fleeting nystagmus, slight hand tremor, ptosis of eyelid, expressionless face, dark circles under eyes, frequent yawning, changes in posture); thick speech with mispronunciation and incorrect words. (*Critical)

Related Factors (r/t)

Sensory alterations: internal (e.g., illness, psychological stress); external (e.g., environmental changes, social cues).

Client Outcomes/Goals

- Wakes up less frequently during night.
- Awakens refreshed and is less fatigued during day.
- Falls asleep without difficulty.
- Verbalizes plan to implement bedtime routines.

Nursing Interventions and Rationales

- Assess client's sleep patterns and usual bedtime rituals and incorporate these into the plan of care.
  Usual sleep patterns are individual; data collected through a comprehensive and holistic assessment are needed to determine the etiology of the disturbance.
- Identify presence of internal or external factors that interfere with sleep (e.g., chronic pain, depression, metabolic diseases such as hyperthyroidism).
- Determine level of anxiety; if client is anxious, refer to nursing interventions and rationales for **Anxiety**.
  Anxiety interferes with sleep; interventions such as relaxation training can help clients reduce anxiety (Hyman et al, 1989).
- Observe client's medications, diet, and caffeine intake.
  Difficulty sleeping can be a side effect of some medications such as bronchodilators; caffeine intake can interfere with sleep.
- Provide measures to assist with sleep such as quiet time before bed, warm milk, or a back massage.
  Simple measures can increase quality of sleep; research on back massage has shown it to be effective (Richards, 1994).
- Provide pain relief measures shortly before bedtime, position client comfortably for sleep.
  Clients have reported that uncomfortable positions and pain are the most likely factors to disturb sleep (Reimer, 1987).
- Monitor for presence of sleep apnea as evidenced by loud snoring and periods of apnea; refer for sleep studies with physician input.
- Keep environment quiet (e.g., avoid use of intercoms, lower volume on radio and television, keep beepers on nonaudio mode, anticipate alarms on IV pumps, talk quietly on unit).
  Excessive noise causes sleep deprivation; sleep deprivation can result in ICU psychosis (Barr, 1993).

- Use soothing sound generators to induce sleep, including sounds of the ocean, rainfall, or waterfall; or use "white noise" such as a fan to block out other sounds.
  The use of ocean sounds was found to promote sleep for a group of postoperative open-heart surgery clients (Williamson, 1992).
- If client is under critical care and is stable, consider instituting the following sleep protocol to foster sleep:
  - **Night shift** Give client the opportunity for uninterrupted sleep from 1:00 AM to 5:00 AM. Keep noise to a minimum in the environment.
  - **Evening shift** Limit napping between 4:00 PM and 9:00 PM. At 10:00 PM turn lights off, provide sleep medication according to individual assessment, and keep noise and conversation on the unit to a minimum.
  - **Day shift** Encourage short naps before 11:00 AM. Enforce a physical activity regimen as appropriate. Schedule newly ordered medications to avoid waking client between 1:00 AM and 5:00 AM.

  Critical care nurses can take effective action to promote sleep (Edwards, Schuring, 1993).

Geriatric

- Observe for underlying illnesses (e.g., nocturia occurring with benign hypertrophic prostatitis).
- Observe elimination patterns; have client decrease fluid intake in the evening; ensure that diuretics are taken early in the morning.
- If client is waking frequently during the night, consider the presence of sleep apnea problems and refer to a sleep clinic for evaluation.
  Sleep apnea in the elderly may be caused by changes in the respiratory drive of the central nervous system, or it may be obstructive and associated with obesity (Foyt, 1992).
- Note boredom; provide changes as necessary (e.g., new decorations or new social activities).
- Suggest light reading or nonexcitable television as an evening activity.
- Increase daytime physical activity.
- Reduce daytime napping; limit naps to short intervals as early in the day as possible.

Client/Family Teaching

- Encourage avoidance of coffee and other caffeinated foods and liquids.
- Teach relaxation techniques, pain relief measures, or the use of imagery before sleep.
- Encourage client to develop a bedtime ritual that includes quiet activities such as reading, television, or crafts.
- Teach the following guidelines for improving sleep habits:
  - Go to bed only when sleepy
  - When awake in the middle of the night, go to another room, do quiet activities, and come back to bed only when sleepy
  - Use the bed only for sleeping, not for reading or snoozing in front of the television
  - Avoid afternoon and evening naps
  - Get up at the same time every morning
  - Recognize that not everyone needs 8 hours of sleep
  - Disassociate lulls in performance and sleeplessness; do not blame sleeplessness for everything that goes wrong during the day

  These guidelines have been found effective in improving quality of sleep (Morin, 1993).

REFERENCES

Barr WJ: Noise notes: working smart, *Am J Nurs* 93:16, 1993.

Edwards GB, Schuring LM: Sleep protocol: a research-based practice change, *Crit Care Nurse* 13:84-88, 1993.

Foyt, MM: Impaired gas exchange in the elderly, *Geriatr Nurs* 13:262-268, 1992.

Hyman RB et al: The effects of relaxation training on clinical symptoms: a meta-analysis, *Nurs Res* 38:216-220, 1989.

Morin C: *J Consult Clin Psychol* 61(1):137-146, 1993.

Reimer M: Sleep pattern disturbance: nursing interventions perceived by patients and their nurses as facilitating nocturnal sleep in hospital. In *Classification of Nursing Diagnoses: Proceedings of the Seventh Conference, North American Nursing Diagnosis Association,* 1987.

Richards KC: Sleep promotion in the critical care unit, *AACN Clin Issues* 5:152-158, 1994.

Williamson J: The effect of ocean sounds on sleep after coronary artery bypass graft surgery, *Am J Crit Care* 1:91-97, 1992.

BIBLIOGRAPHY

Jensen DP, Herr KA: Sleeplessness, *Nurs Clin North Am* 28:385-405, 1993.

Impaired social interaction

Pam Bifano Schweitzer

Definition The state in which an individual participates insufficiently, excessively, or ineffectively in social exchange.

Defining Characteristics

Major Verbalized or observed discomfort in social situations; verbalized or observed inability to receive or communicate a satisfying sense of belonging, caring, interest, or shared history; observed use of unsuccessful social interaction behaviors; dysfunctional interactions with peers, family, or others.

Minor Family report of change in interaction patterns.

Related Factors (r/t)

Knowledge or skill deficit regarding ways to enhance mutuality; communication barriers; self-concept disturbance; absence of significant others or peers; limited physical mobility; therapeutic isolation; sociocultural dissonance; environmental barriers; altered thought processes.

Client Outcomes/Goals

- Identifies barriers that cause impaired social interactions.
- Discusses feelings that accompany impaired and successful social interactions.
- Uses available opportunities to practice interactions.
- Uses successful social interaction behaviors.
- Reports increased comfort in social situations.
- Able to communicate; states feelings of belonging; demonstrates caring and interest in others.
- Family reports effective interactions with client.

Nursing Interventions and Rationales

- Observe for cause of discomfort in social situations; ask client to relate when discomfort began, losses (e.g., loss of health, job, or significant other; aging), and changes (e.g., marriage, birth or adoption of a child, change in body appearance).
  Individualized assessment indicates specific interventions (Warren, 1993).
- Have client list behaviors that are associated with disconnectedness, and discuss alternative responses that may increase comfort.
  Connectedness occurs when a person is actively involved with another person, object, group, or environment; such involvement promotes a sense of comfort, well-being, and anxiety reduction (Hagerty et al, 1993).
- Monitor client's use of defense mechanisms, and support healthy defenses (e.g., client focuses on the present and avoids placing blame on others for his or her own behavior).
  Positive reinforcement of strengths perpetuates them.
- Have client list behaviors that cause discomfort; discuss alternative ways to alleviate discomfort (e.g., focusing on others and their interests, practicing caring statements such as, "I understand you are feeling sad").
- Encourage client to express feelings to others (e.g., "I feel sad also").
  Self-expression invites involvement and increases connectedness (Hagerty et al, 1993).
- Identify strengths of client; have client make a list of strengths and refer to it when experiencing negative feelings. Client may find it helpful to put the list on a 3 × 5 card to carry at all times.
  Being aware of strengths when they are needed can increase successful interactions.

- In a group setting have group members identify each others' strengths.
  This exercise encourages individuals to practice relating to each other on a more intimate level (Drew, 1991).
- Role-play with the client comfortable and uncomfortable social interactions and appropriate responses (e.g., acknowledging a friendly greeting, responding to rude remarks with an "I" statement such as "I understand you may feel that way, but this is how I feel").
  Role-play may help the client develop social interaction skills and identify feelings associated with an isolated state (Warren, 1993).
- Model appropriate social interactions; give positive verbal and nonverbal feedback for appropriate behavior (e.g., make statements such as, "I'm proud that you made it to work on time and did all the tasks assigned to you without saying that your supervisor was picking on you," make eye contact). If not contraindicated, touch the client's arm or hand when speaking.
  One way to learn social skills is to observe the productive interactions of others (Drew, 1991).

Geriatric

- Assess for underlying psychosocial conditions that may be causing isolation.
  Social isolation is not normal for the elderly. Bias of the caregivers and the elderly client leads to a lack of recognition and treatment of the client's mental health needs (Dellasega, 1991).
- Monitor for depression, which is a particular risk in the elderly.
  Age and its accumulated losses may render formerly active people alone; loneliness contributes to depression and to social withdrawal (Warren, 1993).
- Provide group situations for the client.
  Group settings are necessary for the client to practice new skills.

Client/Family Teaching

- Help the client accept responsibility for his or her own behavior; have client keep a journal, and review it together at prescheduled intervals; give client positive feedback for appropriate behaviors, and suggest alternative approaches for those behaviors that did not enhance social interaction.
  Positive reinforcement perpetuates appropriate behaviors.
- Teach social interaction skills for use in actual situations the client is faced with daily.
  Through productive connections with others, social skills are learned and a repertoire of roles for many social situations is developed, which leads to increased self-esteem and the capacity to engage with others (Drew, 1991).
- Practice social skills one-to-one and, when the client is ready, in group sessions.
  Practice improves performance and comfort level.
- Refer to appropriate social agencies for assistance (e.g., family therapy, self-help groups, crisis intervention).

REFERENCES

Dellasega C: Meeting the mental health needs of elderly clients, *J Psychosoc Nurs Ment Health Serv* 29:10, 1991.

Drew N: Combating the social isolation of chronic mental illness, *J Psychosoc Nurs Ment Health Serv,* 29:14, 1991.

Hagerty BM et al: An emerging theory of human relatedness, *Image: J Nurs Sch*, 25:291, 1993.

Warren BJ: Explaining social isolation through concept analysis, *Arch Psychiatr Nurs*, 7:270, 1993.

Social isolation

Gail Ladwig

Definition Aloneness experienced by the individual and perceived as imposed by others and as a negative or threatened state.

Defining Characteristics

Objective *Absence of supportive significant others (e.g., family, friends, group); sad or dull affect; inappropriate or immature interests and activities for developmental age or stage; uncommunicative or withdrawn behavior; lack of eye contact; preoccupation with own thoughts; repetitive meaningless actions; hostility in voice or behavior; desire to be alone; existence in a limited subculture; evidence of physical or mental handicap or altered state of wellness; behavior that is unaccepted by dominant cultural group.

Subjective *Feelings of aloneness imposed by others; feelings of rejection; feelings of difference from others; inadequacy in or absence of a significant purpose in life; inability to meet expectations of others; insecurity in public; expression of values acceptable to the subculture but unacceptable to the dominant cultural group; expression of interests inappropriate to the developmental age or state. (*Critical)

Related Factors (r/t)

Factors contributing to the absence of satisfying personal relationships such as a delay in accomplishing developmental tasks, immature interests, alterations in mental status, unacceptable social behavior, unacceptable social values, altered state of wellness, inadequate personal resources, or an inability to engage in satisfying personal relationships.

Client Outcomes/Goals

- Identifies the reasons for feelings of isolation.
- Practices the social and communication skills needed to interact with others.
- Initiates interactions with others; sets and meets goals.
- Participates in activities and programs at level of ability and desire.
- Describes feelings of self-worth.

Nursing Interventions and Rationales

- Observe for barriers to social interaction (e.g., illness; incontinence; decreasing ability to form relationships; lack of transportation, money, support system, or knowledge).
  Major clinical implication is area of assessment. Each individual may have different etiologies of social isolation; therefore, adequate information must be gathered so appropriate interventions can be planned (Badgor, 1990).
- Note risk factors (e.g., age, ethnic or racial minority, environment, altered state of physical or mental wellness).
  Clients who are at the extremes of the life cycle, in a minority, in a subculture, or in a state of altered physical or mental wellness are at a high risk for social isolation because they differ from the norm.
- Discuss causes of perceived or actual isolation.
  This discussion allows the client to verbalize feelings.
- Promote social interactions; support grieving and verbalization of feelings.
  Mental health includes the ability to express feelings and relate to others; helping the client relate to others and express feelings is a step toward mental health.
- Establish trust one-on-one, and then gradually introduce client to others.
  The first step in reversing social isolation is developing the ability to relate to one person. As this skill is accomplished, the client can gradually learn to relate to others.

- Use active listening skills; establish a therapeutic relationship and spend time with the client.
  Spending time with the client enhances self-esteem.
- Help client to experience success by working together to establish easily attainable goals (e.g., spend 10 minutes conversing with peer).
  Success encourages repetition of behaviors, and setting small achievable goals is more likely to help the client be successful.
- Provide positive reinforcement when client seeks out others.
  Receiving instrumental social support such as practical help, advice, and feedback significantly contributes to positive well-being (White, 1992).
- Help client identify appropriate diversional activities to encourage socialization.
  Active participation by the client is essential for behavioral changes.
- Encourage physical closeness such as touch if appropriate.
  If appropriate, touch can be therapeutic and healing.
- Identify available support systems and involve them in client care.
  Clients cope more successfully with stressful life events if they have support (White, 1992).
- Encourage liberal visitation for hospitalized clients.
  Frequent contact with support persons decreases feelings of isolation.
- Help client identify role models and others with similar interests.
  Sometimes the client needs someone to model appropriate behavior.

Geriatric

- In health-care facility, visit client for at least 10 minutes every 2 to 3 hours.
  The presence of a trusted individual provides emotional security for the client.
- Engage client in dialogue on topics of interest.
  It is difficult to engage in conversation if there is no interest in the topic.
- Help client contact community agencies that provide social services and activities.
  The client may be more willing to participate in services and activities once they have been identified.

Client/Family Teaching

- Teach problem-solving, communication, social interaction, activities of daily living, and positive self-esteem.
  All of these skills are necessary to change isolating behavior.
- Encourage client to initiate contacts with self-help groups, counseling, and therapy.
  If successful adjustment is to occur and be maintained, management of the chronic illness cannot occur in isolation; it requires a complex interaction of resources (White, 1992).
- Provide information to client about senior citizen services, housesharing, pets, day-care centers, church, and community resources.
  The more people and activities the client has to choose from, the more likely it is that the client will find some satisfying way to relieve social isolation.

REFERENCES

Badgor VA: Men with cardiovascular diseases and their spouses, coping health and marital adjustment, *Arch Psychiatr Nurs* 4(4), 1990.

White NE: Coping, social support and adaptation to chronic illness, *West J Nurs Res* 14(2), 1992.

BIBLIOGRAPHY

Johnson BS: *Adaptation and growth: psychiatric-mental health nursing*, Philadelphia, 1993, JB Lippincott.

Townsend M: *Psychiatric mental health nursing: concepts of care,* Philadelphia, 1993, FA Davis.

Spiritual distress (distress of the human spirit)

Gail Ladwig

Definition A disruption in the life principle that pervades a person's being and integrates and transcends one's biological and psychosocial nature.

Defining Characteristics

*Expresses concern with meaning of life and death and with belief systems; expresses anger toward God; questions the meaning of suffering; verbalizes inner conflict about beliefs; verbalizes concern about relationship with deity; questions meaning of own existence; unable to participate in usual religious practices; seeks spiritual assistance; questions moral and ethical implications of therapeutic regimen; uses gallows humor; demonstrates displacement of anger toward religious representatives; describes nightmares and sleep disturbances; shows alterations in behavior or mood evidenced by anger, crying, withdrawal, preoccupation, anxiety, hostility, or apathy. (*Critical)

Related Factors (r/t)

Separation from religious or cultural ties; challenged belief and value system as a result of either intense suffering or the moral and ethical implications of therapy.

Client Outcomes/Goals

- Able to state conflicts or disturbances related to practice of belief system.
- Discusses beliefs about spiritual issues.
- States feelings of trust in self, God, or other belief systems.
- Continues spiritual practices not detrimental to health.
- Discusses feelings about death.
- Displays a mood appropriate for the situation.

Nursing Interventions and Rationales

- Observe client for self-esteem, self-worth, feelings of futility, or hopelessness.
  Verbalizations of feelings of low-self esteem, low self-worth, and hopelessness may indicate a spiritual need.
- Monitor support systems; be aware of own belief systems and accept client's spirituality.
  To effectively help a client with spiritual needs, an understanding of one's own spiritual dimension is essential (Highfield, Carson, 1983).
- Be physically present and available to help client determine religious and spiritual choices.
  Physical presence can decrease separation and aloneness, which clients often fear (Dossey et al, 1988).
- Provide quiet time for meditation, prayer, and relaxation.
  Clients need time to be alone during times of health change.
- Help client make a list of important and nonimportant values.
  Each client is an expert on his or her own path, and knowing a client's values helps in exploring his or her uniqueness (Dossey, 1988).
- Ask how to be most helpful; actively listen, reflect, and seek clarification.
  Active listening promotes reflective communication.
- If client is comfortable with touch, hold client's hand or place hand gently on arm.
  Touch makes nonverbal communication more personal.
- Help client develop short-term goals and tasks; help client accomplish these goals.
  Accomplishing goals increases self-esteem, which may be interrelated to the client's spiritual well-being.

- Help client find a reason for living, and be available for support.
  Some clients associate having meaning in life with spirituality.
- Listen to client's feelings about death; be nonjudgmental; allow time for grieving.
  All grief work takes time and is individual; acceptance of client differences is essential to open communication.
- Help client develop skills to deal with the illness or life-style changes; include client in planning of care.
  Allowing client to make decisions enhances self-worth and spirituality.
- Provide appropriate religious materials, artifacts, or music as requested.
  Helping a client incorporate rituals, sacraments, reading, music, imagery, and meditation into his or her daily life can enhance spiritual health (Conrad, 1985).
- Provide privacy for client to pray with others or to be read to by members of his or her faith.
  This privacy shows respect for and sensitivity to the client.

Geriatric

- Assist client with life review, and help client identify noteworthy experiences.
  Reminiscence is important to the geriatric client.
- Discuss with client personal definitions of spiritual wellness.
  Each person perceives his or her own spirituality differently.
- Discuss the client's perception of God in relation to the illness.
  Different religions view illness from different perspectives.
- Offer to pray with client or caregivers.
  The client or caregiver may find solace in sharing prayer time with the nurse.
- Offer to read from the Bible or other book chosen by client.
  Such a religious ritual may comfort the client.

Client/Family Teaching

- Encourage family and friends to visit and show their concern.
  Social networks support spiritual well-being (Young, Dowling, 1987).
- Encourage family and friends to support client's belief through prayer.
  Positive effects of prayer are rapid recovery and prevention of complications (Byrd, 1988).
- Include directions to the hospital chapel when orienting client and family to the hospital unit.
  Attendance at services and a visit to the chapel may be important to the client and family.
- Refer client to the spiritual advisor of choice; prepare for chosen religious rituals.
  Some religions may have ceremonies associated with healing and illness.
- Refer to counseling, therapy, support groups, or hospice.
  The client may need more support and may need ongoing spiritual assistance.

REFERENCES

Byrd RC: Positive therapeutic effects of intercessory prayer in a coronary care unit population, *South Med J* 81:826, 1988.

Conrad NJ: Spiritual support for the dying, *Nurs Clin North Am* 20:415-426, 1985.

Dossey M et al: *Holistic nursing: a handbook for practice,* Rockville, Md, 1988, Aspen.

Highfield M, Carson C: Spiritual needs of patients: are they recognized? *Cancer Nurs* 6, 1983.

Young G, Dowling W: Dimensions of religiosity in old age: accounting for variation in types of participation. *J Gerontol* 42:376, 1987.

Potential for enhanced spiritual well-being

Gail Ladwig

Definition The process of an individual's developing and unfolding of mystery through harmonious interconnectedness that springs from inner strengths.

Defining Characteristics

Inner strengths as evidenced by a sense of awareness, self-consciousness, sacred source, unifying force, inner core, and transcendence; unfolding mystery regarding one's experience with life's purpose, meaning, mystery, uncertainty, and struggles; harmonious interconnectedness as evidenced by relatedness, connectedness, and harmony with self, others, higher power, God, and the environment.

Client Outcomes/Goals

- States recognition of inner strengths.
- States purpose and meaning for life.
- Expresses feelings of hope.
- Lists values harmonious with inner core.
- States harmony with self, others, higher power, God, and the environment.

Nursing Interventions and Rationales

- Perform a spiritual assessment that includes the client's relationship with God, purpose and direction in life, religious affiliation, and any other significant beliefs.
  A spiritual assessment is a part of holistic evaluation and needs to include the above information (Fehring, Frenn, 1987).
- Assist client with values clarification; have client list the values that are important and on which he or she is willing to consistently act.
  Values clarification is a nursing activity that promotes spiritual health and wellness (Boss, Corbett, 1990).
- Facilitate support from family members and significant others by encouraging family visits, phone calls, and involvement in care.
  These strategies help maintain social support networks to foster hope and spiritual well-being (Farran, McCann, 1989).
- Help arrange visits with the clergy.
  Adults prefer this type of spiritual care (Reed, 1991).
- Allow private time for prayer and family participation in spiritual reading.
  Adults prefer this type of spiritual care (Reed, 1991).
- Set mutual times to sit and talk with client; suggest 30 minutes twice a day; if client does not wish to talk, just sit with client.
  The nurse's presence and willingness to listen contributes to a sense of hope or well-being (Clark, Heidenreich, 1995). Hope is necessary for life; "without hope we begin to die" (Simsen, 1988).
- Offer to pray with or for client.
  Spiritual needs can be met by praying with or for the client (Dettmore, 1984).
- Offer to read to client.
  Some clients cannot read because they are illiterate, have a pathological problem that prevents it, or are taking medications that cause visual problems or drowsiness. Reading, whether or not it is religious, conveys caring because time is being spent with the client (Bolander, 1994).
- Refer to care plan for **Spiritual distress (distress of the human spirit)**.

Client/Family Teaching

- Help client obtain religious rites or spiritual guidance.
  The nurse is rarely the client's primary spiritual caregiver. No single approach to spiritual care is satisfactory for all clients; many kinds of resources are needed (Bolander, 1994).

REFERENCES

Bolander V: *Sorensen and Luckmann's basic nursing: a psychophysiologic approach,* Philadelphia, 1994, WB Saunders.

Boss JA, Corbett T: The developing practice of the parish nurse: an inner-city experience. In Solari-Twadell PA, Djupe AM, McDermott MA, editors: *Parish nursing: the developing practice.* Park Ridge, Ill, 1990, National Parish Nurse Resource Center.

Clark C, Heidenreich T: Spiritual care for the critically ill, *Am J Crit Care* 4:77-81, 1995.

Dettmore D: Spiritual care: remembering your patients' forgotten needs, *Nursing* 14:46, 1984.

Farran CJ, McCann J: Longitudinal analysis of hope in community-based older adults, *Psychiatr Arch Nurs* 3:272-276, 1989.

Fehring RJ, Frenn M: Holistic nursing care: a church and university join forces, *J Christ Nurs* 4:25-29, 1987.

Reed P: Preferences for spiritually related nursing interventions among terminally ill and nonterminally ill hospitalized adults and well adults, *Appl Nurs Res* 4:122-128, 1991.

Simsen B: Nursing the spirit, meeting patients' spiritual needs, *Nurs Times,* 84:31-33, 1988.

Risk for suffocation

Catherine Vincent

Definition Accentuated risk of accidental suffocation (inadequate air available for inhalation).

Defining Characteristics

Presence of risk factors such as

Internal (individual)

Reduced olfactory sensation; reduced motor abilities; lack of safety education; lack of safety precautions; cognitive or emotional difficulties; disease or injury process.

External (environmental)

Pillow placed in infant's crib; propped bottle in infant's crib; vehicle warming in closed garage; children playing with plastic bags or inserting small objects into their mouths or noses; discarded or unused refrigerators or freezers with doors; children left unattended in or near bathtubs, pools, or hot tubs; household gas leaks; smoking in bed; use of fuel-burning heaters not vented to outside; low-strung clotheslines; pacifier hung around infant's head; eating large mouthfuls of food.

Related Factors (r/t)

Refer to risk factors.

Client Outcomes/Goals

- States knowledge of safety measures.
- Demonstrates knowledge of care appropriate for the chronological or developmental age of the client.
- Demonstrates appropriate measures for physically or emotionally challenged clients.
- Identifies potential hazards and verbalizes a willingness to correct them.
- Demonstrates cardiopulmonary resuscitation (CPR).

Nursing Interventions and Rationales

- Assess environment and remove potential hazards.
- Position the mentally altered client so that the tongue is not occluding the airway; provide an artificial airway if necessary.
- Observe for presence of gag reflex before feeding client.
- If the client experiences difficulty swallowing, use semi-solid foods instead of liquids. Refer to nursing interventions and rationales for **Impaired swallowing**.
- Feed client only small amounts of food at a time; hold infant for feeding.
  All of the above interventions help prevent aspiration, which can lead to suffocation.
- Stay with infant, child, or developmentally- or emotionally-delayed client when near water (e.g., bathing, recreational).
  An intense drive for exploration combined with an unawareness of danger makes drowning a threat. A child's high center of gravity and poor coordination make buckets and toilets a threat because the child can look inside and fall over.
- Keep infant's crib away from any environmental hazards in which he or she could become entangled.
- Do not leave plastic bags or small objects in reach of infant or developmentally- or emotionally-delayed client.
- Avoid foods that can be aspirated (e.g., peanuts, popcorn, hard candy, gum, whole or large pieces of hot dog, whole grapes); avoid nonfood items such as balloons and small parts on toys.
  Items that have a rigid consistency, a spherical or cylindrical shape, and a diameter of less than 1 ¼ inches can cause airway occlusion. Mechanical suffocation and asphyxia

resulting from foreign objects in the respiratory tract is the leading cause of death in children under one year of age.

- Do not use powder or lint-containing dressings around clients with tracheostomies; teach client to use cream or a nonelectric razor for shaving.
- Refer to **Airway clearance** or **Sleep pattern disturbance**.

Infant

- Do not tuck blankets.
  Blankets can be caught and make the infant unable to free self.
- Do not use pillows.
  Suffocation occurs when pillow contours to face and blocks airway.
- Do not use plastic bags.
  Plastic is nonporous; if placed over face, infant can suffocate in minutes.
- Do not put cords around neck (e.g., pacifier on cord, toys with strings attached).
  A cord longer than 12 inches can strangulate an infant.

Geriatric

- Observe client for pocketing of food in side of mouth; remove food as needed.
- Position client in high Fowler's position when eating and for one-half hour afterward.

Client/Family Teaching

- Teach safety measures appropriate for the chronological or developmental age of the client; review the nursing interventions.
- Teach overall safety measures (e.g., remove doors before disposing of used refrigerators and freezers, do not smoke in bed or when fatigued, keep garage door open when warming car, have heating systems checked and make sure there is proper ventilation, install working smoke detectors at home).
  These safety measures help prevent suffocation.
- Teach the importance of knowing CPR and how to treat a choking victim; refer to classes.
- Provide information to parents about obtaining the "no choke test tube" if desired.
  This aid teaches parents about the safe size of toys and other small objects (Jones, 1993).
- Caution adults from sleeping with child.
  An adult may roll over and smother the child.
- The distance between crib slats must be 2 ⅜ inches and is a federal regulation.
  An infant's head can be caught between the slats.
- Teach that protruding objects on cribs may catch clothing as child is climbing and may strangle him or her.
- Do not allow children to play with electric garage doors; keep door opener out of reach of children.
  A child may become trapped under a garage door. Children close to the ground may not be large enough to trigger the reverse mechanism on the garage door.

REFERENCES Jones, NE: Childhood residential injuries. *MCN* 18:168-172, 1993.

Impaired swallowing

Roslyn Fine and Betty Ackley

Definition The state in which an individual has a decreased ability to voluntarily pass fluids or solids from the mouth to the stomach via the esophagus.

Defining Characteristics

Observed evidence of a swallowing difficulty (e.g., stasis of food in oral cavity, coughing, choking, wet or gurgly voice, spitting of food, major delay in swallowing, double swallowing, drooling, watering eyes, nasal drainage, evidence of aspiration).

Related Factors (r/t)

Neuromuscular impairment (e.g., decreased or absent gag or swallow reflex, decreased strength or excursion of muscles involved in mastication, perceptual impairment, facial paralysis); mechanical obstruction (e.g., edema, tracheostomy tube, laryngeal or oral cancer); fatigue; limited awareness; reddened or irritated oropharyngeal cavity.

Client Outcomes/Goals

- Demonstrates effective swallowing and swallowing without choking or coughing.
- Free from aspiration (e.g., lungs clear, temperature within normal range).

Nursing Interventions and Rationales

- Assess ability to swallow by feeling client's neck; begin with the submandibular region and end on the top and bottom of larynx while client swallows saliva. Do not rely on the presence of the gag reflex to determine when to feed.
  Normally, the time taken for the bolus to move from the point at which the reflex is triggered to the entry into the esophagus (pharyngeal transit time) is one second or less (Logeman 1983). CVA clients with prolonged pharyngeal transit times have a greatly increased chance of developing aspiration pneumonia (Johnson, McKenzie, Sievers, 1993). Clients can aspirate even if they have an intact gag reflex (Baker, 1993).
- Observe for signs associated with swallowing problems (e.g., coughing, choking, spitting of food, drooling, difficulty handling oral secretions, double swallowing or major delay in swallowing, watering eyes, nasal discharge, wet or gurgly voice, decreased ability to move tongue and lips, decreased mastication of food, decreased ability to move food to the back of the pharynx, slow or scanning speech (Baker, 1993).
- If impaired swallowing is present, refer to a speech and language pathologist for a bedside evaluation, and initiate the dysphagia team.
  The dysphagia team is composed of a rehabilitation nurse, speech and language pathologist, dietician, physician, and radiologist who work together to help the client learn to swallow safely and maintain nutrition.
- If impaired swallowing is present, do not feed client until an appropriate diagnostic workup is completed; ensure nutrition by consulting with physician for enteral feedings.
  Feeding a client who cannot adequately swallow results in aspiration and possibly death.
- If client has an intact swallowing reflex, attempt to feed the client. Observe the following feeding guidelines:
  - Position client upright at a 90-degree angle with the head flexed forward at a 45-degree angle.
    This position forces the trachea to close and the esophagus to open, which makes swallowing easier and reduces the risk of aspiration.
  - Ensure that the client is awake, alert, and able to follow sequenced directions before attempting to feed.
    As the client becomes less alert the swallowing response decreases, which increases the risk of aspiration.

- Begin by feeding client ⅓ teaspoon applesauce; give client increased time to masticate and swallow.
- Place food on unaffected side of the tongue.
- During feeding give the client directions (e.g., "Open your mouth, chew the food completely, and when you are ready, tuck your chin to your chest and swallow").
- Watch for uncoordinated chewing or swallowing, coughing immediately after eating, pocketing of food, wet-sounding voice, sneezing with eating, delay in swallowing more than one second, or a change in respiratory patterns. If any of these signs are present, put on gloves, remove all food from the oral cavity, stop feedings, and consult with a speech and language pathologist and a dysphagia team.
  These actions are signs of impaired swallowing and possible aspiration (Baker, 1993; Donahue, 1990).

- If client tolerates single-textured foods such as pudding, Cream of Wheat, or strained baby food, advance to a soft diet with guidance from the dysphagia team. Some foods such as hamburgers, corn, and pastas are difficult to chew. Also avoid sticky foods such as peanut butter and white bread.
  The dysphagia team should determine the appropriate diet for the client on the basis of progression in swallowing.
- Avoid giving liquids until client is able to swallow effectively; add a thickening agent to liquids to obtain a soft consistency that is similar to nectar, honey, or pudding (depending on degree of swallowing problems).
  Thickened liquids form a cohesive bolus, which the client can swallow with increased efficiency.
- Work with the client on swallowing exercises prescribed by the dysphagia team (e.g., touching palate with tongue, stimulating the tonsillar arch and soft palate with a cold metal examination mirror or cotton swab [thermal stimulation]).
- Keep suction equipment on hand during feeding.
- Check oral cavity for proper emptying after client swallows and after client finishes meal. Provide oral care at the end of the meal.
  It may be necessary to manually remove food from the client's mouth; use latex gloves and keep the client's teeth apart with a padded tongue blade.
- Praise client for successfully eating.
- Keep client in an upright position for 30 to 45 minutes following a meal.
  An upright position aids digestion and prevents aspiration.

Client/Family Teaching

- Teach client and family exercises prescribed by the dysphagia team.
- Teach client step-by-step how to swallow effectively.
- Educate client and family about rationales for food consistency and choices.
- Teach family how to monitor client to prevent aspiration during eating.

REFERENCES

Baker DM: Assessment and management of impairments in swallowing, *Nurs Clin North Am,* 28:793-805, 1993.

Donahue PA: When it's hard to swallow: feeding techniques for dysphagia management, *J Gerontol Nurs* 16:6-9, 1990.

Johnson ER, McKenzie SW, Sievers A: Aspiration pneumonia in stroke, *Arch Phys Med Rehabil* 74:973-976, 1993.

Logemann, JA: *Evaluation and treatment of swallowing disorders,* San Diego, 1983, College Hill.

BIBLIOGRAPHY

Hufler DR: Helping your dysphagic patient eat, *RN*, pp. 36-39, Sept 1987.

Richter JE, Schechter GL: A new, commonsense approach to dysphagia, *Patient Care* 26:87-90, 1992.

Sliwa JA, Lis S: Drug-induced dysphagia, *Arch Phys Med Rehabil* 74:445-447, 1993.

Williams MJ, Walker GT: Managing swallowing problems in the home, *Caring* 11:59-63, 1992.

Risk for altered body temperature

Sandra Cunningham

Definition The state in which an individual is at risk for failure to maintain body temperature within a normal range.

Defining Characteristics

Presence of risk factors such as extremes of age; extremes of weight; exposure to cold/cool or warm/hot environments; dehydration; inactivity or vigorous activity; medications that cause vasoconstriction or vasodilitation; altered metabolic rate; sedation; clothing inappropriate for environmental temperature; illness or trauma that affects body temperature regulation.

Related Factors (r/t)

Refer to risk factors.

Client Outcomes/Goals

- Temperature within normal range.
- Explains measures needed to maintain normal temperature.
- Explains symptoms of hypothermia or hyperthermia.

Nursing Interventions and Rationales

- Check temperature q_____h or use continuous temperature monitoring as appropriate.
  Normal adult body temperature is 96.8°F (36°C) to 100.4°F (38°C). (Black, Matassarin-Jacobs, 1993).
- Take vital signs q______h, noting signs of hypothermia (e.g., decreased pulse, respiration, blood pressure) or hyperthermia (e.g., rapid bounding pulse, increased respiratory rate).
- Monitor client for signs of hypothermia (e.g., shivering, cool skin, piloerection, pallor, slow capillary refill, cyanotic nail beds, decreased mentation, coma).
- Monitor client for signs of hyperthermia (e.g., visual disturbances, headache, nausea and vomiting, muscle flaccidity, absence of sweating, delirium, coma).
- Maintain a consistent room temperature (68-72°F).
  A consistent room temperature limits the environmental effect on thermoregulation.
- Promote adequate nutrition and hydration.
  These factors help maintain a normal body temperature.
- Adjust clothing to facilitate passive warming or cooling as appropriate.
  Clothing adjustments help maintain normal body temperature.
- Avoid sedatives that depress cerebral function and circulation.
  This practice limits the risk factors associated with a risk for altered body temperature.
- Refer to social services and a dietician as appropriate.
  Adequate nutrition, hydration, environment, and clothing decreases the risk of hypothermia or hyperthermia.
  Refer to nursing interventions and rationales for **Hypothermia** or **Hyperthermia** as appropriate.

Geriatric

- Recognize that elderly clients have a decreased ability to adapt to temperature extremes and need proper protection; in cold temperatures, they need extra clothing, bedding, and heat; in hot temperatures, they need extra fluids and air conditioning.
  Older adults have a higher threshold of central temperature for sweating, diminished or absent sweating, impaired warmth or cold perception, impaired shiver response, diminished thermogenesis, abnormal peripheral blood flow response to warmth or cold, and a compromised cardiovascular reserve (Robbins, 1989).

Pediatric

- Recognize that pediatric clients have a decreased ability to adapt to temperature extremes.
  The combination of a relatively larger body surface area, smaller body-fluid volume, immature temperature control mechanisms, and a smaller amount of protective body fat limits the pediatric client's ability to maintain normal temperatures (Henderson, 1990).

Client/Family Teaching

- Teach client and family the actions that prevent hypothermia or hyperthermia.
- Teach client and family the signs of hypothermia and hyperthermia and the appropriate interventions.
  Adequate teaching improves compliance and reduces anxiety.
- Teach client and family the proper method for taking temperature.
  Optimal placement of the appropriate device is essential for accurate monitoring.
- Refer to client/family teaching for **Hypothermia** and **Hyperthermia** as appropriate.

REFERENCES

Black JM, Matassarin-Jacobs E: In Luckmann and Sorensen's *Medical-surgical nursing: a psychophysiologic approach,* Philadelphia, 1993, WB Saunders.

Henderson, DP: Pediatric update: Hypothermia and the pediatric patient. *J Emerg Nurs* 16(6):411-412, 1990.

Robbins, AS: Hypothermia and heat stroke: protecting the elderly patient, *Geriatrics*, vol 44, 1989.

BIBLIOGRAPHY

McCloskey JC, Bulechek GM: *Nursing Interventions Classification (NIC),* St Louis, 1992, Mosby.

Miller CA: *Nursing care of older adults: theory and practice,* Glenview, 1990, Scott, Foresman, Little, Brown Higher Education.

Roncoli M, Medoff-Cooper B: Thermoregulation in low-birth-weight infants, *NAACOG's Clin Issues,* 3:25-33, 1992.

Whaley LF, Wong DL: *Essentials of pediatric nursing,* St Louis, 1989, Mosby.

Ineffective management of therapeutic regimen: families

Margaret Lunney

Definition A pattern of regulating and integrating into family processes a program for treatment of illness and the sequelae of illness that is unsatisfactory for meeting specific health goals.

Defining Characteristics

Major Inappropriate family activities for meeting the goals of a treatment or prevention program.

Minor Lack of family attention to illness and its sequelae; acceleration of illness symptoms of a family member; verbalized desire to manage the treatment of illness and prevent its sequelae; verbalized difficulty with regulation or integration of one or more prescribed regimens; verbalized neglect of family actions to reduce risk factors for progression of illness and sequelae.

Related Factors (r/t)

Refer to **Ineffective management of therapeutic regimen: individual**

Client Outcomes/Goals

- Family members make adjustments in usual activities (e.g., diet, activity, stress management) to incorporate the therapeutic regimens of its members.
- Illness symptoms of family members are reduced.
- Family behaviors to manage the therapeutic regimens of its members are congruent with the desire to do so.
- Family members verbalize a decrease in some of the difficulties of managing therapeutic regimens.
- Family members describe actions to reduce risk factors.

Nursing Interventions and Rationales

- Establish an open and trusting relationship with family members.
  If trust is established with family members, they are more likely to openly share the real difficulties of integrating therapeutic regimens with family process (Lubkin, 1990).
- Review with family members the congruence and incongruence of family behaviors and health-related goals.
  To attain the motivation that is needed for changes in daily habits, family members should understand the relationship of daily habits to health-related goals (Miller, 1992).
- Help family members make decisions regarding ways to integrate therapeutic regimens with daily living. Provide advice or suggestions as solicited and accepted by family.
  Decisions made by the family, rather than by health providers or others, guide everyday actions (Miller, 1992). Advice from others, including nurses, will not be followed unless it is valued and respected by the family.
- Demonstrate respect and trust in family decisions.
  People make decisions that they believe are appropriate for them (Fromer, 1981; Kim, 1983). Families who believe they are respected and trusted by health providers are more likely to collaborate effectively with them.
- Acknowledge the challenge of integrating therapeutic regimens with family behaviors.
  Therapeutic regimens require modifications of daily activities that have already been established based on family values and beliefs (Miller, 1992). Acknowledging the difficulty of changing these previous habits supports families through the process.
- Review symptoms of the illness and help family members develop a greater awareness of symptoms.
  Knowledge and awareness of symptoms improves the ability of the family to adjust behaviors to prevent and manage symptoms (Lubkin, 1990).

- Provide sufficient knowledge to support family decisions regarding therapeutic regimens.
  Knowledge deficits can be a major obstacle to effectively managing therapeutic regimens (Fujita, Dungan, 1994).
- Selectively support family decisions to adjust the therapeutic regimens as indicated.
  Sometimes families do not have access to health providers or need to make independent decisions because of side effects or adverse effects of therapeutic regimens. Family members need to make informed decisions that are in their best interests (Lubkin, 1990; Miller, 1992). Providing support for appropriate decisions improves the ability of the family to make such decisions.
- Advocate for the family in negotiating therapeutic regimens with health providers.
  Illness regimens generally are not arbitrary or absolute; therefore modifications can be discussed as needed to fit with family life-styles (Jackson, Lubkin, 1990; Miller, 1992).
- Help the family mobilize social supports.
  Increased social support helps families meet health-related goals (Miller, 1992; Pender, 1987).
- Help family members modify perceptions as indicated.
  Individual perceptions regarding the seriousness, susceptibility, and threat of illness may be distorted or inaccurate but may be modified with new information (Pender, 1987).
- Use one or more family theories to describe, explain, or predict family dynamics (e.g., Bowen, Satir, Minuchin).
  Family systems are complex and may not be understood by the nurse without adequate knowledge of family theories (Bomar, 1989; Gillis et al, 1989).
- Collaborate with nurses or other consultants regarding strategies for working with families.
  For some families the knowledge and skills of nurses with advanced degrees or of other specialists may be needed to design effective interventions.

Client/Family Teaching

- Teach about all aspects of therapeutic regimens; provide as much knowledge as family will accept; adjust instruction to account for what family already knows; provide information in a culturally congruent manner.
- Teach ways to adjust family behaviors for inclusion of therapeutic regimens.
- Teach safety in taking medication.
- Teach family members to act as self-advocates with health providers who prescribe therapeutic regimens.

REFERENCES

Bomar PJ: *Nurses and family health promotion: concepts, assessment, and interventions,* Baltimore, 1989, Williams & Wilkins.

Fromer MJ: Paternalism in health care, *Nurs Outlook* 29:284-290, 1981.

Fujita LJ, Duncan J: High risk for ineffective management of therapeutic regimen: a protocol study, *Rehabil Nurs* 19:75-79, 1994.

Jackson E, Lubkin I: Advocacy. In Lubkin IM, editor: *Chronic illness: impact and interventions,* ed 2, Boston, 1990, Jones & Bartlett.

Gillis CL et al: *Toward a science of family nursing,* Reading, Mass, 1989, Addison-Wesley.

Kim HS: Collaborative decision making in nursing practice: a theoretical framework, In Chinn PL, editor: *Advances in nursing theory development*, Rockville, Md, 1983, Aspen.

Lubkin IM: *Chronic illness: impact and interventions,* ed 2, Boston, 1990, Jones & Bartlett.

Miller JF: *Coping with chronic illness: overcoming powerlessness,* ed 2, Philadelphia, 1992, FA Davis.

Pender NJ: *Health promotion in nursing practice,* ed 2, Norwalk, Conn, 1987, Appleton-Lange.

Effective management of therapeutic regimen: individual

Suzanne Skowronski

Definition A pattern of regulating and integrating into daily living a program for treatment of illness and sequelae that is satisfactory for meeting specific health goals.

Defining Characteristics

Appropriate choices of daily activities for meeting the goals of a treatment or prevention program; illness symptoms are within a normal range of expectation; verbalized desire to manage the treatment of illness and sequelae; verbalized intent to reduce risk factors for progression of illness and sequelae.

Client Outcomes/Goals

- Follows treatment plan as prescribed.
- States that he or she understands and will follow treatment plan.
- States or writes a schedule that includes treatment plan in activities of daily living.
- States knowledge of risk factors.

Nursing Interventions and Rationales

- Assess cultural, social, and family influences on achievement of health goals or regimen.
  "Cultural lifeways are shared among members of the group and understood, often without persons being aware that their world view differs from another. Symptoms are perceived, labeled, and reacted to in ways that make sense within the culture" (Wenger, 1993, p. 22).
- Assess barriers to understanding steps of the therapeutic regimen (e.g., educational level, developmental age, sensory loss, pain, physical immobility).
  Noncompliance may be the result of factors unrelated to motivation. Physical ability and emotional readiness to perform a task are the basis for implementing a life-style change.
- Monitor client's ability to follow directions, solve problems regarding managing the regimen, and implement skills such as injections, dressing changes, or dietary restrictions.
  Therapeutic regimens consist of a series of actions that directly affect the client's health. Responses to medication and treatments need to be identified as a means to empower the client.
- Observe client's reading and writing ability; provide appropriate teaching aids such as pictures if client is unable to read.
  Reading materials serve to reinforce verbal directions. In the home setting such materials serve to clarify questions when health professionals are not available. Compliance relies heavily on reading skills.
- Identify client's and family's knowledge of illness and treatment.
  Some therapeutic regimens such as diet changes and oxygen therapy have implications for social relationships and support systems. Misunderstanding these implications risks improper implementation of the regimen, which can hinder therapy.
- Develop therapeutic relationship with client by listening to statement of abilities and questions about implementing self-care strategies.
  The meaning of self-care differs for laypersons and professionals. A general theme in nursing and medical literature is that self-care is giving care to oneself that ideally should be given by health care professionals. The layperson sees himself or herself as purchasing a necessary commodity, "knowledge" (Northrup, 1993).

- Encourage client to verbalize feelings about the health alteration (disease state); encourage expressions of anger and loss as appropriate.
  Therapeutic regimens sometimes have side effects such as fatigue, inability to concentrate, and weight loss, which change the client's perception of self as a person with unlimited vitality and resources. There are emotional responses to change and loss.
- Have client repeat instructions in his or her own words.
- Adapt teaching process according to client's learning style; use educational aids (e.g., audiotape, flip charts, printed materials, computer programs).
  Learning is based on sensory perception. An individual's learning style emphasizes mainly a visual, auditory, or psychomotor (experience) modality.
- Develop a written contract with client and regularly evaluate the criteria in the contract.
  A written plan of care (contract) provides a frame of reference for the client and the health professional, and it clarifies expectations.

Geriatric

- Monitor client for memory deficits, signs of sensory loss or depression, and dementia.
  Preexisting disabilities affect retention of learned material.
- Use repetition, verbal cues, and memory aids in teaching the health care regimen.
  Because short-term memory is affected by the aging process, teaching strategies should include repetition, return demonstrations, and routine supervision to ensure compliance.
- Establish a caring relationship with the geriatric client.
  Consistency (same provider), concern, and a nonjudgmental attitude are the most important characteristics of a relationship that promote compliance (Pfister-Minogue, 1993 p. 126).
- Assess the client's knowledge of the health situation and current health habits. Suggest incorporating exercise into current life-style (e.g., parking the car a distance from the doorway, walking at a brisk pace); have client plan extra time for this type of exercise.
  "The client may understand a direction in terms of past experiences. Many older persons never considered physical exercise as a part of 'being active.' To them, physical activity is structured around work, cleaning, and cooking" (Pfister-Minogue, 1993, p. 127).
- Provide for follow-up to determine compliance.
  Long-term compliance requires financial, emotional, and/or social support.

Client/Family Teaching

- Determine whether client and family life-styles, values, and relationships support or hinder compliance.
  Family members may be willing to comply while a health crisis exists but may find the cost in long-term behaviors more difficult. If the dining room is changed to a bedroom for someone with health care monitoring needs, it may affect communication patterns among family members.
- Spend one-to-one time with the child who faces life-style changes. Observe for family systems that help or hinder compliance with a medical or psychotherapeutic regimen.
  "Human behavior is best understood in context. Family patterns can modify individual behavior. Conflict between partners places a child's compliance at risk" (Kuehl, 1993 p. 262).
- Share information about appropriate services that may help with compliance (e.g., dietician, home health agencies, social services, community educational services, peer support groups).

Compliance occurs on many levels simultaneously. Several agencies may be needed to support the treatment regimen; and these services differ from time to time.

- Consider cultural and ethnic issues that promote compliance with the medical regimen. *Clients and families are holistic social units and are affected by role changes (Malone-Rising, 1994).*

REFERENCES

Kuehl B: Child and family therapy: a collaborative approach, *Am J Fam Therapy* 21:260, 1993.

Malone-Rising D: The changing face of long-term care, *Nurs Clin North Am* 29:417-429, 1994.

Northrup D: Self-care myth reconsidered, *Adv Nurs Sci* 15(3):59, 1993.

Pfister-Minogue K: Enhancing patient compliance: a guide for nurses, *Geriatric Nurs* 14:126, 1993.

Wenger F: Cultural meaning of symptoms, *Holistic Nurs Pract* 22:7, 1993.

BIBLIOGRAPHY

Health values: *J Health Beh Ed Promotion* 18(1), 1994. (Entire issue devoted to strategies to stop smoking.)

Leininger M, ed: *Culture care diversity and universality: a theory of nursing,* New York, 1991, National League for Nursing Press.

Powell-Cope G: Family caregivers of people with AIDS: negotiating partnerships with professional health care providers, *Nurs Res* 43:324-329, 1994.

Ineffective management of individual therapeutic regimen

Suzanne Skowronski

Definition A pattern of regulating and integrating into daily living a treatment program for an illness and its aftereffects that is unsatisfactory for meeting specific health goals.

Defining Characteristics

Major Inappropriate choices of daily living for meeting the goals of a treatment or prevention program.

Minor Expected or unexpected acceleration of illness symptoms; desire to treat the illness and prevent sequelae; difficulty with the regulation or integration of regimens for treatment or prevention of complications; treatment regimens not included in daily routines; no action taken to reduce risk factors for the progression of illness and sequelae.

Related Factors (r/t)

Complexity of health care system; complexity of therapeutic regimen; decisional conflicts; economic difficulties; excessive demands on individual or family; family conflict; family patterns of health care; inadequate number and types of cues to action; knowledge deficits; mistrust of regimen or health care personnel; perceived seriousness; perceived susceptibility; perceived barriers; perceived benefits; powerlessness; social support deficits.

Client Outcomes/Goals

- Follows treatment plan as prescribed.
- States, understands, and follows treatment plan.
- Verbalizes possible reasons for not following treatment plan (e.g., finances, lack of understanding).
- States or writes a schedule that includes treatment plan in activities of daily living.
- States knowledge of risk factors.

Nursing Interventions and Rationales

- Assess cultural, social, and family influences on the achievement of health goals and regimens.
  "Cultural lifeways are shared among members of the group and understood, often without persons being aware that their world view differs from another. Symptoms are perceived, labeled, and reacted to in ways that make sense within the culture" (Wenger, 1993, p. 22).
- Assess barriers to understanding steps of the therapeutic regimen such as educational level, developmental age, sensory loss, pain, or physical immobility.
  Noncompliance may be the result of factors unrelated to motivation. Physical ability and emotional readiness to perform a task are the basis for implementing a life-style change.
- Monitor client's ability to follow directions, solve problems, and concentrate.
  Therapeutic regimens consist of a series of actions that directly affect the client's health. Responses to medication and treatments need to be identified.
- Observe client's ability to read and write; provide appropriate teaching aids such as pictures if client is unable to read.
  Reading materials reinforce verbal directions. In the home setting these pamphlets clarify questions when health professionals are not available. Compliance therefore relies heavily on reading skills.

- Identify client's and family's knowledge of illness and treatment.
  Some therapeutic regimens such as diet changes and oxygen therapy have implications for social relationships and support systems. Misunderstandings may result in improper implementation of the regimen, which hinders therapy.
- Develop a therapeutic relationship by listening to client's statements of abilities and questions about implementing self-care strategies.
  The meaning of self-care differs for a layperson and a professional. A general theme in nursing and medical literature is that self-care consists of giving care to oneself that ideally should be given by health care professionals. Laypersons see themselves as purchasing a necessary commodity—"knowledge" (Northrup, 1993).
- Encourage client to verbalize feelings about the disease state; encourage expressions of anger and loss as appropriate.
  Therapeutic regimens sometimes have side effects, which may include fatigue, an inability to concentrate, and weight loss; these effects change the client's perception of self as a person with unlimited vitality and resources. There are emotional responses to change and loss.
- Monitor anxiety as a possible cause of noncompliance.
- Have client repeat instructions in his or her own words.
- Accept client's choices and adapt plan of care accordingly; use educational aids (e.g., audiotape, flip charts, printed materials, computer programs).
  Learning is based on sensory perception. An individual's learning style emphasizes either a visual, auditory, or psychomotor (experience) modality.
- Develop a written contract with client and evaluate its criteria regularly.
  A written plan of care (contract) provides a frame of reference for the client and the health professional, and it clarifies expectations.
- Consult with health care person who prescribed the treatment regimen about possible alterations to encourage compliance.
  Individualized treatment encourages compliance.
- Focus on family time with the child who faces life-style changes. Observe for family systems that hinder or enhance compliance with the medical or psychotherapeutic regimen.
  "Human behavior is best understood in context. Family patterns can modify individual behavior. Conflict between partners places a child's compliance at risk" (Kuehl, 1993, p. 262).

Geriatric

- Monitor client for memory deficits, signs of sensory loss, signs of depression, or dementia.
  Pre-existing disabilities affect retention of learned material.
- Use repetition, verbal clues, and memory aids when teaching the health care regimen.
  To ensure compliance, teaching strategies should include repetition, return demonstrations, and routine supervision.
- Establish a caring relationship with the client.
  "The most important characteristics of a relationship that promote compliance are consistency (same provider), concern, and a nonjudgmental attitude" (Pfister-Minogue, 1993, p. 126).
- Assess client's knowledge of the health situation, and compare present behaviors with required behaviors. Obtain a profile of the client's current health habits. Incorporate exercise into current life-style (e.g., park the car a distance from the door and walk at a brisk pace); plan extra time for this type of exercise.

"The client may understand a direction in terms of past experiences. Many older persons never considered physical exercise as a part of 'being active.' To them physical activity is structured around work, cleaning, and cooking" (Pfister-Minogue, 1993, p. 127).

- Provide for follow-up care to determine compliance.
  Long-term compliance requires financial, emotional, and social support.

Client/Family Teaching

- Assess whether client and family life-styles, values, and relationships are supportive of or a barrier to compliance.
  Family members may be willing to comply while the health crisis exists but may find the cost of long-term behaviors more difficult. If the dining room is changed to a bedroom for someone with health-care monitoring needs, communication patterns among family members may be affected.
- Share information about appropriate services that may help with compliance (e.g., dietician, home health agencies, social services, community educational services, peer support groups).
  Compliance occurs on many levels simultaneously. Several agencies may be needed to support the treatment regimen; the services needed may differ from time to time.
- Consider cultural and ethnic issues when promoting compliance with the medical regimen.
  Clients and families are holistic social units affected by role changes.

REFERENCES

Kuehl B: Child and family therapy: a collaborative approach, *Am J Fam Therapy* 21:260, 1993.

Northrup D: Self-care myth reconsidered, *Adv Nurse Sci* 15(3):59, 1993.

Pfister-Minogue K: Enhancing patient compliance: a guide for nurses, *Geriatr Nurs* 14:126, 1993.

Wenger F: Cultural meaning of symptoms, *Holistic Nurs Pract* 22:7, 1993.

BIBLIOGRAPHY

Health values: *J Health Beh Educ Promotion* 18, 1994. (Entire issue devoted to strategies to stop smoking.)

Leininger M, editor: *Culture care diversity and universality: a theory of nursing*, New York, 1991, National League for Nursing Press.

Ineffective thermoregulation

Sandra Cunningham

Definition The state in which an individual's temperature fluctuates between hypothermia and hyperthermia.

Defining Characteristics

Major Fluctuations in body temperature above or below the normal range.

Refer to major and minor defining characteristics for **Hypothermia** and **Hyperthermia.**

Related Factors (r/t)

Trauma; illness; immaturity; aging; fluctuating environmental temperature.

Client Outcomes/Goals

- Maintains temperature within a normal range.
- Explains measures needed to maintain normal temperature.
- Explains symptoms of hypothermia or hyperthermia.

Nursing Interventions and Rationales

- Monitor temperature every 2 hours as appropriate.
  Normal temperature lies between 96.8°F (36°C) to 100.4°F (38°C) (Black, Matassarin-Jacobs, 1993).
- Take vital signs q_____h, noting signs of hypothermia (e.g., decreased pulse, respiration, blood pressure) or hyperthermia (e.g., rapid or bounding pulse, increased respiratory rate).
  These signs allow for early identification of ineffective thermoregulation.
- Monitor for signs of hypothermia (e.g., shivering, cool skin, piloerection, pallor, slow capillary refill, cyanotic nail beds, decreased mentation, coma).
  These signs allow for early identification of ineffective thermoregulation.
- Assess for signs of hyperthermia (e.g., visual disturbances, headache, nausea and vomiting, muscle flaccidity, absence of sweating, delirium, coma).
  These signs allow for early identification of ineffective thermoregulation.
- Adjust environmental temperature to client's needs.
  An appropriate temperature limits the environmental effects on thermoregulation (Robbins, 1989, Meyer-Pahoulis et al, 1993).
- Adjust clothing to facilitate passive warming or cooling appropriate to client needs.
  Clothing adjustments help maintain a normal body temperature.
- Refer to social services or a dietician as appropriate.
  Preventive approaches (e.g., adequate environment, nutrition, hydration, clothing) decrease the risk of hypothermia or hyperthermia.

Refer to **Hypothermia** and **Hyperthermia** for additional nursing interventions.

Client/Family Teaching

- Teach client and family an age-appropriate method for taking temperature.
- Teach client and family the importance of thermoregulation and the possible negative effects of excessive heat or cold.
- Teach client and family ways to recognize, prevent, and treat hypothermia or hyperthermia.
  Appropriate teaching improves compliance and reduces anxiety.

REFERENCES Black JM, Matassarin-Jacobs E: In Luckmann and Sorensen's *Medical-surgical nursing: a psychophysiologic approach*, Philadelphia, 1993, WB Saunders.

Meyer-Pahoulis E et al: The pediatric patient in the post anesthesia care unit, *Nurs Clin North Am* 28:519-529, 1993.

Robbins AS: Hypothermia and heat stroke: protecting the elderly patient, *Geriatrics* 44(1):73-80, 1989.

BIBLIOGRAPHY Bliss-Holtz J: Determination of thermoregulatory state in full-term infants, *Nurs Res,* 42:204-207, 1993.

McCloskey JC, Bulechek GM: *Nursing interventions classification (NIC),* St Louis, 1992, Mosby.

Miller CA: *Nursing care of older adults: theory and practice,* Glenview, Ill, 1990, Scott, Foresman/Little.

Roncoli M, Medoff-Cooper B: Thermoregulation in low-birth-weight infants, *NAACOG's Clin Issues,* 3:25-33, 1992.

Whaley LF, Wong DL: *Essentials of pediatric nursing,* St Louis, 1989, Mosby.

Altered thought processes

Helen Kelley

Definition The state in which an individual experiences a disruption in cognitive operations and activities.

Defining Characteristics

Inaccurate interpretation of environment; cognitive dissonance; distractibility; memory deficits or problems; hypervigilance; hypovigilance; inappropriate or nonreality-based thinking.

Related Factors (r/t)

Head injury; mental disorder; personality disorder; organic mental disorder; substance abuse; severe interpersonal conflict; sleep deprivation; sensory deprivation or overload; impaired cerebral perfusion; metabolic or electrolyte imbalances.

Client Outcomes/Goals

- Oriented to time, place, and person; demonstrates improved cognitive function.
- Free from physical harm.
- Performs activities of daily living appropriately and independently.
- Identifies community resources for help after discharge.

Nursing Interventions and Rationales

- Observe for causes of altered thought processes; refer to related factors.
- Monitor and record client's neurological status (level of consciousness, increased intracranial pressure), mental status (memory, cognition, judgment, concentration), vital signs, lab values and ability to follow commands.
  This examination helps to determine pathophysiological or psychiatric symptoms.
- Report any new onset or sudden increase in confusion.
- Assess client's understanding, and adjust communication accordingly; speak slowly and calmly; use short phrases and concrete and nontechnical words; use written words if appropriate; allow time for thinking; use face-to-face communication; listen carefully; seek clarification.
  Effective communication promotes understanding.
- Assess pain and promptly provide comfort measures.
  The confused client cannot accurately report pain; untreated pain increases anxiety and agitation (Foreman, 1989).
- Provide safety measures (e.g., bed in low position, siderails, available call light, close and frequent observations, limited activities, assistance with ambulation as needed, limited use of sedatives and central nervous system depressants).
  These precautions reduce the risk of injury to the client.
- Use soft restraints with discretion and with physician's order.
  Restraints may exacerbate confusion (Yorker, 1988).
- Provide orientation for client (e.g., call client by name; introduce self on each contact; frequently orient client to time, date, and place; prominently display an easily read clock and calendar in room and refer to them; request family to bring in familiar pictures and articles from home).
  These steps help reinforce reality and provide cues that maintain orientation.
- Stay with client if he or she is agitated and likely to be injured.
- Establish predictable care routines; maintain continuity of client's nursing staff.
  Routines promote feelings of security.
- Frequently check on client and have brief interactions to prevent sensory deprivation.
- Avoid an overstimulated or sensory-deprived environment; provide adequate lighting (not too bright); alternate short, frequent contacts with defined rest periods; monitor noise levels.

Excessive environmental stimuli can adversely affect the client's level of orientation and increase disorganization.

- Assist client with daily hygiene as needed; encourage self-care.
  Good hygiene and self-care increase self-esteem and autonomy.
- Provide support to family during client's period of disorientation; involve family in current care and in the planning of postdischarge care.
  Family involvement provides for continuity of care.
- Initiate a social service referral to find help for client following discharge.
- Limit use of sedatives and central nervous system depressants.
- Observe for hallucinations as evidenced by inappropriate laughter, slow verbal responses, lip movements without sound, smiling at inappropriate times, or grimacing.
- Ask direct questions such as, "Are you seeing or hearing something now?" or "Do you sometimes hear or see things that other people don't hear or see?"
- Do not attempt to argue or change client's beliefs; do not imply agreement.
  These actions encourage the client to hold more rigidly to beliefs.
- Accept that the client is seeing or hearing things that are not there, but tactfully tell the client that only he or she is hearing or seeing these things; focus on the feelings that accompany the hallucinations and delusions rather than their content (e.g., "You look frightened").
  Acceptance promotes a sense of trust and understanding.
- Set limits on delusional conversations (e.g., "We discussed that; let's talk about what is happening now on the unit").
- Ask for clarification when necessary.
- Help client to state needs and to ask for assistance.
- Involve client in short activities.
- Refer to **Risk for violence** for further nursing interventions and rationales.

Geriatric

- Monitor for dementia as evidenced by a gradual onset and progressive deterioration or for delirium as evidenced by an acute onset and generally reversible course.
  States of confusion require careful assessment (Vermeersch, 1990).
- Focus on feelings presented in hallucinations and delusions rather than the content.
  Tuning into the disoriented client's feelings is more important than rigidly insisting that he or she share the nurse's reality; give comfort and understanding when client experiences processing difficulties (Bleathman, Morton, 1992).

Client/Family Teaching

- Teach family reorientation techniques and the need to frequently repeat instructions.
- Help family identify coping skills, environmental supports, and community services for dealing with chronically mentally ill clients.
- Discuss the caregiver's need for respite; offer support, encouragement, and information for meeting those needs.

REFERENCES

Bleathman C, Morton I: Validation therapy: extracts from 20 groups with dementia sufferers, *J Adv Nurs* 17:658-666, 1992.

Foreman M: Complexities of acute confusion, *Geriatr Nurs,* 3:136-42, 1989.

Vermeersch PE: Clinical assessment of confusion, *Appl Nurs Res* pp. 28-33, 1990.

Yorker BC: The nurses's use of restraint with a neurologically impaired patient, *J Neurosci Nurs* 20:390-392, 1988.

BIBLIOGRAPHY

Algase DL, Beel-Bates CA: Everyday indicators of impaired cognition: development of a new screening scale, *Res Nurs Health* 16:57-66, 1993.

Coyle MK: Organic illness mimicking psychiatric episodes, *J Gerontol Nurs* 13:31-35, 1987.

Inaba-Roland T, Maricle S: Assessing delirium, *Heart Lung* 19:45-55, 1992.

Wilson HS, Kneisel CR: *Psychiatric nursing*, Menlo Park, Calif, 1992, Addison-Wesley.

Impaired tissue integrity

Diane Krasner

Definition The state in which an individual experiences damage to tissues such as subcutaneous tissue, fascia, or muscle.

Defining Characteristics

Destruction of skin surface (full thickness); disruption or destruction of body tissues.

Related Factors (r/t)

Altered circulation; nutritional deficit or excess; fluid deficit or excess; knowledge deficit; impaired physical mobility; chemical irritants (including body excretions, secretions, medications); thermal factors (temperature extremes); mechanical factors (pressure, shear, friction); irradiation (including therapeutic irradiation).

Client Outcomes/Goals

- Reports any altered sensation or pain at site of tissue impairment.
- Demonstrates understanding of plan to heal tissue and prevent injury.
- Describes measures to protect and heal the tissue, including wound care.

Nursing Interventions and Rationales

- Assess site of impaired tissue integrity and determine etiology (e.g., acute or chronic wound, burn, dermatological lesion, pressure ulcer, leg ulcer).
  Prior assessment of wound etiology is critical for proper identification of nursing interventions (Krasner, 1990).
- Determine size and depth of wound, (e.g., full thickness wound, stage-III or stage-IV pressure ulcer).
  Wound assessment is more reliable when performed by the same caregiver, when the client is in the same position, and when the same measures are used.
- Classify pressure ulcers in the following manner:
  - **Stage III** Full-thickness skin loss involving damage to or necrosis of subcutaneous tissue that may extend down to, but not through, underlying fascia. The ulcer appears as a deep crater with or without undermining of adjacent tissue.
  - **Stage IV** Full-thickness skin loss with extensive destruction, tissue necrosis, or damage to muscle, bone, or supporting structures (e.g., tendons, joint capsules). (Adapted from the National Pressure Ulcer Advisory Panel Consensus Development Conference Statement, 1989).
- Monitor site of impaired tissue integrity at least once daily for color changes, redness, swelling, warmth, pain, or other signs of infection. Determine if client is experiencing changes in sensation or pain.
  Systematic inspection can identify impending problems early (Bryant, 1993).
- Monitor status of skin around the wound; monitor client's skin care practices, noting type of soap or other cleansing agents used, temperature of water, and frequency of skin cleansing.
  Individualize plan according to client's skin condition, needs, and preferences. Avoid harsh cleansing agents, hot water, extreme friction or force, or too frequent cleansing (Panel for the Prediction and Prevention of Pressure Ulcers in Adults, 1992).
- Monitor client's continence status and minimize exposure of the skin impairment site and other areas to moisture from incontinence, perspiration, or wound drainage.
  If client is incontinent, implement an incontinence management plan to prevent exposure to chemicals in urine and stool that can strip or erode the skin; refer to a physician (e.g., urologist, gastroenterologist) for an incontinence work-up (Doughty,

1991; Urinary Incontinence Guideline Panel, 1992; Wound, Ostomy and Continence Nurses Society, 1992, 1994).

- Monitor for correct placement of tubes, catheters, and other devices; assess skin and tissue affected by the tape that secures these devices.
  Mechanical damage to skin and tissues as a result of pressure, friction, or shear is often associated with external devices.
- In orthopedic clients, check every 2 hours for correct placement of footboards, restraints, traction, casts, or other devices, and assess skin and tissue integrity. Be alert for symptoms of compartment syndrome. Refer to care plan for **Risk for peripheral neurovascular dysfunction**.
  Mechanical damage to skin and tissues (pressure, friction, or shear) is often associated with external devices.
- For clients with limited mobility, use a risk assessment tool to systematically assess immobility-related risk factors.
  A validated risk assessment tool such as the Norton Scale or the Braden Scale should be used to identify clients at risk for immobility-related skin breakdown (Panel for the Prediction and Prevention of Pressure Ulcers in Adults, 1992).
- Implement a written treatment plan for topical treatment of the skin impairment site.
  A written treatment plan ensures consistency in care and documentation (Maklebust, Sieggreen, 1991). Topical treatments must be matched to the client, the wound, and the setting (Krasner, 1990).
- If necrotic tissue (eschar or slough) is present, and if consistent with overall client management goals, identify a plan for debridement.
  Healing does not occur in the presence of necrotic tissue (Pressure Ulcer Treatment Guideline Panel, 1994).
- Select a topical treatment that maintains a moist wound-healing environment and balances with the need to absorb exudate and fill dead space.
  Caution should always be taken to not dry out the wound (Pressure Ulcer Treatment Guideline Panel, 1994).
- Position the client off the site of impaired tissue integrity. If consistent with overall client management goals, turn and position client at least every 2 hours, and carefully transfer client to avoid the adverse effects of external mechanical forces (pressure, friction, and shear).
  If the goal of care is to keep the client comfortable (e.g., a terminally ill client), turning and repositioning may not be appropriate. Maintain the head of the bed at the lowest degree of elevation possible to reduce shear and friction, and use lift devices, pillows, foam wedges, and pressure-reducing devices in the bed (Panel for the Prediction and Prevention of Pressure Ulcers in Adults, 1992).
- Avoid massaging around the site of impaired tissue integrity and over bony prominences.
  Research suggests that massage may lead to deep-tissue trauma (Panel for the Prediction and Prevention of Pressure Ulcers in Adults, 1992).
- Assess client's nutritional status; refer for a nutritional consult and/or institute dietary supplements.
  Inadequate nutritional intake places the client at a risk for skin breakdown, and it compromises healing (Krasner, 1990).

Client/Family Teaching

- Teach skin and wound assessment and ways to monitor for signs and symptoms of infection, complications, and healing.
  Early assessment and intervention helps prevent the development of serious problems.
- Teach use of a topical treatment that is matched to the client, the wound, and the setting.
  The topical treatment needs to be adjusted as the status of the wound changes.
- If consistent with overall client management goals, teach how to turn and reposition client at least every 2 hours.
  If the goal of care is to keep the client comfortable (e.g., a terminally ill client), turning and repositioning may not be appropriate (Panel for the Prediction and Prevention of Pressure Ulcers in Adults, 1992).
- Teach the use of pillows, foam wedges, and pressure-reducing devices to prevent pressure injury.

REFERENCES

Bryant R: *Acute and chronic wounds,* St Louis, 1993, Mosby.

Consensus Development Conference Statement. Buffalo, NY, 1989, National Pressure Ulcer Advisory Panel.

Doughty D: *Urinary and fecal incontinence: nursing management,* St Louis, 1991, Mosby.

Krasner, D: *Chronic wound care: a clinical source book for healthcare professionals*, King of Prussia, Pa, 1990, Health Management.

Maklebust J, Sieggreen M: *Pressure ulcers: guidelines for prevention and nursing management*, West Dundee, Ill, 1991, S-N.

Panel for the Prediction and Prevention of Pressure Ulcers in Adults: *Pressure ulcers in adults: prediction and prevention.* Clinical Practice Guideline No 3. Rockville, Md, May 1992, Agency for Health Care Policy and Research, Public Health Service, US Department of Health and Human Services, AHCPR Publication No. 92-0047.

Urinary Incontinence Guideline Panel. *Urinary incontinence in adults:* Clinical Practice Guideline. Rockville, Md, March 1992, Agency for Health Care Policy and Research, Public Health Service, US Department of Health and Human Services, AHCPR Publication No. 92-0038.

Wound, Ostomy, and Continence Nurses Society: *Standards of care: dermal wounds: pressure ulcers,* Costa Mesa, CA, 1992, WOCN.

Wound, Ostomy, and Continence Nurses Society: *Standards of care: patient with fecal incontinence,* Cosa Mesa, CA, 1994, WOCN.

Wound, Ostomy, and Continence Nurses Society: *Standards of care: patient with urinary incontinence,* Costa Mesa, CA, 1992, WOCN.

Altered tissue perfusion (specify type): cerebral, renal, cardiopulmonary, GI, peripheral

Betty Ackley

Definition The state in which an individual experiences a decrease in nutrition and oxygenation at the cellular level as a result of a deficit in capillary blood supply.

Defining Characteristics

Cold extremities; dependent, blue, or purple skin color; *leg is pale when elevated, and color does not return when leg is lowered; *diminished arterial pulsations; shiny skin; lack of lanugo; round scars covered with atrophied skin; gangrene; slow-growing, dry, thick, and brittle nails; claudication; blood pressure changes in extremities; bruits; slow-healing lesions. (*Critical)

Related Factors (r/t)

Interruption of arterial flow; interruption of venous flow; exchange problems; hypovolemia; hypervolemia.

Client Outcomes/Goals

- Demonstrates adequate tissue perfusion as evidenced by palpable peripheral pulses, warm and dry skin, adequate urinary output, and the absence of respiratory distress.
- Verbalizes knowledge of treatment regimen, including medications and their actions and possible side effects.
- Lists any suggested life-style changes.
- Identifies factors causing decreased tissue perfusion.
- Demonstrates adequate cerebral perfusion as evidenced by improved mentation, normal vital signs, and freedom from neurological dysfunction.

Nursing Interventions and Rationales

Cerebral Perfusion

- Monitor level of consciousness, ability to follow commands, and appropriateness of behavior.
  A change in level of consciousness is generally the first sign of neurological deterioration (Mitchell, Ackerman, 1992).
- Note new onset of confusion, dizziness, or syncope.
  Decreased cerebral perfusion is associated with these symptoms.
- Take vital signs q____min/h.
  Characteristic vital sign changes seen with increased intracranial pressure include increased pulse pressure, slow and bounding pulse, decreased respiratory rate, and increased temperature resulting from pressure damage on vasomotor centers of brain; these changes are later *signs of increased pressure. Elevated temperatures increase the cerebral metabolic rate, which increases intracranial pressure (Vos, 1993).*
- Watch client's respirations for any abnormal patterns such as Cheyne-Stokes respiration; apneustic, cluster, or ataxic breathing patterns; or hyperventilation.
  Characteristic respiratory patterns develop depending on the location of the cerebral insult (Mitchell, Ackerman, 1992).
- Monitor motor function by checking grasping and leg strength and client's ability to move all four extremities; at lower levels of consciousness determine client's response to pain by applying nailbed pressure at all four extremities.
- If intracranial pressure monitoring is in place, monitor cerebral perfusion pressure, and maintain it at the prescribed level. Notify physician of an increase or decrease in cerebral perfusion pressure. Refer to care plan for **Decreased adaptive capacity, intracranial.**

To ensure adequate perfusion of the brain, cerebral perfusion should be maintained within a prescribed range.

- Limit suctioning if possible; if suctioning is necessary, preoxygenate and hyperventilate client, and limit to two suction passes that last no longer than 15 seconds.
  Research has shown a strong association between suctioning and increased intracranial pressure (Mitchell, Ackerman, 1992). Careful suctioning can help prevent sustained increases in intracranial pressure (Rudy, Turner, Baun, 1992).
- When positioning client, avoid any neck flexion or head rotation; keep head in a neutral position.
  Neck flexion and head rotation decrease venous return, which increases intracranial pressure (Williams, Coyne, 1993).
- Position client as ordered, generally in a semi-Fowler's position with a 30-degree elevation. Always watch client's response to position changes; if cerebral perfusion pressure decreases after elevating head of bed, consider keeping bed flat and obtain physician's input.
  Elevated intracranial pressure can be lowered by raising the head of the bed, but an elevated head of the bed may compromise cerebral perfusion pressure (Winkelman, 1994).
- Avoid any knee flexion; do not raise knee gatch.
  Knee flexion traps venous blood in the intra-abdominal space, which first increases abdominal and then thoracic pressure and reduces venous return from the head (Vos, 1993).
- Sequence nursing care so that rest periods alternate with noxious activities such as suctioning and position changing; allow intracranial pressure to return to baseline before initiating any other nursing activities (Mitchell, Acklerman, 1992).
  These measures help prevent sustained increases in intracranial pressure, which can cause neurological damage.
- Touch client gently and talk quietly while giving care.
  Gentle touching and talking can have a therapeutic effect on the client with increased intracranial pressure (Mitchell, Johnson, Habermann-Little, 1985).

Peripheral Perfusion

- Check peripheral pulses bilaterally; if unable to find them, use a Doppler stethoscope.
  Diminished or absent peripheral pulses indicate decreased or absent arterial flow.
- Note skin color and temperature.
  Skin pallor or mottling, cool or cold skin temperature, or an absent pulse can signal arterial obstruction, which is an emergency that requires immediate intervention. Rubor (reddish-blue color accompanied by dependency) indicates dilated or damaged vessels. Brownish discoloration of skin indicates chronic venous insufficiency (Bright, Georgi, 1992).
- Check capillary refill.
  Nailbeds usually return to a pinkish color within 3 seconds after nailbed compression.
- Note skin texture and the presence of hair, ulcers, or gangrenous areas on the legs or feet.
  Thin, shiny, dry skin with hair loss and brittle nails is seen with arterial insufficiency along with gangrene, or ulcerations on toes and anterior surfaces of the foot. If ulcerations on the side of the leg, usually venous in nature.
- Note presence of edema in extremities and rate it on a 4-point scale. Measure circumference of extremities at same time each day in the early morning.
- Assess for pain in extremities, noting severity, quality, timing, and exacerbating and alleviating factors.

Arterial insufficiency is associated with pain during walking (claudication) that is relieved by rest. Clients with severe arterial disease have feet pain while at rest, which keeps them awake at night. Venous insufficiency is associated with aching, cramping, and discomfort (Bright, Georgi, 1992).

- If venous insufficiency is present with edema, elevate legs as ordered and ensure that there is no pressure under the knee, which decreases venous circulation.
- If arterial insufficiency is present, do not elevate legs above the level of the heart.
  With arterial insufficiency, leg elevation decreases arterial blood supply to the legs.
- If arterial insufficiency is present, keep client warm and have him or her wear socks and sheepskin-lined slippers when mobile. Do not apply heat.
  Clients with arterial insufficiency complain of being constantly cold; therefore keep extremities warm to maintain vasodilation and blood supply. Heat application can easily damage ischemic tissues (Creamer-Bauer, 1992).
- Provide meticulous foot care. Refer to podiatrist if a foot or nail abnormality is present.
  Ischemic feet are very vulnerable to injury; careful foot care can prevent further injury.
- If venous insufficiency is present, apply support hose as ordered.
  Support hose encourage increased venous return.

Geriatric

- Change positions slowly when getting client out of bed.
  The elderly have increased postural hypotension resulting from age-related losses of cardiovascular reflexes.

Client/Family Teaching

- Explain the importance of good foot care; recommend that the diabetic client wear padded socks, special insoles, and jogging shoes.
  Cushioned footwear can decrease pressure on feet, decrease callus formation, and save the feet (George, 1993).
- Stress importance of not smoking, following a weight loss program (if client is obese), carefully controling diabetic condition, controling hyperlipidemia and hypertension, and reducing stress.
  All of these risk factors for atherosclerosis can be modified (Bright, Georgi, 1992).
- Teach to avoid exposure to cold, limit exposure to brief periods if going out in cold weather, and wear warm clothing.
- Teach to recognize the signs and symptoms that need to be reported to a physician (e.g., change in skin temperature, color, or sensation).

NOTE: If client is receiving anticoagulant therapy, refer to care plan for **Altered protection**.

REFERENCES

Bright LD, Georgi S: Peripheral vascular disease, is it arterial or venous?, *Am J Nurs* 92(8):34-47, 1992.

Creamer-Bauer C: Tissue perfusion, altered peripheral. In Gettrust KV, Brabec PD, editors: *Nursing diagnosis in clinical practice: guidelines for planning care*, Albany, NY, 1992, Delmar.

George NE: Give 'em the old soft shoe: working smart, *Am J Nurs* 93(2):16, 1993.

Mitchell PH, Ackerman LL: Secondary brain injury reduction. In Bulechek GM, McCloskey JC, editors: *Nursing interventions: essential nursing treatments*, ed 2, Philadelphia, 1992, WB Saunders.

Mitchell PH, Johnson FB, Habermann-Little BH: Promoting physiologic stability: touch and ICP, *Commun Nurs Res* 18:93, 1985 (abstract).

Rudy EB, Turner BS, Baun M: Endotracheal suctioning in adults with head injury, *Heart Lung* 20:667-674, 1992.

Vos HR: Making headway with intracranial hypertension, *Am J Nurs* 93(2):28-39, 1993.

Williams A, Coyne SM: Effects of neck position on intracranial pressure, *Am J Crit Care* 2:68-71, 1993.

Winkelman C: Advances in managing increased intracranial pressure: a decade of selected research, *AACN Clin Issues* 5:9-14, 1994.

BIBLIOGRAPHY

Rising CJ: The relationship of selected nursing activities to ICP, *J Neurosci Nurs* 25:302-308, 1993.

Risk for trauma

Gail Ladwig

Definition Accentuated risk of accidental tissue injury (e.g., wound, burn, fracture).

Defining Characteristics

Presence of risk factors such as

Internal (individual)

Weakness; balancing difficulties; reduced temperature or tactile sensation; reduced large- or small-muscle coordination; reduced hand-eye coordination; lack of safety education; lack of safety precautions; insufficient finances to purchase safety equipment or effect repairs; cognitive or emotional difficulties; history of previous trauma.

External (environmental)

Slippery floors (e.g., wet or highly-waxed); snow or ice collected on stairs or walkways; unanchored rugs; bathtub without hand grips or antislip equipment; unsteady ladders or unanchored electrical wires; litter or liquid spills on floors or stairways; high beds; children playing without gates at the top of the stairs; obstructed passageways; unsafe window protection in homes with young children; inappropriate call-for-aid mechanisms for bedresting client; pot handles facing toward front of stove; very hot bathwater (e.g., unsupervised bathing of young children); potentially ignitable gas leaks; delayed lighting of gas burner or oven, experimentation with chemicals or gasoline; unscreened fires or heaters; plastic aprons or flowing clothes around an open flame; children playing with matches, candles, or cigarettes; inadequately stored combustible items or corrosives (e.g., matches, oily rags, lye); contact with rapidly moving machinery, industrial belts, or pulleys; coarse bed linen; struggles within bed restraints; faulty electrical plugs, frayed wires, or defective appliances; contact with acids or alkalis; fireworks; radiotherapy; use of cracked dishware or glasses; knives stored uncovered; guns or ammunition stored unlocked; large icicles hanging from the roof; exposure to dangerous machinery; children playing with sharp-edged toys; high-crime neighborhood and vulnerable clients; driving a mechanically unsafe vehicle; driving under the influence of alcoholic beverages or drugs; driving at excessive speeds; driving without necessary visual aids; children riding in the front seat in car; smoking in bed or near oxygen; overloaded electrical outlets; grease waste collected on stoves; use of thin or worn potholders; misuse of necessary headgear for motorized cyclists; carrying young children on adult bicycles; unsafe road or road-crossing conditions; playing or working near vehicle pathways (e.g., driveways, laneways, railroad tracks); nonuse or misuse of seatbelts.

Related Factors (r/t)

Refer to risk factors.

Client Outcomes/Goals

- Free from trauma.
- Explains actions that can be taken to prevent trauma.

Nursing Interventions and Rationales

- Provide vision aids for visually impaired clients.
  A client with a sensory loss must be protected from injury; therefore the visually impaired client must wear vision aids (Potter, Perry, 1993).
- Assist client with ambulation.
- Have family member evaluate water temperature for client.
  A client with a tactile sensory impairment resulting from age or psychological or physiological factors needs to be protected from burns.

- Assess client for causes of impaired cognition.
  Confusion from delirium and depression is reversible, but dementia is not reversible and has implications for long-term safety (Holt, 1993).
- Use reality orientation to improve client's cognition.
  Focusing on what is real helps decrease the client's delusions and hallucinations and helps prevent the client from acting out and injuring himself or herself.
- Make a social service referral for financial assistance.
- Teach safety measures to prevent trauma; ensure that the client can read if using written materials.
  Health care professionals have a legal and ethical obligation to provide clients with self-care instructions they can understand (Wong, 1992).
- Keep walkways clear of snow, debris, and household items.
  Such measures prevent trauma from falls.
- Provide assistive devices in bathrooms (e.g., handrails, nonslip decals on floor of shower and bathtub).
  Such measures help to prevent trauma from falls.
- Ensure that call-light systems are functioning and that client is able to use them.
  Often hospital injuries result from a client's attempt to get self out of bed and use the bathroom if he or she cannot contact the caregiver.
- Never leave young children unsupervised around water or cooking areas.
  Young children are at risk for drowning even in small amounts of water. Heat and fire from cooking are a hazard to young children.
- Keep flammable and potentially flammable articles out of the reach of young children.
- Lock up harmful objects such as guns.
  Accidental discharge of guns is a major cause of trauma.
- Teach to observe safety in high-crime neighborhoods (e.g., lock doors, do not leave home at night without a companion, keep entry ways well lit).
  Adequate lighting helps protect the home and its inhabitants from crime (Potter, Perry, 1993).
- Instruct clients not to drive under the influence of alcohol or drugs. Assess for problems and refer to appropriate resources regarding drug and alcohol education.
  A well supported relationship exists between alcohol consumption and traumatic deaths from falls, fires, burns, and motor vehicle crashes.
- Refer to nursing interventions and rationales for **Risk for injury**.
- Refer to nursing interventions and rationales for **Impaired home maintenance management**.
- Refer to care plan for **Risk for poisoning, Risk for aspiration,** and **Risk for suffocation**.

Geriatric

- Perform a home safety assessment.
  Nurses provide care to the clients at home and need to know what contributes to a safe environment and how to help the client achieve one (Potter, Perry, 1993).
- Mark stove knobs with bright colors; outline step borders.
  Easily visible markings are helpful for clients with decreased depth perception (Potter, Perry, 1993).
- Increase lighting in hallways and other dark areas; place a light in the bathroom.
- Discourage driving at night.
  A decline in depth perception, slower recovery from glare, and night blindness are common in the elderly and make night driving a difficult and unsafe task (Ringsven, Bond, 1991).

Client/Family Teaching

- Educate family regarding age-appropriate child safety, environmental safety precautions, and how to intervene in an emergency.
- Teach family to assess day-care center's or babysitter's knowledge regarding child safety, environmental safety precautions, and assisting a child in an emergency.
- Discuss various ways an adolescent can protect self from trauma while maintaining peer relationships.

Refer to care plans for **Risk for poisoning, Risk for aspiration, Risk for suffocation, Risk for injury,** and **Impaired home maintenance management**.

REFERENCES

Holt J: How to help confused patients, *Am J Nurs* 93:32-36, 1993.

Potter A, Perry A: *Fundamentals of nursing: concepts, process & practice,* St Louis, 1993, Mosby.

Ringsven M, Bond D: *Gerontology and leadership skills for nurses,* Albany, NY, 1991, Delmar.

Wong M: Self-care instructions: do patients understand educational materials?, *Focus Crit Care* 19:47-49, 1992.

Unilateral neglect

Leslie Kalbach and Betty Ackley

Definition The state in which an individual is perceptually unaware of and inattentive to one side of the body.

Defining Characteristics

Major Consistent inattention to stimuli on an affected side.

Minor Inadequate self-care; positioning or safety precautions in regard to affected side; failure to look toward affected side; food left on plate on affected side.

Related Factors (r/t)

Effects of disturbed perceptual abilities (e.g., hemianopsia, one-sided blindness, neurological illness, trauma).

NOTE: Because the right hemisphere is dominant in directing attention, unilateral neglect is more common if neurological pathology occurs in this hemisphere of the brain, which results in left-sided neglect (Kalbach, 1991).

Client Outcomes/Goals

- Demonstrates techniques that can be used to minimize unilateral neglect.
- Both sides of the body are cared for appropriately, and the affected side is free from harm.
- Free of injury, skin breakdown, or contractures.

Nursing Interventions and Rationales

- Monitor client for signs of unilateral neglect (e.g., not washing or shaving one side of the body, sitting or lying inappropriately on affected arm or leg, failing to respond to stimuli on the contralateral side of lesion, eating food on only one side of plate, or failing to look to one side of the body).
  Looking, listening, touching, and searching deficits occur on the affected side of the body and may or may not be associated with a loss of vision, sensation, or motion on the affected side (Kalbach, 1991).
- Provide a safe, well lit, and clutter-free environment; place call light on unaffected side; keep side rails up when client is in bed; cue client to environmental hazards when mobile.
  Cognitive impairment may accompany neglect; thus safety is of paramount importance.

NOTE: Nursing interventions for clients with unilateral neglect should be implemented in the following stages as the client progresses:

Stage I—Focus attention mainly on the nonneglected side

- Set up environment so that most activity is on the unaffected side
- Keep client's personal items within view and on the unaffected side
- Position client's bed so that activity is on the unaffected side
  The initial priority is client safety (Kalbach, 1991).

Stage II—Help client develop an awareness of the neglected side

- Gradually focus client's attention to the affected side
- Gradually move personal items and activity to the affected side
- Stand on client's affected side when assisting with ambulation or activities of daily living
  The goal is now for the client to develop an awareness of the neglected side.

Stage III—Help client develop the ability to compensate for the neglect

- Encourage client to bathe and groom the affected side first
- Focus touch and talking on the affected side; use a positive approach (e.g., "Mary, turn your head to the left and you'll see your grandchildren" (Carnevali, Patrick, 1993)

- Use constant and positive reminders to keep the client scanning the entire environment
- Use bright yellow or red stickers on outer margins in reading or writing exercises; have the client look for the sticker before reading or writing
  Use cues and anchors to promote attention to the neglected side and help the client develop compensatory mechanisms to deal with neglect syndrome (Kalbach, 1991).

- Refer to a rehabilitation nurse specialist or occupational therapist for continued help in dealing with unilateral neglect; include visual stimuli and eye-patching techniques. *Monocular patching with lateralized visual stimulation may significantly reduce neglect in daily activities (Butter, Kirsch, 1992).*

Client/Family Teaching

- Explain the pathology and symptoms of unilateral neglect.
- Teach the client how to scan to regularly check the position of his or her body parts and how to regularly turn his or her head from side to side, especially for safety when ambulating.
- Teach the caregivers positive cueing (reminders to help the client remember to interact with entire environment).

REFERENCES

Butter CM and Kirsch N: Combined and separate effects of eye patching and visual stimulation on unilateral neglect following stroke, *Arch Phys Med Rehabil*, 73:1133-1139, 1992.

Carnevali DL, Patrick M: *Nursing management for the elderly,* ed 3, Philadelphia, 1993, JB Lippincott.

Kalbach LR: Unilateral neglect: mechanisms and nursing care, *J Neurosci Nurs*, 23:125-129, 1991.

Altered urinary elimination

Kathie Hesnan

Definition The state in which an individual experiences a disturbance in urine elimination.

NOTE: This is a general diagnosis that is relevant when the pattern or source of the problem has not been identified. The author has chosen to use the nursing diagnosis mainly for referring to urinary tract infection. Please refer to more specific nursing diagnoses on urinary elimination for other alterations in urinary elimination as needed such as **Stress incontinence, Urge incontinence, Reflex incontinence, Functional incontinence, Urinary retention,** or **Total incontinence.**

Defining Characteristics

Dysuria; frequency; hesitancy; incontinence; nocturia; retention; urgency.

Related Factors (r/t)

Anatomical obstruction; sensory motor impairment; urinary tract infection; pregnancy; postpartum trauma; swelling; pain.

Client Outcomes/Goals

- Voids 1000 to 1500 ml of clear, amber-colored urine without difficulty daily and in an appropriate receptacle.
- Explains measures to prevent a urinary tract infection (UTI).

Nursing Interventions and Rationales

- Assess for incontinence or urine retention, and refer to the appropriate nursing diagnosis if necessary.
- Monitor patterns of voiding and characteristics of urine, and keep records of input and output.
- Observe if alteration is physiological, psychological, or environmental, and intervene accordingly.
- If dysuria, urgency, or frequency are present, obtain order for a urine culture and monitor temperature, blood pressure, and pulse q4h; watch for signs of sepsis shock.
  Urgency and involuntary loss of urine may be symptoms of a UTI (Silverblatt, 1988).
- Provide and encourage intake of fluids; avoid citrus juices, tomato juices, or caffeinated fluids.
  These items may be bladder irritants to some individuals, which can lead to frequency, urgency, and incontinence.
- Clients who have pain accompanied by frequency, urgency (even at night), and bladder fullness that may or may not resolve after voiding, may have interstitial cystitis and should be referred to a health care professional who specializes in its treatment.
  Interstitial cystitis is a chronic inflammatory condition of the bladder (Fletcher, 1988). For clients with suspected interstitial cystitis, dietary changes such as eliminating alcohol, caffeine, artificial sweeteners, citrus fruits, and acidic foods may be helpful (Ratner, 1992).
- Provide unobstructed access to the bathroom or toilet.
- Help client plan a voiding schedule that fits into his or her life-style and yields voids of approximately 300 ml.
- Ensure that pericare is done daily and as needed.
- Encourage verbalization of feelings about problems with urination.

Geriatric

- For toileting problems, determine factors that interfere with self-care and remove any barriers that exist.
- Gear interventions toward maintaining continence, functional independence, and self-care.

- Watch for signs of UTI, but do not expect to see the usual symptoms; the elderly may have a change in mentation, a new onset of incontinence, or even an absence of symptoms.
  Physiological and cognitive changes make it difficult to diagnose a UTI from symptoms alone. A urinalysis is a basic test for clients with urinary incontinence or changes in voiding function (Urinary Incontinence Guideline Panel, 1992).
- If not contraindicated, encourage postmenopausal women to drink one 10 ounce glass of cranberry cocktail per day to prevent UTIs.
  Drinking one glass of cranberry juice cocktail daily has been shown to significantly reduce the incidence of UTIs in elderly women (Avorn et al, 1994).

Client/Family Teaching

- Teach the need to finish taking the prescribed UTI medication and the need for follow-up urine specimens.
- Teach symptoms of UTIs.
- Teach methods to prevent UTIs such as voiding every 3 to 4 hours, drinking adequate amounts of fluid, showering instead of bathing, voiding after intercourse, and wiping perineum from front to back.

REFERENCES

Avorn J et al: Reduction of bacteriuria and pyuria after ingestion of cranberry juice, *JAMA* 271:751-754, 1994.

Fletcher S: Interstitial cystitis: painful bladder syndrome, *Nurs Pract* 13:7-12, 1988.

Ratner V et al: Interstitial cystitis: A bladder disease finds legitimacy, *J Women Health* 1:63-68, 1992.

Silverblatt FM: Incontinence and bacteriuria in elderly patients, *Hosp Pract* 23(9):77-90, 1988.

Urinary Incontinence Guideline Panel. *Urinary Incontinence in Adults:* Clinical practice guideline. Rockville, Md, March 1992, Agency for health care policy and research, Public health service, US Department of Health and Human Services, AHCPR Publication No. 92-0038.

BIBLIOGRAPHY

Petit J: Urinary tract infections in older adults, *Nurs Pract* 13:21-29, 1988.

Urinary retention

Kathie Hesnan

Definition The state in which an individual experiences incomplete emptying of the bladder.

Defining Characteristics

Major — Bladder distention; frequent voiding of small amounts (less than 100 ml); absence of urine output.

Minor — Sensation of bladder fullness; dribbling; residual urine; dysuria; overflow incontinence; hesitancy.

Related Factors (r/t)

High urethral pressure caused by weak detrusor; inhibition of reflex arc; strong sphincter; blockage of urethra; medications that affect voiding; postpartum perineal trauma; swelling; pain; neurological damage.

Client Outcomes/Goals

- Urinates 1200 to 1500 ml of clear straw-colored urine in a 24-hour period and has less than 100 ml residual urine; performs intermittent self-catheterization independently with volumes less than 500 ml.
- States relief from pain of full bladder; suprapubic area is free of bladder distension.
- Describes measures to prevent and treat urinary retention.
- Free from upper urinary tract damage.

Nursing Interventions and Rationales

- Use indwelling catheter only as a last resort.
  Long-term use of an indwelling catheter (more than 2 to 4 weeks) can lead to secondary problems such as bacteriuria, UTIs, and encrustations that cause blockage, unprescribed removal, pain, or bladder spasms (Urinary Incontinence Guideline Panel, 1992).
- Evaluate for medications that could cause retention such as tricyclic antidepressants, phenothiazines, anticholinergics, antihistamines, antihypertensives, drugs for parkinsonism, and some analgesics.
  These medications can cause bladder relaxation or increased urethral sphincter tone.
- Assess for retention of postvoid residual with either a bladder scan or catheterization; if this method yields an amount greater than 200 ml, notify physician.
- Instruct client to double void, relax the pelvic muscles in between voiding attempts, and not strain because straining contracts the pelvic musculature.
  In clients with mild to moderate obstruction, more complete bladder emptying may be accomplished with double voiding (Gross, 1992).
- Monitor client for dystonia, urgency, or frequency.
- Assess for fecal impaction or constipation.
  The distended rectum can cause pressure on the bladder and lead to urgency, incontinence, or retention of urine (Urinary Incontinence Guideline Panel, 1992).
- Provide privacy for voiding.
- Help male client stand during a void; help female client onto commode for a void.
- Run water in the sink and pour a measured amount of warm water over the perineum.
- Increase daily fluid intake to 2000 ml within the cardiac and renal reserve.
- Play recorded sounds of waterfalls or the ocean prn.
- Offer medication prn for pain, which can interfere with voiding.
- Trigger reflex arc by lightly touching the perineal area.

- If clean intermittent catheterization is to be used, teach client how to care for the catheter and other supplies.
  Proper care of the supplies decreases the chance of clinical bacteriuria or infection. Plastic urethral catheters can be used if the client is knowledgeable and the environment is appropriate (Moore et al, 1993).
- Do not routinely teach Credé's methods.
  A urological evaluation must be done to ensure that the sphincter and bladder are coordinated so that reflux does not occur.
- Regulate fluid intake according to the catheterization schedule.
  Drinking a large volume of fluid before going to bed may cause the client to get up during the night to catheterize.

Geriatric

- Help elderly male sit on commode to void.
- Assess for fecal impaction if present, and treat according to protocol.

Client/Family Teaching

- Teach use of relaxation techniques such as deep breathing and visualization (e.g., visualize standing beside a waterfall).
- Teach intermittent self-catheterization with physician approval if retention continues.
- Instruct in a plan for home care that includes a voiding routine, fluid intake, knowledge regarding symptoms of retention or UTI, knowledge regarding when to notify physician, awareness of available community resources.
- Teach client to respond to the voiding urge.
- If constipation or fecal impaction is associated with urine retention, teach client and family an individualized bowel program. Refer to care plan for **Constipation**.

REFERENCES

Gross J: Bladder dysfunction after stroke, *Urol Nurs* 12:55-63, 1992.

Moore K et al: Bacteriuria in intermittent catheterization users: the effect of sterile versus clean reused catheters, *Rehabil Nurs* 18:306-309, 1993.

Urinary Incontinence Guideline Panel. *Urinary Incontinence in Adults:* Clinical practice guideline. Rockville, Md, March 1992, Agency for health care policy and research, Public health service, US Department of Health and Human Services, AHCPR Publication No. 92-0038.

BIBLIOGRAPHY

Williams M et al: Urinary retention in hospitalized elderly women, *J Gerontol Nurs* 19:7, 1993.

Inability to sustain spontaneous ventilation

Leslie Lysaght

Definition The state in which a response pattern of decreased energy reserves results in an individual's inability to maintain breathing adequate for supporting life.

Defining Characteristics

Major Dyspnea; increased metabolic rate; increased heart rate; decreased PO_2; increased PCO_2.

Minor Increased restlessness; apprehension; increased use of accessory muscles; decreased tidal volume; decreased cooperation; decreased SaO_2.

Related Factors (r/t)

Metabolic factors; respiratory muscle fatigue.

Client Outcomes/Goals

- Arterial blood gases within safe parameters for client.
- Free of dyspnea or restlessness.

Nursing Interventions and Rationales

- Assess and respond to changes in client's respiratory status. Monitor client for dyspnea, including respiratory rate, use of accessory muscles, intercostal retractions, flaring of nostrils, and subjective complaints.
  It is essential to monitor for these signs of impending respiratory failure (McCord, Cronin-Stubbs, 1992).
- Administer indicated diuretics, analgesics, or antianxiety medications; titrate supplemental oxygen as indicated.
  Interventions to decrease workload on the heart, maintain comfort, minimize anxiety, or increase the available oxygen for gas exchange are necessary interventions in respiratory failure.
- Collaborate with physician, client, and family regarding care plan and interventions; consider client's wishes, overall health, and reversibility of the medical condition.
  Many clients and their families make decisions about the level of aggressiveness of therapy they desire. Health care providers have a responsibility to allow the client to participate in care decisions.
- Recognize that confusion accompanied by a progression to somnolence may be an ominous sign of respiratory failure with carbon dioxide narcosis.
- If client has unresolved dyspnea, deteriorating arterial blood gases, changes in level of consciousness, or panic, prepare the client for intubation and placement on ventilator.
  Immediate intervention is necessary for signs and symptoms of acute respiratory failure.
- Administer sedation for client comfort during intubation per physician's order.

Ventilator Support

- Tape endotracheal tube securely, auscultate breath sounds, and get a chest x-ray examination to confirm endotracheal tube placement.
  These interventions are necessary to maintain an adequate airway (Hudak, Gallo, 1994).
- Suction as needed and hyperoxygenate and hyperventilate per protocol; note frequency, type, and amount of secretions.
  These steps assure adequate oxygenation (Dam, Wild, Baun, 1994).
- Prevent unplanned extubations.
  Endotracheal tube placement must be maintained in order to ventilate the client.
- Analyze and respond to arterial blood gas results.
  Ventilatory support must be closely monitored to ensure adequate oxygenation and an acid-base balance.

- Support client comfort and keep client and family involved in plan of care.
- Help client identify and use a communication method such as a letter board, paper and pencil, or mouthing of words.
  Alternative strategies of communication prevent isolation and loss (Menzel, 1994).
- Rotate endotracheal tube from side to side every 24 hours. Assess and document skin condition, and note tube placement at lip line. Provide oral care q4h and prn.
  These steps prevent skin breakdown at the lip line that results from endotracheal tube pressure.
- Assess bilateral anterior and posterior breath sounds q4h and prn; respond to any relevant changes.
- Monitor respiratory rate and identify ventilator-assisted and independent respiratory efforts.
  These methods evaluate the client's respiratory efforts.
- Assess tolerance to ventilatory assistance and monitor for dysynchronous chest movement, subjective complaints of breathlessness, and high-pressure alarms. Collaborate with interdisciplinary team in resolving problems with changes in ventilatory settings, sedation, analgesia, relaxation techniques, or neuromuscular blockers.
- Respond to ventilator alarms; if unable to rapidly locate source of alarm, ambu bag client while awaiting respiratory therapist. Common causes of a high-pressure alarm include client resistance or the need for suction; a common cause of a low-pressure alarm is ventilator disconnection.
  Bagging the client with an ambu bag connected to oxygen safely supports ventilation until the mechanical problem can be resolved. Ensure that the ambu bag is available, and know how to use it.
- Collaborate with interdisciplinary team in treating and responding to the cause of underlying acute respiratory failure.
  The mechanical ventilator is usually a ventilation support used temporarily until the underlying pathology can be treated.
- Implement appropriate interventions to maintain client comfort, mobility, nutrition, and skin integrity.
  These interventions prevent functional losses (Gift et al, 1992).

REFERENCES

Dam V, Wild C, Baun B: Effect of oxygen insufflation during endotracheal suctioning on arterial pressure and oxygenation of coronary artery bypass graft patients, *Am J Crit Care* 3:191-197, 1994.

Gift A, Austin D: The effects of a program of systematic movement of COPD patients, *Rehabil Nurs* 17:6-10, 1992.

Hudak C, Gallo B: *Management modalities: respiratory system.* In *Critical care nursing: a holistic approach,* ed 6, Philadelphia, 1992, Mosby.

McCord M, Cronin-Stubbs D: Operationalizing dyspnea, *Heart Lung* 21:167-179, 1992.

Menzel L: Need for communication-related research in mechanically ventilated patients, *Am J Crit Care* 3:165-167, 1994.

BIBLIOGRAPHY

Ackerman M: The effect of saline lavage prior to suctioning, *Am J Crit Care* 2:326-330, 1993.

Campbell R, Branson R: How ventilators provide temporary O_2 enrichment: what happens when you press the 100% suction button?, *Respir Care* 37:933-937, 1992.

Dysfunctional ventilatory weaning response (DVWR)

Leslie Lysaght

Definition The state in which a client cannot adjust to lowered levels of mechanical ventilator support, which interrupts and prolongs the weaning process.

Defining Characteristics

Mild DVWR

Major — Restlessness; respiratory rate slightly increased above baseline.

Minor — Responds to lowered levels of mechanical ventilator support with expressed feelings of increased need for oxygen, breathing discomfort, fatigue, warmth, queries about possible machine malfunction, or an increased concentration on breathing.

Moderate DVWR

Major — Responds to lowered levels of mechanical ventilator support with a slight increase from baseline blood pressure (<20 mm Hg), a slight increase from baseline heart rate (<20 beats/min), or a baseline increase in respiratory rate (<5 breaths/min).

Minor — Hypervigilence to activities; inability to respond to coaching; inability to cooperate; apprehension; diaphoresis; eye widening; decreased air entry on auscultation; color changes (e.g., pale complexion, slight cyanosis); slight respiratory accessory muscle use.

Severe DVWR

Major — Agitated response to lowered levels of mechanical ventilator support; deterioration in arterial blood gases from current baseline; increase in blood pressure from baseline (>20 mm Hg); significant increase in respiratory rate from baseline.

Minor — Profuse diaphoresis; full respiratory accessory muscle use; shallow and gasping breaths; paradoxical abdominal breathing; discoordinated breathing with the ventilator; decreased level of consciousness; adventitious breath sounds; audible airway secretions; cyanosis.

Related Factors (r/t)

Physical — Ineffective airway clearance; sleep pattern disturbance; inadequate nutrition; uncontrolled pain or discomfort.

Psychological — Knowledge deficit of the weaning process and patient role; perceived inefficacy about the ability to wean; decreased motivation; decreased self-esteem; moderate or severe anxiety; fear; hopelessness; powerlessness; insufficient trust in the nurse.

Situational — Uncontrolled episodic energy demands or problems; inappropriate pacing of diminished ventilator support; inadequate social support; adverse environment (e.g., noise, activity, negative events in the room, low nurse-client ratio, extended nurse absence from bedside, unfamiliar nursing staff); history of ventilator dependence (>1 week); history of multiple unsuccessful weaning attempts.

Client Outcomes/Goals

- Weaned from ventilator and maintains adequate arterial blood gases.
- Return of blood pressure, pulse, and respiration to baseline.
- Free of dyspnea and restlessness.

Nursing Interventions and Rationales

- While on the ventilator, coach client to increase strength of respiratory muscles; say to the client, "Feel the difference between the machine's breaths and your own. Work to make your own breaths as deep and full as the machine's."
- Assess client's readiness for weaning evidenced by an adequate nutritional status or balance, adequate rest and comfort, resolution of the initial medical problem that resulted in ventilator dependence, control and stability of any chronic health problems, hemodynamic stability, psychological readiness, alertness, stable vital signs, adequate respiratory parameters, an inspiratory force >20 cm, and an airway free of secretions.

To ensure the best outcome, it is important that the client be in an optimal physiological and psychological state before introducing the stress of a wean (Weilitz, 1993).

- Identify any reasons for previous unsuccessful weaning attempts, and include that information in development of the weaning plan.
  Analyzing client responses after each weaning attempt prevents repeatedly unsuccessful weans.
- Promote rest and comfort throughout the weaning period (e.g., administer analgesics, position client in bed or chair).
  NOTE: Avoid analgesics that suppress respirations.
- Help client identify personal strategies that result in relaxation and comfort (e.g., television, reading, visualizing, relaxation techniques, family visits); support implementation of these strategies.
  Personal strategies for relaxation are effective (Gift, Moore, Soeken, 1992).
- Negotiate with client to set goals for weaning; push client to accomplish more within his or her capabilities.
  Goals promote client rehabilitation (Weaver, Narsagage, 1992).
- Help client identify the desired amount of information about or participation in the weaning plan; help client identify progress.
  Control of the situation allows the client to participate to his or her fullest interest and capability.
- Collaborate with interdisciplinary team (physician and respiratory therapist) in identifying a weaning plan, timeline, and goals; revise plan throughout the wean.
- Provide a safe and comfortable environment. Make call light readily available and assure client that his or her needs will be met; provide all necessary levels of ventilator support.
  A client who feels safe and trusts the health care providers can focus on the higher level work of weaning.
- During the wean, monitor client's physiological and psychological responses; acknowledge and respond to fears and subjective complaints.
- Focus on achievement of small goals throughout the wean; maintain client's self-esteem and self-efficacy.
- Ensure that client is free of pain before weaning; teach relaxation and imagery as alternatives to narcotic use.
- Do not give narcotics immediately before weaning; carefully schedule pain medications and weaning; wean after the effects of the sedatives but not the analgesics have worn off.
- Suction airway prn and auscultate lung sounds to assess for changes throughout the wean.
  Continued assessment and maintenance of airway clearance throughout the wean supports client comfort, safety, and trust.
- Schedule weaning periods in the morning when client is rested; cluster care activities to promote successful weaning; avoid doing other procedures during weaning; keep environment quiet and promote rest between weaning periods.
- Limit visitors during the wean to close and supportive persons; have a visitor leave if he or she is negatively affecting the weaning process.

- Coach client through episodes of increased anxiety. Remain with client or place a supportive and calm significant other in this role. Give positive reinforcement, and with permission use touch and hold client's hand.
  It is not unusual for a client with lung disease to experience self-limiting episodes of increased shortness of breath. Supporting and coaching a client through such episodes allows the wean to continue.
- Avoid pharmacological sedation if possible; consult with physician about selecting a sedative drug with minimal muscle-relaxing effects.
- Terminate the wean with physician collaboration when signs and symptoms of fatigue or intolerance appear as evidenced by a blood pressure increase or decrease of 20 mm Hg, pulse rate increase or decrease of 20 beats/min, respirations >25 or <8, dysrhythmias (especially premature ventricular contractions), decreased oxygen saturation levels, panic, dyspnea, use of accessory muscles, intercostal retraction, flaring of nostrils, changes in level of consciousness, or a subjective inability to continue.
  Immediately responding to and intervening in weaning intolerance limits client fatigue and discomfort and promotes the ability for later success.
- If the dysfunctional ventilatory weaning response is severe, slow down the weaning process and consider weaning in 5-minute periods.

REFERENCES

Gift A, Moore T, Soeken K: Relaxation to reduce dyspnea and anxiety in COPD patients, *Nurs Res* 41:242-250, 1992.

Weaver T, Narsagage G: Physiological and psychological variables related to functional status in chronic obstructive pulmonary disease, *Nurs Res* 41:286-290, 1992.

Weilitz P: Weaning a patient from mechanical ventilation, *Crit Care Nurse* 13:33-41, 1993.

BIBLIOGRAPHY

Hudak C, Gallo B: Management modalities: respiratory system, in *Critical care nursing: a holistic approach*, ed 6, Philadelphia, 1992, Mosby.

Risk for violence: self-directed or directed at others

Judy Rizzo

Definition

The state in which an individual experiences behaviors that can be physically harmful either to the self or others.

Defining Characteristics

Major Body language (e.g., clenched fists, tense facial expression, rigid posture, tautness indicating effort to control); hostile or threatening verbalizations (e.g., boasting of or prior abuse of others); increased motor activity (e.g., pacing, excitement, irritability, agitation); overt and aggressive acts (e.g., goal-directed destruction of objects in environment); possession of destructive objects (e.g., gun, knife, weapon); rage; self-destructive behavior; active aggressive suicidal acts; suspicion of others; paranoid ideations, delusions, or hallucinations; substance abuse or withdrawal (e.g., verbalized warnings of losing control, increased perspiration, dilated or constricted pupils).

Minor Increased anxiety levels; fear of self or others; inability to verbalize feelings; repetition of verbalizations (e.g., continued complaints, requests, and demands); anger; provocative behavior (e.g., argumentive, dissatisfied, overreactive, hypersensitive); vulnerable self-esteem; depression (specifically active, aggressive, or suicidal acts); inability to see other options; poor impulse control; low frustration tolerance; poor coping skills.

Related Factors (r/t)

Antisocial character; battered women; catatonic excitement; child abuse; manic excitement; organic brain syndrome; panic states; rage reactions; suicidal behavior; temporal lobe epilepsy; toxic reactions to medications; personality disorder; dyscontrol syndrome.

Client Outcomes/Goals

- Does not harm self or others.
- Relaxed body language; decreased motor activity.
- No aggressive activity.
- Able to demonstrate control or states feelings of control.
- Expresses decreased anxiety and control of hallucinations.
- Able to talk about feelings; expresses anger appropriately.
- No access to harmful objects.

Nursing Interventions and Rationales

Violence Toward Others

- Identify behaviors that indicate impending violence against self or others.
  Knowing, recognizing, and promptly intervening in early precipitating factors prevents violence.
- Allow and encourage client to verbalize anger.
  "Talking replaces action." Talking about anger displaces it and prevents the client from acting on it.
- Identify stimuli that instigate violence.
- Help client identify when anger occurs; have client keep an anger diary, and together discuss alternative responses.
- Maintain a calm attitude (anxiety is contagious).
- Provide a low level of stimuli in client's environment; place client in a quiet, safe place, and speak in slow, quiet tones.
  A safe, quiet environment decreases the outside stimuli that may be precipitating violent behavior.

- Redirect possible violent behaviors into physical activities if client is physically able (e.g., punching bags, hitting pillows, walking, jogging).
- Provide sufficient staff if a show of force is necessary to demonstrate control to the client.
- Use chemical restraints as ordered; obtain an order for medication and administer immediately.
  Medications should be offered before restraints or seclusion is considered; the medications used most often are haloperidol (Haldol) and lorazepam (Ativan).
- Use mechanical restraints if ordered and as necessary.
- Follow the institution's protocol for releasing restraints; observe client closely; remain calm and provide positive feedback as client's behavior becomes controlled.
- Know and follow institution's policies and procedures concerning violence.
  Being familiar with and following the policies and procedures of the department prevents violence.
- Protect other clients in the environment from harm; follow safety protocols of the department.
  Others could be injured during a violent outburst, and their safety must be considered.

Violence Toward Self

- Monitor and document client's potential for suicide.
- Monitor suicidal behaviors or verbalizations (e.g., giving away possessions, stating "I'm going to kill myself" or "My parents won't have to worry about having me around anymore").
  Take verbalizations of suicide seriously until assessment and intervention proves otherwise.
- Monitor seriousness of intent; say to client, "Do you have a plan?", "How will you do it?", and "Do you have the means?"
  Always use a planned intervention model to assess suicide risk and intent.
- Observe client's behavior every 15 minutes; stagger times of observation.
  Staggering observations ensures that the client does not memorize a pattern.
- Remove all dangerous objects from the client's environment.
- Use suicide precautions if indicated such as one-to-one staffing (constant attendance) and removal of all dangerous objects.
- Make a verbal or written contract with client; have client state or write "I will notify staff if I have suicidal or violent thoughts" or "I will not act on my thoughts."
  Written contracts are not legal documents and should be used only as an adjunct to other interventions, never as the primary treatment intervention.

NOTE: If suicidal client is demonstrating violent behavior, nursing interventions and rationales for **Violence toward others** may be appropriate.

Geriatric

- Monitor for suicidal risk.
- Observe for dementia and depression.
- Monitor for paradoxical drug reactions.
  Violent behavior can be stimulated when the desired action is actually to calm the client.
- Assess for polypharmacy, medication toxicity, and untoward reactions to over-the-counter or prescribed drugs; assess for other brain insults such as recent falls or injuries, strokes, or transient ischemic attacks.
  An elderly client's untoward responses to medications and brain injury may appear to be mental illness.
- Decrease environmental stimuli if violence is directed at others.

Client/Family Teaching

- Teach relaxation and exercise as ways to release anger.
- Refer to individual or group therapy.
- Teach family how to recognize an increased risk for suicide as evidenced by changes in behavior, changes in verbal and nonverbal communication, withdrawal, depression, or lifting of depression.
  Client is at peace because a plan has been made and because the client has the energy to carry out plan; thus when depression lifts, super vigilance is necessary.
- Teach use of appropriate community resources in emergency situations (e.g., hotline, community mental health, emergency room).
- Encourage use of self-help groups in nonemergency situations.

BIBLIOGRAPHY

Aguilera D, Messick J: *Crisis intervention: theory and methodology,* St Louis, 1990, Mosby.

Lehmann L et al: Training personnel in the prevention and management of violent behavior, *Hosp Community Psychiatry* 34:40-43, 1983.

Morrison E: Theoretical modeling to predict violence in hospitalized psychiatric patients, *Res Nurs Health,* 12:31-41, 1989.

O'Brien P, Caldwell C, Transwau G: Destroyers: written treatment contracts can help cure self-destructive behaviors of the borderline patient, *J Psychosoc Nurs*, 23:19-23, 1985.

Schwartz J, Kettley J, Rizzo J: *Suicide, principals and practice of emergency medicine,* Philadelphia, 1992, Lea & Febiger.

Worthington K: Taking action against violence in the workplace, *The American Nurse,* pp 11-13, June 1993.

Appendixes

Appendix A

Nursing diagnoses arranged by Maslow's Hierarchy of Needs*

Because human beings adapt in many ways to establish and maintain the self, health problems are much more than simple physical matters. Maslow's Hierarchy of Needs (see diagram) is a system of classifying human needs. Maslow's hierarchy is based on the idea that lower-level physiological needs must be met before higher-level abstract needs can be met.

For nurses, Maslow's hierarchy has special significance in decision making and planning for care. By considering need categories as you identify client problems, you will be able to provide more holistic care. For example, a client who demands frequent attention for a seemingly trivial matter may require help with self-esteem needs. Need levels vary from client to client. If a client is short of breath, he or she is probably not interested in or capable of discussing his or her spirituality. In addition, a client's need level may change throughout planning and intervention, so you will need to be vigilant in your assessment.

Read the descriptions of each category in the diagram, and see how you would relate them to nursing diagnoses. Compare your evaluation with how the authors categorized the nursing diagnoses according to this hierarchy. Be sure to assess clients for potential problems at all levels of the pyramid, regardless of their initial complaint.

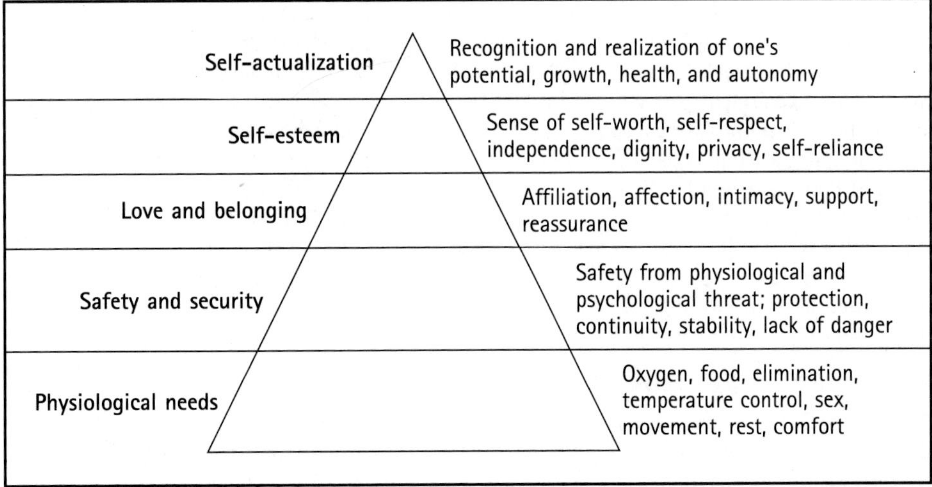

*Adapted from Sparks SM, Taylor CM: *Nursing Diagnosis Reference Manual,* Springhouse, Pa, 1991, Springhouse.

Physiological Needs

Activity Intolerance
Airway Clearance, Ineffective
Aspiration, Risk for
Breast-feeding, (Effective, Ineffective, Interrupted)
Breathing Pattern, Ineffective
Cardiac Output, Decreased
Constipation (Colonic, Perceived)
Confusion, Acute
Confusion, Chronic
Diarrhea
Environmental Interpretation Syndrome, Impaired
Fatigue
Fluid Volume Deficit
Fluid Volume Excess
Gas Exchange, Impaired
Hyperthermia
Hypothermia
Incontinence (Bowel, Functional, Reflex, Stress, Total, Urge)
Infant Behavior, Disorganized
Infant Behavior, Potential for Enhanced
Infant Behavior, Risk for Disorganized
Infant Feeding Pattern, Ineffective
Intracranial, Decreased Adaptive Capacity
Memory, Impaired
Mobility Impairment
Nutrition, Altered
Oral Mucous Membranes, Altered
Pain (Chronic)
Protection, Altered
Self-Care Deficit (Specify)
Sensory-Perceptual Alteration
Sexual Dysfunction
Sexuality Pattern, Altered
Sleep Pattern Disturbance
Swallowing Impairment
Temperature, Risk for Altered Body
Thermoregulation, Impaired
Thought Process, Altered
Tissue Integrity, Impaired
Urinary Elimination Pattern, Altered
Urinary Retention
Ventilation, Inability to Sustain Spontaneous
Ventilatory Weaning Response, Dysfunctional

Safety and Security Needs

Communication, Impaired Verbal
Disuse Syndrome, Risk for
Dysreflexia
Fear
Grieving (Anticipatory, Dysfunctional)
Health Maintenance, Altered
Home Maintenance Management, Impaired
Infection, Risk for
Injury, Risk for
Knowledge Deficit
Perioperative Positioning Injury, Risk for
Peripheral Neurovascular Dysfunction, Risk for
Therapeutic Regimen, Ineffective Management
Therapeutic Regimen, Ineffective Management: Families
Therapeutic Regimen, Ineffective Management: Community
Unilateral Neglect

Love and Belonging Needs

Caregiver Role Strain
Coping, Ineffective Family
Loneliness, Risk for
Parent/Infant/Child Attachment, Risk for Altered
Parental Role Conflict
Parenting, Altered
Relocation Stress Syndrome
Social Interaction, Impaired
Social Isolation

Self-Esteem

Adjustment, Impaired
Alcoholism, Altered Family Process
Body Image Disturbance
Community Coping, Ineffective
Community Coping, Potential for Enhanced
Coping (Defensive, Ineffective Individual)
Decisional Conflict
Denial
Diversional Activity Deficit
Hopelessness
Noncompliance
Personal Identity Disturbance
Post-Trauma Response
Powerlessness
Rape-Trauma Syndrome
Self-Esteem (Chronic Low, Self Mutilation, Risk for Situational Low, Disturbance)
Violence, Risk for

Self-Actualization Needs

Effective Management of Therapeutic Regimen: Individual
Energy Field Disturbance
Growth and Development, Altered
Health-Seeking Behaviors
Knowledge Deficit
Potential for Enhanced Spiritual Well-Being
Spiritual Distress

Appendix B

Nursing diagnoses arranged by Gordon's functional health patterns*

Health Perception-Health Management

Health-Seeking Behaviors (Specify)
Altered Health Maintenance (Specify)
Ineffective Management of Therapeutic Regimen (Specify Area)
Effective Management of Therapeutic Regimen
Ineffective Family Management of Therapeutic Regimen
Ineffective Community Management of Therapeutic Regimen
Noncompliance (Specify Area)
Risk for Infection (Specify Type/Area)
Risk for Injury
Risk for Trauma
Risk for Perioperative Positioning Injury
Risk for Poisoning
Risk for Suffocation
Altered Protection (Specify)
Energy Field Disturbance

Nutritional-Metabolic

Altered Nutrition: More than Body Requirements or Exogenous Obesity
Altered Nutrition: Risk for More than Body Requirements or Risk for Obesity
Altered Nutrition: Less than Body Requirements or Nutritional Deficit (Specify Type)
Ineffective Breast-feeding
Interrupted Breast-feeding
Effective Breast-feeding
Ineffective Infant Feeding Pattern
Impaired Swallowing (Uncompensated)
Risk for Aspiration
Altered Oral Mucous Membranes (Specify Alteration)
Fluid Volume Deficit
Risk for Fluid Volume Deficit
Fluid Volume Excess
Risk for Impaired Skin Integrity or Risk for Skin Breakdown
Impaired Skin Integrity
Impaired Tissue Integrity (Specify Type)
Risk for Altered Body Temperature
Ineffective Thermoregulation
Hyperthermia
Hypothermia

Elimination

Colonic Constipation
Perceived Constipation
Intermittent Constipation Pattern
Diarrhea
Bowel Incontinence
Altered Urinary Elimination Pattern
Functional Incontinence
Reflex Incontinence
Stress Incontinence
Urge Incontinence
Total Incontinence
Urinary Retention

Activity-Exercise

Activity Intolerance (Specify Level)
Risk for Activity Intolerance
Fatigue
Impaired Physical Mobility (Specify Level)
Risk for Disuse Syndrome
Self Bathing—Hygiene Deficit (Specify Level)
Self Dressing—Grooming Deficit (Specify Level)
Self Feeding Deficit (Specify Level)
Self Toileting Deficit (Specify Level)
Diversional Activity Deficit
Impaired Home Maintenance Management (Mild, Moderate, Severe, Potential, Chronic)
Dysfunctional Ventilatory Weaning Response (DVWR)
Inability to Sustain Spontaneous Ventilation
Ineffective Airway Clearance
Ineffective Breathing Pattern
Impaired Gas Exchange
Decreased Cardiac Output
Altered Tissue Perfusion (Specify)

*Adapted from Gordon M: *Manual of Nursing Diagnosis, 1995-1996*, St Louis, 1995, Mosby.

Dysreflexia
Disorganized Infant Behavior
Risk for Disorganized Infant Behavior
Potential for Enhanced Organized Infant Behavior
Risk for Peripheral Neurovascular Dysfunction
Altered Growth and Development

Sleep-Rest

Sleep-Pattern Disturbance (Specify Type)

Cognitive-Perceptual

Pain (Specify Type and Location)
Chronic Pain (Specify Type and Location)
Sensory/Perceptual Alterations
Unilateral Neglect
Knowledge Deficit (Specify Area)
Altered Thought Processes (Specify)
Acute Confusion
Chronic Confusion
Impaired Environmental Interpretation Syndrome
Impaired Memory
Decisional Conflict (Specify)
Decreased Intracranial Adaptive Capacity

Self-Perception—Self-Concept

Fear (Specify Focus)
Anxiety
Risk for Loneliness
Hopelessness
Powerlessness (Severe, Moderate, Low)
Self-Esteem Disturbance
Chronic Low Self-Esteem
Situational Low Self-Esteem
Body Image Disturbance
Risk for Self-Mutilation
Personal Identity Disturbance

Role-Relationship

Anticipatory Grieving
Dysfunctional Grieving
Altered Role Performance (Specify)
Social Isolation or Social Rejection
Social Isolation
Impaired Social Interaction
Relocation Stress Syndrome
Altered Family Processes (Specify)
Altered Family Processes: Alcoholism
Altered Parenting (Specify Alteration)
Risk for Altered Parenting (Specify Alteration)
Parental Role Conflict
Risk for Altered Parent/Infant/Child Attachment
Caregiver Role Strain
Risk for Caregiver Role Strain
Impaired Verbal Communication
Risk for Violence

Sexuality-Reproductive

Altered Sexuality Patterns
Sexual Dysfunction
Rape Trauma Syndrome
Rape Trauma Syndrome: Compound Reaction
Rape Trauma Syndrome: Silent Reaction

Coping-Stress Tolerance

Ineffective Coping (Individual)
Defensive Coping
Ineffective Denial or Denial
Impaired Adjustment
Post-Trauma Response
Family Coping: Potential for Growth
Compromised Family Coping
Disabling Family Coping
Ineffective Community Coping
Potential for Enhanced Community Coping

Value-Belief

Spiritual Distress (Distress of Human Spirit)
Potential for Enhanced Spiritual Well-Being

Appendix C

Nursing diagnoses arranged by human response patterns*

Exchanging

Altered Nutrition: More than Body Requirements
Altered Nutrition: Less than Body Requirements
Altered Nutrition: Potential for More than Body Requirements
Risk for Infection
Risk for Altered Body Temperature
Hypothermia
Hyperthermia
Ineffective Thermoregulation
Dysreflexia
Constipation
Perceived Constipation
Colonic Constipation
Diarrhea
Bowel Incontinence
Altered Urinary Elimination
Stress Incontinence
Reflex Incontinence
Urge Incontinence
Functional Incontinence
Total Incontinence
Urinary Retention
Altered (Specify Type) Tissue Perfusion (Renal, Cerebral, Cardiopulmonary, Gastrointestinal, Peripheral)
Fluid Volume Excess
Fluid Volume Deficit
Risk for Fluid Volume Deficit
Decreased Cardiac Output
Impaired Gas Exchange
Ineffective Airway Clearance
Ineffective Breathing Pattern
Inability to Sustain Spontaneous Ventilation
Dysfunctional Ventilatory Weaning Response (DVWR)
Risk for Injury
Risk for Suffocation
Risk for Poisoning
Risk for Trauma
Risk for Aspiration
Risk for Disuse Syndrome
Altered Protection
Impaired Tissue Integrity
Altered Oral Mucous Membranes
Impaired Skin Integrity
Risk for Impaired Skin Integrity
Decreased Adaptive Capacity: Intracranial
Energy Field Disturbance

Communicating

Impaired Verbal Communication

Relating

Impaired Social Interaction
Social Isolation
Risk for Loneliness
Altered Role Performance
Altered Parenting
Risk for Altered Parenting
Risk for Altered Parent/Infant/Child Attachment
Sexual Dysfunction
Altered Family Processes
Caregiver Role Strain
Risk for Caregiver Role Strain
Altered Family Process: Alcoholism
Parental Role Conflict
Altered Sexuality Patterns

Valuing

Spiritual Distress (Distress of the Human Spirit)
Potential for Enhanced Spiritual Well Being

Choosing

Ineffective Individual Coping
Impaired Adjustment
Defensive Coping
Ineffective Denial
Ineffective Family Coping: Disabling
Ineffective Family Coping: Compromised
Potential for Enhanced Community Coping
Ineffective Community Coping
Family Coping: Potential for Growth

*From North American Nursing Diagnosis Association: *Nursing Diagnoses: Definitions and Classification 1995-1996*, Philadelphia, author.

Ineffective Management of Therapeutic Regimen (Individuals)
Noncompliance (Specify)
Ineffective Management of Therapeutic Regimen: Families
Ineffective Management of Therapeutic Regimen: Community
Effective Management of Therapeutic Regimen: Individual
Decisional Conflict (Specify)
Health-Seeking Behaviors (Specify)

Moving

Impaired Physical Mobility
Risk for Peripheral Neurovascular Dysfunction
Risk for Perioperative Positioning Injury
Activity Intolerance
Fatigue
Risk for Activity Intolerance
Sleep Pattern Disturbance
Diversional Activity Deficit
Impaired Home Maintenance Management
Altered Health Maintenance
Feeding Self-Care Deficit
Impaired Swallowing
Ineffective Breast-feeding
Interrupted Breast-feeding
Effective Breast-feeding
Ineffective Infant Feeding Pattern
Bathing/Hygiene Self-Care Deficit
Dressing/Grooming Self-Care Deficit
Toileting Self-Care Deficit
Altered Growth and Development
Relocation Stress Syndrome
Risk for Disorganized Infant Behavior
Disorganized Infant Behavior
Potential for Enhanced Organized Infant Behavior

Perceiving

Body Image Disturbance
Self-Esteem Disturbance
Chronic Low Self-Esteem
Situational Low Self-Esteem
Personal Identity Disturbance
Sensory/Perceptual Alterations (Specify) (Visual, Auditory, Kinesthetic, Gustatory, Tactile, Olfactory)
Unilateral Neglect
Hopelessness
Powerlessness

Knowing

Knowledge Deficit (Specify)
Impaired Environmental Interpretation Syndrome
Acute Confusion
Chronic Confusion
Altered Thought Processes
Impaired Memory

Feeling

Pain
Chronic Pain
Dysfunctional Grieving
Anticipatory Grieving
Risk for Violence: Self-directed or Directed at Others
Risk for Self-Mutilation
Post-Trauma Response
Rape-Trauma Syndrome
Rape-Trauma Syndrome: Compound Reaction
Rape-Trauma Syndrome: Silent Reaction
Anxiety
Fear

Appendix D

Pain: Assessment guide and equianalgesic chart

Margo McCaffery

Assessment: Use of Pain Rating Scales

Nursing Assessment/Diagnosis of the Pain Sensation. Ask the client, if at all possible. The client's self-report of pain is the single most reliable indicator of how much pain the client is experiencing. The rating given by the client is always what is recorded in the client's record.

Basic Measures of Pain. The hierarchy of importance of basic measures of pain are as follows (AHCPR, Quick Ref. Acute Pain in Children, 1992; Report of the Consensus Conference on the Management of Pain in Childhood Cancer. Schechter, Altman, Weisman, editors: *Pediatrics* 86:813-834, 1990):

1. Client's self-report
2. Report of parent, family, or others close to client
3. Behaviors (e.g., facial expressions, body movements, crying)
4. Physiological measures; "neither sensitive nor specific as indicators of pain" (AHCPR, Quick Ref. Acute Pain in Children, 1992, p. 7)

Client/Family Teaching

NOTE: When it is obvious that pain is severe (e.g., following trauma or major surgery), a pain rating scale need not be used initially. Give an analgesic and wait until the client is better able to cooperate.

1. Explain the primary purposes of a pain rating scale. Show the client/family the scale.
   a. Provides quick, consistent communication between client and caregiver/nurse/ physician. Emphasize that the client must volunteer information since caregivers do not necessarily know when the client has pain.
   b. Helps establish pain relief goal satisfactory to client.
2. Explain the specific pain rating scale (e.g., 0 to 10; 0 = no pain and 10 = worst possible pain). When a numerical scale is used, verify that the client can count up to the number used. If the client does not understand whatever scale is "standard" in that clinical setting, select another scale.
3. Discuss the word pain. Explain that pain is discomfort that may occur anywhere in the body; may have various characteristics such as aching, hurt, pulling, tightness, burning, or pricking; and may be mild to severe. If the client prefers some other term such as hurt, use that word.
4. To verify that the client understands how the word pain (or other word preferred by client) is used, ask the client to give two examples of pain he or she has now or has experienced.
5. Ask the client to practice using the pain rating scale by rating his or her current or past painful experiences.
6. Ask the client what pain rating would be acceptable or satisfactory to him or her while at rest and active. This helps set a realistic, initial goal. Zero pain is not always possible. Once the initial goal is achieved, the possibility of better pain relief can be considered. Emphasize to the client that satisfactory pain relief is a level of pain that is

noticeable but not distressing and enables the client to sleep, eat, and perform other required or desired physical activities.

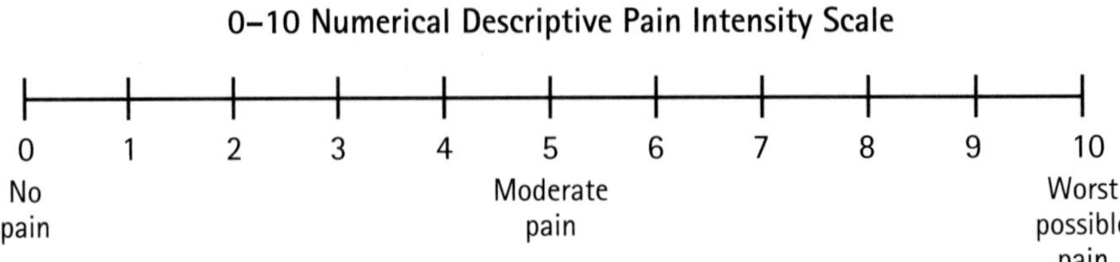

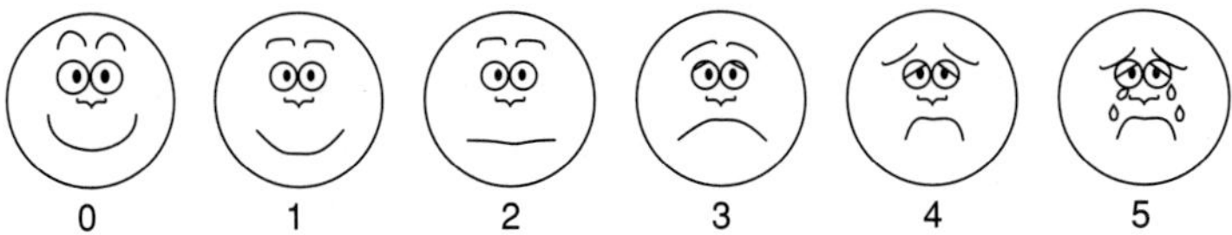

Recommended for persons age 3 years and older. Explain to the person that each face is for a person who feels happy because he or she has no pain (hurt) or sad because he or she has some or a lot of pain. Face 0 = very happy because he doesn't hurt at all. Face 1 = hurts just a little bit. Face 2 = hurts a little more. Face 3 = hurts even more. Face 4 = hurts a whole lot. Face 5 = hurts as much as you can imagine, although you don't have to be crying to feel this bad. Ask the person to choose the face that best describes how he or she is feeling. (From Wong D: *Nursing Care of Infants and Children*, ed. 5, 1995, p. 1085. Copyrighted by Mosby–Year Book. Reprinted by permission. The Wong/Baker FACES Pain Scale may be reproduced for clinical use provided the copyright information is retained with the scale. Research reported in Wong, D and Baker, C: Pain in children: comparison of assessment scales. *Pediatric Nursing* 14:9-17, 1988.)

Dose equivalents for opioid analgesics in opioid-naive adults and children ≥ 50 kg body weight[1]

Drug	Approximate equianalgesic dose		Usual starting dose for moderate to severe pain	
	Oral	Parenteral	Oral	Parenteral
Opioid agonist[2]				
Morphine[3]	30 mg q 3-4 h (repeat around-the-clock dosing) 60 mg q 3-4 h (single dose or intermittent dosing)	10 mg q 3-4 h	30 mg q 3-4 h	10 mg q 3-4 h
Morphine, controlled-release[3,4] (MS Contin, Oramorph)	90-120 mg q 12 h	N/A	90-120 mg q 12 h	N/A
Hydromorphone[3] (Dilaudid)	7.5 mg q 3-4 h	1.5 mg q 3-4 h	6 mg q 3-4 h	1.5 mg q 3-4 h
Levorphanol (Levo-Dromoran)	4 mg q 6-8 h	2 mg q 6-8 h	4 mg q 6-8 h	2 mg q 6-8 h
Meperidine (Demerol)	300 mg q 2-3 h	100 mg q 3 h	N/R	100 mg q 3 h
Methadone (Dolophine, other)	20 mg q 6-8 h	10 mg q 6-8 h	20 mg q 6-8 h	10 mg q 6-8 h
Oxymorphone[3] (Numorphan)	N/A	1 mg q 3-4 h	N/A	1 mg q 3-4 h
Combination opioid/NSAID preparations[5]				
Codeine[6] (with aspirin or acetaminophen)	180-200 mg q 3-4 h	130 mg q 3-4 h	60 mg q 3-4 h	60 mg q 2 h (IM/SC)
Hydrocodone (in Lorcet, Lortab, Vicodin, others)	30 mg q 3-4 h	N/A	10 mg q 3-4 h	N/A
Oxycodone (Roxicodone, also in Percocet, Percodan, Tylox, others)	30 mg q 3-4 h	N/A	10 mg q 3-4 h	N/A

From Jacox A et al. *Management of Cancer Pain*: Clinical Practice Guideline No. 9. Rockville, Md, March 1994. Agency for Health Care Policy and Research, Public Health Services, US Department of Health and Human Services (AHCPR Publication No. 94-0592).

[1]Caution: Recommended doses do not apply for adult patients with body weight less than 50 kg.

[2]Caution: Recommended doses do not apply to patients with renal or hepatic insufficiency or other conditions affecting drug metabolism and kinetics.

[3]Caution: For morphine, hydromorphone, and oxymorphone, rectal administration is an alternate route for patients unable to take oral medications. Equianalgesic doses may differ from oral and parenteral doses because of pharmacokinetic differences.

[4]Transdermal fentanyl (Duragesic) is an alternative option. Transdermal fentanyl dosage is not calculated as equianalgesic to a single morphine dose. See the package insert for dosing calculations. Doses above 25 μg/h should not be used in opioid-naive patients.

[5]Caution: Doses of aspirin and acetaminophen in combination opioid/NSAID preparations must also be adjusted to the patient's body weight. Aspirin is contraindicated in children in the presence of fever or other viral disease because of its association with Reye's syndrome.

[6]Caution: Codeine doses above 65 mg often are not appropriate because of diminishing incremental analgesia with increasing doses but continually increasing nausea, constipation, and other side effects.
Note: Published tables vary in the suggested doses that are equianalgesic to morphine. Clinical response is the criterion that must be applied for each patient; titration to clinical responses is necessary. Because there is not complete cross-tolerance among these drugs, it is usually necessary to use a lower than equianalgesic dose when changing drugs and to retitrate to response.
Codes: q=query. N/A=not available. N/R=not recommended. IM=intramuscular. SC=subcutaneous.

Index

Index

Entries in **boldface** refer to official NANDA diagnoses; *italics* indicate page numbers in nursing care plans

I

Q

R

T

U